AF526343

BEHAVIOR DISORDERS IN INFANTS, CHILDREN, AND ADOLESCENTS

BEHAVIOR IN INFANTS, AND

RANDOM HOUSE  NEW YORK

DISORDERS CHILDREN, ADOLESCENTS

Edited by
JOHN M. REISMAN
DEPAUL UNIVERSITY

First Edition
987654321
 All inquiries should be addressed to Newbery Award Records, Inc., 201 East 50th Street, New York, N.Y. 10022. Published in the United States by Newbery Award Records, Inc., a subsidiary of Random House, Inc., New York and simultaneously in Canada by Random House of Canada Limited, Toronto. Distributed by Random House, Inc.

Library of Congress Cataloging in Publication Data
Main entry under title:

Behavior disorders in infants, children, and adolescents.

Includes index.
1. Child psychopathology. I. Reisman, John M.
RJ499.B387 1986 618.92′89 86-509
ISBN 0-394-35576-8

Manufactured in the United States of America

Acknowledgments

We acknowledge with appreciation permission to quote from Golden, G. S. (1974), Gilles de la Tourette's syndrome following methylphenidate administration, *Developmental Medicine and Child Neurology, 16,* 76–78.

We are grateful to the American Psychiatric Association for permission to quote from DSM-III.

TO OUR FRIENDS

Contributors

Penelope H. Brooks is Director of the Mental Retardation Research Training Program at the John F. Kennedy Center of Peabody College, Vanderbilt University.

Edward C. Budd is a Member of Community Mental Health Services of Medina County, Medina, Ohio.

Brian D. Carter is Assistant Professor of Psychology in Psychiatry and Behavioral Sciences, Bingham Child Guidance Clinic, University of Louisville School of Medicine.

Rosalind D. Cartwright is Professor and Chairman, Department of Psychology and Social Sciences, and Director of the Sleep Disorder Service and Research Center, Rush-Presbyterian-St. Luke's Medical Center, Chicago.

Sheldon Cotler is Professor and Chairman, Department of Psychology, DePaul University.

Geraldine Dawson is Director of the Child Clinical Psychology Program at the University of Washington.

Loretta Haroian is Dean of Professional Studies, Department Chair in Child/Adolescent Sexuality, Advanced Study of Human Sexuality, San Francisco.

Richard J. Lawlor is Assistant Professor of Clinical Psychology, Department of Psychiatry, University of Indiana Medical School, and is Chairman of the Indiana State Board of Examiners.

Charles Mahone is Professor of Psychology, Texas Tech University.

John Paul McKinney is Professor, Department of Psychology and Department of Pediatrics and Human Development, Michigan State University.

Gary B. Mesibov is Associate Professor of Psychology, Departments of Psychiatry and Psychology, University of North Carolina, Chapel Hill, and is Associate Director of Division TEACCH.

James E. Patton is School Psychologist, Grant Wood Area Education Agency, Cedar Rapids, Iowa.

Mary Ann Reinhart is Assistant Professor, Office of Medical Education Research and Development, College of Human Medicine, Michigan State University.

John M. Reisman is Professor of Psychology, De Paul University.

Donald K. Routh is Professor of Psychology, University of Iowa.

David A. Sabatino is Dean, School of Education and Human Services, University of Wisconsin-Stout.

Robert A. Sedlak is Professor and Director of the Office of Research and Services, University of Wisconsin-Stout.

C. Eugene Walker is Professor of Psychology and Director of Pediatric Psychology, Department of Psychiatry and Behavioral Sciences, Health Sciences Center, University of Oklahoma at Oklahoma City.

Steven Weber is Laboratory Director of the Milwaukee Regional Sleep Disorders Center, Columbia Hospital, Milwaukee.

Pamela Doxsey West is Coordinator of Clinical Services, Family and Child Study Center, John F. Kennedy Center of Peabody College, Vanderbilt University.

Preface

As a former practicing clinical child psychologist and as a current teacher of child psychopathology at the undergraduate and graduate levels I have felt the need for a text that would address the disorders of children with understanding and a high degree of scholarliness. It is my belief that this aim can best be achieved by asking experts in a particular field of child psychopathology to share their knowledge with us. At the same time I have seen it as my job as editor to ensure a certain uniformity of style and that the contributions are distinctive and readable.

This book can serve as either an undergraduate or graduate level text. It takes as its basic framework the latest classification system of the American Psychiatric Association (DSM-III), not because it is the best or final word on the subject, but because it is the official nomenclature and so is the one most likely to be used in the United States. A number of its chapters are unusual and rarely presented, such as "Sleep Disorders" and "Psychosexual Disorders." We trust that you will wonder, as I did, how such topics could have been neglected in the past.

We hope you will find this book informative and helpful. Things change, and the certain convictions of one time become the dated beliefs of another. What does not change is the quest for understanding, humility about what we know, and respect for views that differ from our own. We trust that those attitudes are reflected in this book and that they will be enduring.

John M. Reisman

Contents

PART II
DISORDERS

PART I

OVERVIEW

Introduction

This book is in two parts. The first provides a consideration of issues important to an understanding of the field of child psychopathology. Chapter 1 presents, within a historical context, the major theories used to explain why children misbehave (etiology). Chapter 2 discusses concerns related to categorization (diagnosis) and critically evaluates the official psychiatric classification system (DSM-III) for disorders in childhood. Chapter 3 examines the prevalence and outcomes of disorders, with special attention given to results of their treatment. The second part of the book is devoted to detailed examinations of particular disorders, and how they are identified and defined in DSM-III. In each of these eleven chapters, prevalence, assessment, etiology, treatment and outcome for the specific problems are discussed.

Part I makes clear why there is so much disagreement in psychopathology and how it is that estimates of the prevalence of disorder can vary so widely. It also makes clear that DSM-III has use insofar as it serves as a stable frame of reference for communication, but that it is best regarded as a flawed and temporary expedient. This is to say that while DSM-III provides a framework for this book and diagnostic criteria are endorsed, they are not given an unqualified approval and in many instances are given no approval at all.

Within this section there are no chapters devoted to psychologial testing and treatment. Instead, it was thought preferable to present matters of assessment and treatment in relation to the disorders. Of course in a broad and true sense this book is devoted to nothing but assessment and treatment.

CHAPTER 1

Models of Child Psychopathology

John M. Reisman

Throughout history people have been puzzled and concerned about the misbehaviors of children and have endeavored to understand and explain them as best they could. Why are children disobedient? Why don't they learn? Why don't they listen to the good advice of their parents? Why do they act silly or sad or peculiar? These questions have been asked repeatedly, though never in any prior age with the scientific rigor, energy, and comprehensiveness of our own.

That there are even distinctive periods in human life known as childhood and adolescence, which extend over the years from birth until sexual maturity and the assumption of adult responsibilities, is a relatively recent development in human history. Two major forces acted to bring about this modern awareness and demarcation of youth. The first involved economic and industrial changes brought about by the growth of technologies and machines. This reduced the demand for labor and the need for children to enter the work force, with the result that the period of childhood could be prolonged, both voluntarily and through compulsory education. Within the United States the first compulsory school attendance legislation was enacted in Massachusetts in 1852, and it was not until 1918 in Mississippi that all the states had such laws (Cremin, 1961).

The second major force was the advance in medical science. Prior to this century infant mortality rates were very high and children died from a variety of illnesses—diphtheria, polio, smallpox—whose virulence only within recent years was substantially reduced, if not almost totally eliminated. For example, the infant mortality rate in England toward the end of the nineteenth century was about 142 deaths per 1,000 births (Despert, 1970, p. 93); by 1980 the rate was about 12 deaths per 1,000 (Lunde, 1983). As a result of medical progress the likelihood of a child's survival appreciably increased, with a consequent increase in parental involvement and concern about the welfare of their children (Aries, 1962).

In industrial societies, such as the United States, the increased duration of dependence of children upon parents and adults and the increased proportion of children born who were expected to grow into maturity sharpened governmental awareness of the psychological and educational problems of youth and made socially compelling the search for their understanding and treatment. Unlike previous periods in history, ours regards childhood as of enormous importance, perhaps of the greatest importance, in development. We know little children can have big psychological problems, that they can be emotionally conflicted, terribly unhappy, and seriously cut-off from reality. We acknowledge the validity of their concerns and opinions. Moreover, we believe there is a community responsibility to do all that can be done to help them have satisfying and productive lives. So accepting are we of these attitudes and values that it is difficult to appreciate their newness and the accomplishments they represent.

The purpose of this chapter is to describe the various models proposed concerning the psychological disturbances of children. These models constitute recurrent themes whenever treatment and etiology, the study of origins or causes, of a specific disorder are discussed. These explanations are models, in the sense that they broadly describe the origins of psychopathology, which vary somewhat in the individual case depending upon its peculiar circumstances. We shall be considering five models: (1) nature, (2) medical or biogenic,(3) psychodynamic, (4) behavioral, and (5) ecological or systems model. In the sections that follow we shall see how each of them has influenced, and continues to influence, how people view and deal with children's disorders.

The Nature Model

One of the oldest explanations is that children behave as they do because they were born to so behave or because their personalities are expressive of their inherent natures. Children who are slow to learn, it is argued, are born with certain defects of reason or intellect; aggressive children are born with pugnacious qualities; kindly children have gentle natures, and so on. Or, it may be contended, it is inherent in all humans to exhibit certain personality characteristics at certain times in their development. Or, it is in the nature of the human organism to be selfish, impulsive, obstinate, and curious.

The nature model is expressed at one extreme in the traditional reproach of one parent to another that any objectionable behavior of their child "must have come from your side of the family" and, at the other extreme, in the sciences of genetics and sociobiology.

Historical Development of the Nature Model

In Biblical times it seems to have been assumed that many behaviors or traits were inborn, particularly those that appeared to be intractable or not easily modified. A common behavior of children, disrespect and disobedience of parents, was of special concern, and led to a drastic and straightforward prescription for its elimination:

> If a man have a stubborn and rebellious son, which will not obey the voice of his father, or the voice of his mother, and *that*, when they have chastened him, will not hearken unto them: Then shall his father and his mother lay hold on him, and bring him out unto the elders of his city, and unto the gate of his place; And they shall say unto the elders of his city, This our son *is* stubborn and rebellious, he will not obey our voice; *he* is a glutton, and a drunkard. And all the men of his city shall stone him with stones, that he die: so shall thou put evil from among you; and all Israel shall hear, and fear (Deuteronomy 21: 18–21).

Among the ancient Greeks and Romans, and many other early peoples, infanticide was practiced. Infants born with obvious physical defects were killed. Older children, whose behavior developed into markedly deviant patterns, were thought to be idiots: incurable, stupid, hopeless. They were not pitied, and no obligation was felt to rear them. Viewed with contempt, they were at best tolerated, and if too burdensome, were abandoned.

Hippocrates (460–377 B.C.) and Galen (130–200 A.D.) are credited with developing one of the first temperament classification systems (Watson, 1963, pp. 14–15, 80). *Temperament* refers to inherent tendencies to exhibit certain qualities of personality as a result of one's physical structure, glandular and nervous system functioning, or bodily functioning in general. Hippocrates thought that there were four liquid secretions, or *humors*, in the body—blood, black bile, yellow bile, and phlegm—and that diseases and disorders were due to imbalances of these fluids.

About 600 years later Galen related excesses of the humors to definite types of personality. An excess of blood was assumed to be responsible for an ardent, optimistic, warm temperament (sanguine). Too much yellow bile predisposed the person to irritability and flashes of anger (choleric). Abundant black bile led to a temperament dominated by moodiness and depressed affect (bilious). And an oversupply of phlegm accounted for a personality characterized by sluggishness and indifference (phlegmatic).

Although this system must have had some appeal, since its types have found their way into our language, a more popular view down through the centuries was that it was in the nature of children to be willful, stupid, and disobedient. The more obstinate and deviant the behavior of the child, the greater the stupidity, and up to a point, the more vigorously adults had to combat it. Adults did this by inflicting punishments.

In the days of the Roman empire teachers routinely made use of the lash, the rod, and the whip to bring unruly children under control. The state exercised major responsibility for the education and rearing of most children, as it did in the days of ancient Greece when children were conscripted and trained for military service (Despert, 1970).

The emergence of early Christianity as a powerful religion and force had two relevant effects. First, it gave support to the need of children for strict discipline by its concept of original sin. Second, since it was thought to be in the very nature of humans to be impulsive, morally weak, and easily led astray by temptations, the church encouraged parents to be watchful over their children and to play a more responsible and significant role in their upbringing.

No doubt the church also played some role in softening the attitudes of people toward the deviant and retarded. Among the educated and the nobility in medieval Europe, the "stupid" came to be regarded with pity and for a time were perversely considered to be humorous, witty, and profound in the gibberish they uttered (Rosen, Clark, & Kivitz, 1976, pp. *xiii–xxiv*). Dwarfs and "fools" not only found livelihoods as court jesters, but also, as in Shakespeare's *King Lear*, their comments were seen as singularly honest and wise.

During the eighteenth century among the aristocracy and upper classes of Europe, babies and children came to be viewed as innocent, especially insofar as their knowledge of sexual matters was concerned. Up until then it had not been uncommon to engage in sexual practices in the company of children and to fondle them and initiate them into sex prior to adolescence. It had also been assumed that due to their corruptible natures they engaged in masturbation without guilt and were quite eager to be led astray. The "new" attitude was that children were born pure and uncorrupted: "This [childhood] is the age of innocence . . . the age when one can forgive anything, the age when hatred is unknown, when nothing can cause distress; the golden age of human life, the age which defies Hell, the age when life is easy and death holds no terrors, the age to which the heavens are open. Let tender and gentle respect be shown to these young plants of the Church. Heaven is full of anger for whosoever scandalizes them" (Aries, 1962, p. 110, quoting the caption to an engraving of that period).

Contributing to this change in attitudes was the French philosopher René Descartes (1596–1650). An intellectual who sought to establish what could be known with certitude by doubting everything, Descartes was led to believe that we are born with certain ideas, among which is the idea of God (Boring, 1950, p. 165). In opposition to Descartes's notion of innate ideas came the arguments of the British empiricists, such as John Locke (1632–1704), who contended that all our ideas come to us from our experiences. In either case, the notion of children being born bad was greatly modified, and the groundwork was prepared for an exhilarating and revolutionary point of view.

Within the eighteenth century Jean-Jacques Rousseau (1712–1778) vigorously and eloquently advocated a radically different conception of children, though one which had derivations from Descartes and Locke. Rousseau claimed that children were born good and had an innate apprehension of God and a sense of what is right and wrong. They became bad, not because they were born bad, but because of the corrupting influences and evils of their society. Social injustices, the artificialities of class distinctions, and an overemphasis upon intellect and reason, rather than on natural expression, were held accountable by Rousseau for distorting innate goodness into the shabby and despicable (Reisman, 1982, pp. 3–4).

Rousseau's writings set the stage for a dramatic event. In 1799 a bruised and naked boy of eleven or twelve was discovered in the woods in the district of Aveyron, France. Because he was unable to speak, it was supposed the child had been abandoned and had grown wild, a true child of nature. Once the fears of the lad were overcome, there was hope he would provide conclusive answers to what had heretofore been philosophical speculations (Lane, 1976). Would he be kindly and good in his dealings with others? When he learned to speak, would he give utterance to the ideas of God and conscience or would these ideas have to be taught?

A physician, Jean Itard, who had experience in the education of the deaf, was engaged to teach the Wild Boy of Aveyron, or Victor, as he was soon called. For five years Itard devoted almost all his energies to this endeavor, and in the process developed a number of ingenious techniques for training the retarded, many of which continue to be employed. His labors demonstrated conclusively that with diligence and skill improvements in behavior can be achieved in even very severely retarded children.

However, there were disappointing limits to what was accomplished. Victor's natural behavior was offensive to Itard and to some of his sponsors. At a dinner party, Victor made improper advances to a woman, and when rebuffed, ran into the garden and climbed a tree. This did not seem consistent with what people had been led to expect by Rousseau, and although his deportment improved, Itard feared the social consequences as Victor grew into adolescence and adulthood.

Moreover, Victor never learned to speak so that no answer could be provided to the question of the existence of innate ideas. Itard concluded that Philippe Pinel, the French psychiatrist who had examined Victor and diagnosed him an idiot, was essentially right. Instructional efforts were abandoned, and Victor lived the remainder of his life in a cottage provided for him by the French government and under the care of Itard's former housekeeper.

Despite Itard's discouragement, many were heartened by the modest successes achieved. Certainly his results gave hope where there had earlier been only totally gloomy appraisals, such as that of the psychiatrist Jean Esquirol, who in writing of idiots, stated: "Everything in them betrays a constitution that is imperfect, life-forces misapplied. They are incurable. . . . There is no way of giving them a larger amount of reason or intelligence, even for a few moments" (Lane, 1979, p. 262).

Edward Seguin studied under Itard, established the first school for retardates in Paris in 1837, emigrated to the United States in 1848, and continued for the next thirty years to encourage the education of the retarded. On the European continent, Maria Montessori (1870–1952) built upon Itard's work and carried it further. The legacy of Victor and his teacher was rich and has served to stimulate others to do what can be done to help children (Reisman, 1982).

Current Manifestations of the Model

Today the nature model continues to find popular expression in explanations that emphasize "breeding," the child "takes after" someone in the family, or a youngster is a "bad seed." Among scientists it is generally agreed that certain disorders, for example, Down syndrome (mongolism or trisomy-21), are primarily genetically determined, while many disorders are significantly influenced in their age of onset and probability of occurrence by genetic variation (Kallman, 1953; Schwarz, 1979). Given children with certain genetic predispositions and given the proper circumstances or experiences, particular behaviors will be exhibited.

After carefully weighing the evidence of familial studies of intelligence, Bouchard and McGue (1981) concluded that the partial genetic determination of intelligence was indisputable. This was based on the demonstration of study after study of a greater correspondence between intelligence test scores with those of greater genetic similarity. Moreover, it has been argued that a number of disorders—schizophrenia, depression, neurosis—seem to have genetic linkages since they occur more frequently among relatives more closely related to known patients.

Advances in staining and microscopy

have led to the identification and direct investigation of chromosomes and important implications for the understanding of behavior. An extra Y chromosome was found, more often than would be the case in the general male population, among adult male criminals with known homocidal tendencies (Jarvik, Kloda, & Matsuyama, 1973). This finding suggested that the frequently observed greater aggressiveness of boys as compared to girls could have something to do with the Y chromosome that determines maleness, rather than solely being a function of cultural roles and expectations.

One of the most significant implications of the nature model is that of inherent limits, a restriction at variance with many of our values. We are cautioned that while it may be possible to modify or restrain innate inclinations, this would be counter to what is natural and hence could have harmful effects. What adults should do, according to the proponents of this model, is recognize that children are not infinitely malleable and that what can be achieved must depend upon the child's inherent make-up. What attributes appear to be inherent? According to some workers at the Gesell Institute of Child Development, far more than many adults recognize.

Ilg and Ames (1955) have argued the child's physical structure or physique predisposes the youngster to characteristic behaviors that parents cannot readily change to their opposite. They noted three types of physique, originally described by Kretschmer in 1921 and subsequently revised by Sheldon in 1940 (Reisman, 1982, pp. 174, 281–283): the thin *ectomorph*, associated with shy, quiet, retiring behaviors; the corpulent *endomorph*, who tends to be jolly, friendly, sociable, easy-going, and noncompetitive; and the muscular, strong *mesomorph*, who is inclined toward activity, competitiveness, and aggressive pursuits.

In addition, Ilg and Ames (1955, 1972) counseled adults to be aware of the fairly uniform and predictable changes associated with growth or maturation. As the child develops, skills and behaviors appear, such as walking, talking, reading, and abstract thought. Efforts to train the child in order to accelerate the process or to promote the acquisition of a skill before the child is ready are regarded by them as generally frustrating, possibly damaging, and certainly unwise. Furthermore, the personalities of children change in a rhythmic ebb and flow that is somewhat associated with chronological age (Ilg & Ames, 1972).

A period of calm, cooperative, agreeable behavior is supposed to be followed by a time of agitation, storminess, rebelliousness, and emotional lability, which is often followed by a phase of pleasantness and quiet. These phases or stages appear to have a tempo of several months early in the child's life and may last a year or more in childhood and adolescence. For Ilg and Ames this is an orderly course of natural events in which the periodic shifts are of much greater import than the specific ages at which the alterations in behavior commonly take place. By being aware of these expected changes, adults may anticipate disruptions in the behavior of the conforming child and improvements in the behaviors of children who seem quite agitated and disturbed. Although superficially the child may impress adults as inconsistent and bewildering, there is an underlying predictability and harmony. Accordingly, patience and understanding, acceptance and firmness in dealing with extreme disruptions, and consistency and a valuation of the child's unique endowments are extolled as the adult qualities that should be developed when dealing with children.

Chess, Thomas, and Birch (1965) have been involved in a painstaking longitudinal study of 231 children that sought to isolate those characteristics of infants that were sufficiently stable and consistent to be regarded as temperament. Their observations led them to identify nine clusters of behavior: (1) *activity level:* some infants tend to be more active and energetic than others; (2) *regularity in habits:* having bowel movements, going to sleep, and eating at about the same time each day; (3) *response to novel stimuli:* whether interested in and attracted to new things, or frightened and withdrawn when something new is introduced; (4) *ease in adjusting to changes in routine;* (5) *sensitivity to various kinds of stimulation:* some infants appeared more aware of lights and sounds than others; (6) *mood:* some infants seemed usually happy and agreeable, while others seemed usually cranky and irritable; (7) *intensity of response to stimulation,* whether high or low; (8) *ease with which the infant becomes distracted;* and (9) *ability to sustain attention and persist in the performance of a task.*

In subsequent reports of their research, Thomas, Chess, and Birch (1968, 1970) isolated three temperamental categories of children from the nine clusters of behavior. About 10 percent of youngsters appeared to comprise the **difficult child** type: irritable, bossy, demanding, whining, overactive, irregular in their habits, prone to throw temper tantrums, distressed by the novel, and slow in adapting to change. A large proportion of the children of the difficult type, about 70 percent, later evidenced psychological problems that required professional attention. In marked contrast was the **easy child** type, which fortunately for parents constituted about 40 percent of the sample: children with friendly and pleasant dispositions, regularity in habits, and interest in and readily adaptable to what was new. The remainder of the group, some 50 percent, comprised a mixed or **slow-to-warm-up child** type; these children were somewhat cautious and reserved, though they eventually did respond positively, and had some desirable and some undesirable characteristics.

Thomas and Chess (1977) cautioned, however, that the correlations between the ratings of infants and children, though significant, were low. Correlations ranged from .21 to .54, with most below .40, and "there are significant correlations from one year to the next for all (9) categories except approach/withdrawal, distractability, and persistence. As the time span for the comparison (between one rating and another) is increased, from one year to two, three or four years, the number of significant correlations decreases" (Thomas & Chess, 1977, pp. 160–161). Similar cautions were raised about the stability of temperament ratings made of infants at one month, three months, and six months of life (Kronstadt, et al., 1980), and about the influence of experiential factors, such as child-rearing practices and attitudes, upon temperament characteristics (deVries & Sameroff, 1984).

Despite these reservations, the nature model affords a precautionary balance to unbridled enthusiasm about the plasticity of human behavior. Look, it seems to say, many of the troublesome actions of infants and children are neither their willful disobedience nor the fault of adult mismanagement. They are merely functions of the way children are and how they develop; they are the correlates of inborn physical structures whose consequences must be recognized and respected; they are the result of innate predispositions and vulnerabilities impacting against an unfortunate environment. Be aware of the limits and the currents of development. Recognize the child's unique endowments and their implications and appreciate them. For while some modification of behavior is possible, children cannot be shaped into whatever is desired without due concern for inherent abilities, tendencies, and processes.

The Medical Model

A second explanation for psychological disturbances is that they are products of affliction, illness, or disease. It follows from this model that a disorder is treated best when means are found to remedy the cause. It also follows that a disturbed child is no more accountable for troublesome behaviors than a person with a cold is responsible for sneezing. Medications and other forms of treatment may be prescribed to attack the ailment or to alleviate symptoms.

This model can be traced back to prehistoric times, when the punching of holes in skulls—trephines—is presumed to have been done in order to allow evil spirits that afflicted the person to escape (Lahey & Ciminero, 1980, p. 9). Although Hippocrates and Galen represented more enlightened interludes, a belief in possession persisted through the centuries. The Bible attributed King Saul's jealousy, depression, and murderous impulses toward David to an evil spirit, and by the Middle Ages in Europe beliefs in devils and demons were widely accepted as ordinary truths (Zilboorg & Henry, 1941). The question was not whether possession existed, but how one distinguished between possession by good or bad forces and what one was to do about them.

Quite sensibly it was believed that the nature of the possession or vision was crucial in determining the significance of the influence. If a child saw visions of angels and heavenly beings or was scrupulous in religious observances, favorable influences were at work and a life devoted to God might be indicated. However, if a child saw visions of the devil and his kind or engaged in mischief and evil doings, then exorcism and purging were indicated.

With the growth of empiricism and science, beliefs in spirits diminished and were supplanted by demonstrations of the existence of other organisms and factors which can bring about illness: infections, parasitic invasions, damage to cortical structures, and so on. Pinel, in 1798, in his *Philosophical Nosology* specified four types of mental disease: mania, melancholia, dementia, and idiocy. The last, idiocy, was considered the major form of psychiatric disturbance in infancy and childhood, and Pinel contended it was brought about by a variety of noxious agents: terrors or fears experienced by the mother during pregnancy or birth, convulsions from verminous infections, extremely painful first or second dentitions, and complications from epilepsy and rickets (Lane, 1976). While Pinel believed idiocy was incurable, he insisted that all the mentally ill should be treated with understanding, compassion, kindness, and respect. This approach to the afflicted came to be known as *moral treatment.*

Pinel's contemporary in the United States, Benjamin Rush, regarded as the father of American psychiatry, did not believe children could suffer serious mental illnesses, aside from idiocy, because by their very natures they were too unstable and labile for their ideas to have lasting effects. But he did recognize that children misbehaved and that they were often beaten severely for it. In an article in 1790 Rush urged teachers to refrain from inflicting physical punishments upon their pupils and to employ less drastic methods of discipline: "Had I influence enough in our legislature to obtain only a single law, it should be to make the punishment for striking a school-boy, the same as for assaulting and beating an adult member of society. The world was created in love. . . . Nations and families that are happy, are made so only by love. . . . Children are capable of loving in a high degree. They may therefore be governed by love" (Brenner, 1970, pp. 222–223). Rush is also credited with fostering the development of moral treatment during the first half of the nineteenth century (Kauffman, 1981, p. 34).

Moral treatment, which included humane living conditions and suitable recreational and occupational activities, achieved some degree of popularity and became a major method for dealing with mental illness during the early nineteenth century. Many psychiatrists argued the mentally ill were victims of the stresses of living and needed the safety of "asylums" for their recovery. Yet, in part because of the successes claimed for moral treatment, the method fell into disrepute. The reasons given for its decline are many, including the exaggeration of its rates of cure and the overenthusiasm of its proponents. But unquestionably the growth of the sciences and the vision of a medical model built upon the promise of great scientific advances were also significant.

The nineteenth century German psychiatrist W. Griesinger (1817–1868) asserted that all mental illnesses were caused by physiological disturbances. In order for psychiatry to progress, the physiological cause of every disorder had to be determined and its specific cure found. There were, indeed, early successes to indicate the validity of this model. Certain disorders were traced to the effects of chronic alcoholism. Others were found to be due to neurological damage. Still others were associated with syphilitic infection.

These demonstrations of the biological origins of psychic disturbances suggested a true science of psychiatry was imminent. By isolating and treating the specific cause, the alcoholism (or vitamin B deficiency) in Korsakoff's psychosis and the syphilitic infection in general paresis, precise, informed help could be given patients. Emil Kraepelin (1855–1926), the father of descriptive psychiatry, urged his colleagues to adopt a deliberate, careful approach to their subject. Psychiatrists should identify those symptoms that were associated with a particular disease, the *syndrome,* and they should patiently observe the natural course of the illness in their patients. Kraepelin's study of dementia praecox (schizophrenia), a severe disorder whose onset was thought to be in adolescence, led him to conclude it was incurable, and thus contributed to an attitude of futility and resignation about its treatment (Reisman, 1982, pp. 32–33).

Germany at this time occupied an unprecedented position of respect for its cultural and scientific achievements, so its directions in psychiatry commanded attention and exerted a profound influence throughout Europe and the Western Hemisphere. The medical model advocated that all mental disorders be understood as illnesses or diseases, that their physiological origins be determined, that their natural courses and outcomes be studied, and that appropriate treatments through medical procedures be found and applied. Simultaneously, a broadened understanding of what constituted mental illness was taking place which brought many of the troublesome behaviors of children within the province of psychiatry.

Some early publications gave currency to the notion of mental illness in childhood: In 1867 there appeared a chapter, "Insanity of Early Life," written by the British psychiatrist Maudsley for his book *Physiology and Pathology of Mind;* in 1887 a text by Emminghaus was published on the mental disorders of children; and in 1898 a book by Ireland was entitled *The Mental Afflictions of Children* (Kanner, 1962). Surprisingly, one of the significant forces in promoting the medical model came from the personal document of a former patient in a mental hospital, Clifford Beers (1876–1943).

A Yale graduate, Beers had suffered from delusions, depression, and such despair that he attempted suicide. After his recovery, he resolved to write a book which would report the deplorable conditions he experienced in mental hospitals and which would "serve as the opening gun in a permanent campaign for the improvement in the care and treatment of mental sufferers, and the prevention, whenever possible, of mental illness itself" (Beers, 1970, p. 255).

His book, *A Mind That Found Itself,* originally published in 1908, helped make Beers the leader of the *mental hygiene* movement. Eminent members of the medical profession, notably the distinguished American psychiatrist Adolf Meyer, had been waiting for just such a catalyst. With the support of enlightened philanthropists, a National Committee for Mental Hygiene was founded in 1909 to inform the public and stimulate the provision of services.

That same year the Juvenile Psychopathic Institute opened in Chicago, The Institute, a branch of the Juvenile Court, had as its purpose the study of delinquents so more effective recommendations for their treatment and judicial disposition could be determined. William Healy, a psychiatrist, was the first director of this agency. He believed delinquency indicated the presence of some illness, and in 1915 published *The Individual Delinquent: A Text-Book of Diagnosis and Prognosis for All Concerned in Understanding Offenders,* which through its compelling case histories of children who ran afoul of the law illustrated that among the factors contributing to criminality were: drinking too much tea and coffee, exposure to adventurous novels and motion pictures, and "bad habits" or masturbation (Healy, 1927, pp. 278–280, 304–310, 559–567). Despite its shortcomings by contemporary standards, this book was highly successful in getting judges to consider delinquent children medical as well as legal problems and to establish additional clinics similar to Healy's.

By the 1920s the Juvenile Psychopathic Institute was renamed the Institute for Juvenile Research and the National Committee for Mental Hygiene embarked on a program to establish child guidance clinics throughout the United States. The American Orthopsychiatric Association, an organization of psychiatrists, psychologists, and social workers interested in the treatment of children, had its first convention in 1924 at the Institute and elected William Healy its first president. That association continues to function as a powerful force for the mental health of children.

The appellation "emotionally disturbed" was introduced in 1932 by a pediatrician, Sullivan (Despert, 1970, p. 27). Shortly thereafter, in 1933, Potter delineated the symptoms that he believed pointed to the severe form of mental illness, schizophrenia, in childhood: bizarre thinking and acting, disturbances of speech and emotions; and, the major sign of the disorder, a profound withdrawal: "The drive for integration with the environment, so characteristic of normal children and so essential for their personality development is outstandingly absent" (Potter, 1933).

Potter's article made explicit that children could suffer from psychiatric ailments fully as serious as those of adults. It joined with a mounting body of evidence and professional opinion to regard abnormal behaviors in children as expressions of a range of illnesses, diseases, and disorders. Accordingly, the misbehaviors of children came to be seen as more or less serious forms of disturbance for which the children needed appropriate kinds of medical treatment. The disobedient child, the child who could not learn, the withdrawn or aggressive youngster, was thus regarded as afflicted with some form of malady.

The medical model encompasses genetic and intrauterine events. In recognition of how broadly it is to be understood, it is sometimes referred to as the biogenic or the biogenetic model, but its more simple designation is usually employed. Those who espouse the medical model tend also to embrace the nature model, though not all who espouse the nature model accept the medical model.

Within our society the medical model is the most influential, yet it is not without its critics (Szasz, 1960). Their concerns, their alternative explanations, and their claims for legitimacy will be examined shortly.

The Psychodynamic Model

A psychodynamic model sees disorders as expressions of conflict. The conflict may be within the individual, between opposing values, beliefs, and inclinations. It may be wholly, or in part, unconscious; that is, the person may not be able to articulate or explain fully why distress is experienced or why disturbing behaviors occur. It may be expressed in disruptive and unsatisfying relationships with others.

The elements of this model can be traced back at least as far as ancient Greece, when Socrates argued that a major task for man is to attain harmony between his appetites or drives and his reason (Robinson, 1981, p. 61). However, it took 2,400 years before that view was vigorously championed and gained wide acceptance as a continuous and unending problem in human development. Credit for that achievement is due largely to the efforts and stimulation of one man, Sigmund Freud. Freud's genius persuasively illustrated how: (1) psychological conflicts originate in early childhood and are never finally resolved; (2) the individual is seldom fully aware of the feelings and wishes determining complex behaviors, so to a large extent unconscious forces influence us all; and (3) many disorders, and in particular those known as *neurotic,* are unsuccessful attempts to control and to gratify childlike wishes.

Since Freud's psychodynamic theory, *psychoanalysis*, is the most complete, comprehensive, and influential example of this model and since its implications have commanded attention, it will be presented in some detail. Over the years psychoanalysis has been extended, modified, and amplified until it has become to all intents and purposes a theory of general psychology, which continues to evolve (Blanck & Blanck, 1979). This discussion will be confined to its relevance in explaining psychological disturbances in childhood and to its most distinctive features, the psychosexual (Freud) and the psychosocial (Erikson) theories of development.

Psychoanalysis focuses upon the age-appropriate expression of pleasurable impulses and aggressive feelings and the acquisition of certain beliefs. Essentially it stresses the person's accommodations in gaining self-satisfactions without incurring the displeasure of others. Freud started with the fact that while most adults achieve sexual satisfaction in intercourse with a person of the other sex, there are many who derive pleasure from a wide variety of sexual practices: from looking, fondling, sucking, fetishes, sado-masochistic activities, and so on. Based upon his observations and the reports of his patients, he concluded sexual or pleasurable experiences of a sexual nature occur throughout infancy and childhood in a predictable fashion as part of human growth toward adult sexuality (Fancher, 1973).

Freud identified a definite sequence of stages in development, though he recognized that people make progress at different rates and that everyone remains slightly impeded (*fixated*) within each particular stage. Many psychological disorders are presumed to once have been ordinary behaviors in growth. In other words, *it is hypothesized that almost all forms of psychopathology occur normally in development. Therefore, what constitutes psychopathology usually involves a judgment or determination of the age-inappropriateness of behavior. An uncommon persistence of behaviors beyond the age at which they are appropriate (fixation) or a resumption of immature behaviors (regression) constitute two major forms of psychopathology.*

For example, infants typically wet their beds and soil themselves. Urinating and making bowel movements in their diapers is normal. However, by the ages of four or five years most children learn to go to the toilet and to remain dry at night. Those who do not are, assuming there is no organic problem, fixated and exhibiting a disorder called functional enuresis or/and encopresis. If there were a child who did appear to be toilet-trained for a time and who did, after some stress, begin to bedwet again, this would constitute a regression. Of course, an immediate question is why fixations and regressions take place.

Freud believed the natural tendency toward the rapid expression and satisfaction of sexual and aggressive impulses was of the greatest psychological significance. The infant wishes gratification as soon as possible and comes to learn that the world does not stand ready to provide or allow instant satisfaction. To some extent unavoidably, but also often deliberately, parents discipline and frustrate their child. The result is that conflict is often experienced by the youngster between gaining gratification and fearing disapproval or punishment.

Psychoanalysis argues such conflicts are a necessary and desirable price to be paid for human growth and socially acceptable behavior. Without the frustration of impulses the child would not learn to become inhibited and to delay translating wishes into immediate action. Without the gratification of impulses the child would not learn to be self-trusting and trusting of others.

Psychoanalysis contends progress in development depends upon this proper balance between frustration and gratification. Excesses or deficiencies of either produce abnormalities. If there is too much satisfaction and too little frustration, it is predicted the child will be excessively fixated and will be interested largely in the gratification of impulses found in the state when indulgences occurred. If there is too little satisfaction and too much frustration, it is predicted the child will become angrily preoccupied in wresting gratifications for the impulses that have been thwarted.

Moreover, the child who is too greatly

fixated will be handicapped in meeting the challenges and demands of the next stage. As a consequence, more mature and socially desirable avenues of impulse satisfaction will not be fully explored and attained. In some cases, the child may appear to be progressing normally, but encounter so much failure and threat that a retreat or regression to an earlier, safer, more satisfying stage of impulse expression occurs.

Freud's theory begins its description of human development when the infant is unaware of self or others, of what is real and what is not, of where the body ends and the outside world begins. This phase *primary narcissism,* covers the first month of life. Clearly an overfixation or regression to this stage would be indicative of a very serious disorder. The entire body surface provides pleasure in a relatively undifferentiated way during narcissism through being fondled, stroked, and caressed. However, gradually the infant becomes aware of a mothering person and pleasurable activities and contact with the world become focused on the mouth.

Simultaneously the infant begins to acquire feelings of trust and mistrust in the mothering person, the *oral stage.* Based upon these early experiences of being cared for and fed, the infant forms a feeling and belief about whether people and events are basically safe, decent, generous, predictable, concerned, and worthy of confidence. The frustrations that inevitably accompany the intervals between the infant's cries for care and the arrivals of satisfaction make complete trust virtually impossible. And it would be of dubious adaptive value to the person if by some herculean effort it could be fashioned. Gullibility is no asset in the real world. Nevertheless the balance of trust and suspicion is thought to be ideally tipped in favor of trust.

The pleasurable activities of the oral stage are not entirely abandoned upon progress to the next stage; in fact, *people normally remain fixated to a slight degree at every stage.* This is evidenced by the pleasure derived from tactile and oral stimulations: petting, snuggling, cuddling, eating, chewing, sucking. But when these activities are excessive, persistent, or exclusionary, a disturbance is indicated. The school-age child who is forever eating or chewing on pencils, who frequently demands to be given things and then is dissatisfied with whatever is given and received, who often solicits adults for care and protection, is behaving in patterns suggestive of overfixation at the oral stage.

The *anal stage* coincides with that time in growth when the child is able to run about and "get into everything." During this period, parents are compelled to restrict and limit the child's movements, toilet training is being carried on with vigor, precious and dangerous objects have to be safeguarded from the child's eagerness to explore them, and rules and regulations have to be established for the protection and well-being of all concerned. The child may rip, tear, and throw things, pull on animals, hit people with whatever is handy, and butt into conversations and pieces of furniture. Many harried parents feel they are forever saying, "*No!*" and the child soon learns that the use of this simple two-letter word has great power to upset grown-ups and to send them scurrying about with much distress.

In this process of training, parents, both by accident and by design, communicate what is good and bad and when their child is good and bad. Since a child's understanding is limited and colored in a different way from that of adults, many of the parents' evaluative comments are interpreted as personal criticisms, regardless of how impersonally they may attempt to make them. Going to the bathroom is good, and when one goes to the bathroom, one is good. Urine and feces are dirty, smelly, and bad. Cleanliness and neatness are good. Being messy and sloppy are bad. Doing what parents tell you is good. Not doing what parents tell you is bad. The world is organized and structured into dichotomies, and there is no compromise or shading between opposites.

Characteristic of this state is an early kind of morality in which the child learns what is right and wrong but feels these standards are imposed by adults and does not internalize or accept them. Therefore the child may agree with an adult that a certain act is wrong and yet commit the prohibited act as soon as the adult steps out of the room or stops watching.

Desirable carryovers from the anal stage are socially accepted interests in arts, crafts, gardening, collecting, science, neatness, and orderliness. Overfixations at this stage would be evidenced in soiling, bedwetting, constipation, negativism, obstinacy, compulsions, overactivity, inhibitions of motor movements, cruelty, and difficulties in following directions despite an apparent understanding of them.

The *phallic stage* spans the nursery and early school years. Impulses of a pleasurable and aggressive sort center on the penis or clitoris and involve the parent of the other sex. Boys wish to have exclusive possession of their mothers, and girls are supposed to desire their fathers. Jealousy and competitiveness occur in connection with the same-sex parent; that is, boys are jealous of and compete with their fathers and a similar situation obtains with girls and their mothers. This conflict is what analysts call the Oedipus complex, or, more poetically, "the family romance."

A little four-year-old may boast about the day when he will be stronger and bigger than his father and that he wishes to marry his mother when he grows up; a little girl may announce that she wishes her mother would go away and leave control of the house to her. In addition, there is often strutting, flexing of muscles, playing house, dressing up in adult clothing, and smearing on cosmetics.

Some parents are flattered by these attempts of their children to possess and to emulate them. However, ordinarily the child's attentions and wishes are discouraged. Eventually, the child renounces the conflict out of love for the same-sex parent and out of fear of the retribution that might be inflicted if the Oedipal wishes were put into action. To the extent that the parents encourage the child's fantasies and behave in accordance with them, the complex is less easily resolved. One of Freud's earliest cases, Little Hans (Freud, 1909), dealt with the analysis of the fears of this five-year-old, which were related to Oedipal concerns. The usual outcome is repression of the complex, an improved relationship between the child and both parents, and an internalization or acceptance by the child of many parental values, prohibitions, and standards.

As the child grows older these concepts of morality come to be influenced by a broadening circle of people outside the family and by information gained from books and other media of communication. These different points of view act to modify the child's moral beliefs and make them less dichotomous and rigid. Gradually, acts come to be judged upon the basis of the contexts in which they occur, intentions count for more in determining rightness or wrongness than the mere act itself, and the child acquires a greater tolerance and appreciation for radically different standards and practices.

Ordinary fixations at this stage are expressed in friendships and intimate relationships with people who are reminiscent of the parents, in associations that gain parental approval, and in personal satisfactions derived from contacts with those who share familiar attitudes and beliefs.

Unusual fixations are indicated by inappropriate gender behaviors, flirtatious and seductive crushes on adults, extreme rivalry with peers for adult attention, and excessive anxiety or phobias.

Phobic reactions are explained by the theory as unconscious displacements from the feared parent to innocuous objects or situations. Thus, the child may be fearful of animals, leaving home and going to school, or of meeting new adults. Analysts would recommend these fears be reduced by resolving the conflict within the child and promoting a harmonious relationship within the family.

The next stage was called *latency* by Freud since he believed there was no new zone of psychosexual development but rather a consolidation and strengthening of the child's ability to deal with impulses. Latency coincides with the child's elementary school education and is presumed to end with the physical changes associated with puberty. Therefore major tasks facing the child are adjustments to the demands of education, getting along with classmates, and dealing with teachers.

For many children, the contrast between school and home is marked. Positively, some find a freedom, an acceptance, and an intellectual stimulation outside their homes that they have not previously enjoyed. However, others encounter unpleasant restrictions and regulations at school that make this environment exceedingly distasteful and aversive.

Similarly, the teacher can represent only one more adult to whom the child must adjust. Behaviors that might have been tolerated and praised at home may be met with strong disapproval in the classroom. A boy's zest for living and sense of humor may be favored less than his keeping left-hand margins 1½-inches wide and staying put in his seat. Children are expected to obey arbitrary rules and to sense the subtle benefits conferred by following directions.

Children are also challenged in the classroom by having to compete against and make friends with a variety of other children. Peer interactions inevitably involve comparisons and may result in feelings of competence and accomplishment—Erikson's concept of *industry*—or of inadequacy. The host of satisfactions and problems associated with peer acceptance and rejection are well known (Bower, 1969).

As emphasized by Alfred Adler (Ansbacher & Ansbacher, 1956), a sense of inadequacy is probably an unavoidable consequence of the fact that children are born small, weak, and dependent upon adults for their survival. But what they experience, particularly in school, are repeated messages about their performance and themselves which can serve as constructive or destructive influences. Ideally, the child should find education an enhancement to self-esteem, but realistically a sense of failure is all too frequently what is communicated.

Although boys like girls and girls like boys, in this stage there is reluctance to acknowledge it, and more than at any other period the sexes tend to be segregated in their choice of friends. Consequently same-sex attachments develop. Normal fixations are suggested by preferences for companionship with members of one's own sex and by an emphasis upon competition with peers.

The key to overfixations at this and subsequent stages of development lies in the determination of the extent or exclusiveness of the behaviors more so than in the behaviors themselves or their mere persistence. For example, competitiveness, in and of itself, is regarded as the most distinctive aspect of our culture and its economic system; competition is valued, extolled, and held to be the best means for the motivation of human beings. Within our society what would make competition excessive would be an evaluation of the individual's preoccupation with it, to the extent that close and cooperative relationships are precluded.

Similarly, close relationships with members of one's own sex are only thought to be of concern when they hinder or prevent the development of heterosexual attachments. If intimacy with members of the other sex cannot be achieved, the analytic or psychodynamic model would regard this as less mature since it fails to follow the ideal pattern of psychosexual development.

Freud did not merely state that heterosexual attachments are expected to take place during adolescence. He specified that these relationships occur between peers. When they do not, if the adolescent forms crushes or becomes romantically involved with adults, recapitulations of the Oedipal conflict would be suspected.

Moreover, in later adolescence pressures increase to make plans about vocational and career goals. Certain job opportunities have to be realistically considered in light of scholastic achievements and one's abilities. A history of a lack of accomplishment may now preclude the very careers that at that moment appear most desirable to one's parents, one's peers, and oneself. Further, the variety of jobs in our society exceeds the abilities of anyone gaining sufficient familiarity with all of them so as to make an informed choice. Doubts and uncertainties are to be expected. Only one thing seems certain: American culture encourages the adolescent to select a career which will give expression to his or her own individuality.

A feeling of knowing who you are—identity—is regarded as the central issue of adolescence, though it is understood that such knowledge is acquired from birth and affirmed throughout life. However, it is the adolescent's task to decide about a vocation, one of the important pieces in the mosaic of identity and one of a number of decisions about self made at this time. Among the other significant choices are sexual preferences, religion, generational differences in values, and challenges concerning leaving the comforts and safety of family for a relatively independent existence.

The discontinuities and disruptions in patterns of living during this period are so great and the apprehensions and uncertainties they arouse so prevalent that for centuries it has been characterized as a time of "storm and stress." While the hard facts of research argue that this picture of tumult is not true of most adolescents (Douvan & Adelson, 1966; Weiner, 1970, pp. 21–31) and while one of the few studies conducted to test Erikson's theory suggested the major problem articulated by children has to do with autonomy and feelings of self-acceptance and self-respect (Ciaccio, 1971), the model has retained its importance for understanding the conflicts confronted by many youngsters in their development.

Also note that Erikson's psychosocial model postulates the continuation of age-specific conflicts through adulthood. This means that parents and teachers are normally engaged in problems of their own, at best associated with the issues relevant to their chronological ages, which may hamper them in their ability to deal with the problems of children. For example, a child's failures at school may be a bitter and galvanizing reminder to a father of his own failures and concerns about achieving success.

The oft-repeated theme of the psychodynamic model is of conflicts and issues operating at an unconscious level to disrupt functioning. Symptoms are relatively unimportant in this model, and often are not treated directly. What is important are unconscious conflicts. Psychopathology is expressive of these conflicts, and so it is to be expected that the child or adolescent will *not* be able to affirm their existence in casual conversation. Only with patience and understanding, and probably only after overcoming some resistance, will the child be able to recognize and confirm their existence and begin the task of dealing with them effectively.

Since many psychoanalysts are also physicians, they do not see the psychodynamic and medical models as mutually exclusive, but as the former being included within the latter. Analysts who are not physicians consider the psychodynamic model as separate from the medical. There is less confusion about the behavioral model's integrity and distinctiveness since its proponents are critical of the other two positions.

The Behavioral Model

As we have seen, even before there was a behaviorism, there were philosophers who argued that all we know derives from sensory stimuli informing us about the world (Locke) and these sensory stimuli or environments can shape human behaviors for good or ill (Rousseau). One result of this line of reasoning has been a very practical one: Inherent limitations of the child are not conceded until social improvements in the child's condition have been made and educational efforts have been attempted and exhausted. Even then, limitations might not be conceded. For who can provide an ideal environment or be certain that the best education has been offered or that efforts were not within a hair's breadth of achieving success?

Optimism and pragmatism are in the spirit of this model, as are reform and experimentation, and a willingness to see how much can be accomplished given proper training and care. This is the spirit with which Jean Itard worked to teach the Wild Boy of Aveyron. This is the spirit with which Seguin continued his mentor's task of training retardates. This is also the spirit with which clinical psychology was launched as a profession.

The founder of clinical psychology was Lightner Witmer, who established the first psychological clinic at the University of Pennsylvania in 1896 and who immediately initiated training for psychologists in this field of endeavor. At that time clinical psychology was clinical child psychology, and it was Witmer's conviction that many of the problems of children were consequences of their lack of training or of their improper training. Accordingly, to be helped, children had to be taught how to behave appropriately (Witmer, 1907, 1908–1909).

However, this educational point of view was soon swept aside by the considerable excitement and controversy generated by psychoanalysis. The analytic contention of unconscious emotional problems afflicting children had great appeal. The case of Little Hans, for example, illustrated that the phobias of children were complex affairs, representing the displacement of fears from parental figures to innocuous objects. It was this argument that John Watson, father of behaviorism, vigorously disputed (Watson, 1928).

The major tenet of the behavioral model was illustrated in 1920: *Symptoms are learned, and hence they can be unlearned or the person can be taught new and better ways of behavior.* Shortly after World War I Watson sought to demonstrate the conditioning of fears in children, and thus by inference to demonstrate that phobias too could be conditioned and need not be explained by unconscious conflicts. In a series of studies with infants he found children showed an unconditioned fear response to a loud noise produced by the banging of two iron bars. Then he paired the presentation of a white rat, which presumably did not elicit any fear response, with the loud clanging noise to an infant whom he called Albert. In short order Albert not only evidenced fear of the rat, but also seemed afraid of other white furry objects that had not been in the experiment, that is, the fear had *generalized* (Watson & Raynor, 1920). It was Watson's contention that those who were ignorant of Albert's conditioning would have assumed his fears were innate or products of unconscious conflict. But they were not. They had been taught.

A further study along the same lines illustrated how such fears might be reduced or extinguished. A child given the pseudonym of Peter feared rabbits, and Mary Cover Jones (1924) alleviated that fear by presenting a rabbit at a safe distance from Peter during his mealtimes. The pleasurable, relaxing responses associated with eating were stronger than the competing fear responses. Gradually the rabbit was brought closer and closer to Peter, without Peter feeling afraid, until finally he was able to touch and play with it.

As subsequently elaborated, the behavioral model ignored questions of why children behave as they do and focused upon the question, "Under what conditions does a child exhibit this particular behavior?" The emphasis shifted to a specific behavior, to determining those environmental conditions associated with its maintenance, and to the manipulation of those conditions so the behavior could be predicted and controlled (Ross, 1980, p. 3). This process, involving careful observation and measurement of the problem behavior before, during, and after its manipulations is called a *functional analysis*.

The principles of learning employed to modify a response are assumed to have been at work when the response was acquired. Foremost among these principles is that of reinforcement.

"A positive reinforcer strengthens any behavior that produces it: a glass of water is positively reinforcing when we are thirsty, and if we then draw and drink a glass of water, we are more likely to do so again on similar occasions. A negative reinforcer strengthens any behavior that reduces or terminates it: when we take off a shoe that is pinching, the reduction in pressure is negatively reinforcing, and we are more likely to do so again when a shoe pinches" (Skinner, 1974, p. 46). Similarly, the absence of a reinforcer or the administration of a punishing or aversive stimulus reduces the likelihood of a response being made—if we draw water from a well and come up dry or the water is foul-tasting, we are less inclined to draw water from that well again.

Almost anything can constitute a reinforcer. *Primary reinforcers* are those that appear to be unlearned and which are essential for survival, such as food and water. *Secondary reinforcers* are those that have been associated with rewards and have acquired rewarding properties, such as smiles, words of approval, and money. It has also been suggested by Premack (1959) that allowing someone to perform a high probability behavior can be rewarding for the performance of a low probability behavior; for example, if a boy often runs about a room and shouts, he can be rewarded for sitting still for a certain time by being allowed briefly to run around a room and shout.

Although the behavioral model assumes the performance of pathological behaviors because of the rewards associated with them, there are behavior therapists who recognize it is not always easy to specify reinforcers, particularly in connection with cognitive and social learning. The former contends that involved in much psychopathology is the learning of incorrect cognitions or beliefs ("I am a bad person" or "I have to be perfect") and thus the task of therapy is to teach the person to stop thinking those thoughts and to think reasonable ones (Ellis, 1973; Meichenbaum, 1977). Social learning emphasizes observational learning, vicarious learning, the acquisition of expectations, modeling, and what makes a person an effective model; within this realm attention is directed to the influences of television and significant persons in the child's life who exhibit, and thus inadvertently teach, disturbed behaviors, feelings, and beliefs (Bandura, 1978).

What is shared by those who subscribe to the behavioral model are: an aversion to unconscious processes and the need to illuminate the patient's remote past; convictions about the learned, rather than illness, nature of psychopathology; the importance of a functional analysis of the behavior or symptom; and the use of training procedures to bring about improvement. At the present time this model enjoys a position of considerable prominence among psychologists and growing favor among psychiatrists as well.

The Ecological or Systems Model

Ecology refers to the study of organisms in relation to their environments, so this model has two facets: one, it argues that a child's pathology is a function of the family system or the particular network of significant interpersonal interactions; and two, it argues that pathology has to be understood within the context of the society or culture and its practices (Moos, 1975).

Taking the family aspect first, the model states the child's psychopathology is a product of family pathology, usually disturbed communications within this system. The child may be singled out as a scapegoat within the family (Ackerman, 1966), who is sacrificed so that the other members of the system may gratify their needs. Or the child may be the recipient, as well as the sender, of a steady stream of disturbing behaviors or messages, which bring about emotional distress, conflict, and turmoil (Satir, 1967). In either case the child's disturbance is seen as a price paid by the family for maintaining some stability. Therefore, to change the child, the system must be changed. If the child alone is changed, resistance from others in the system may result or some other member's breakdown may occur.

To illustrate, Freud mentioned in a postscript to the case of Little Hans that after the boy's improvement, "His parents had been divorced and each of them had married again. In consequence of this he [Little Hans] lived by himself; but he was on good terms with both of his parents, and only regretted that as a result of the breaking-up of the family he had been separated from the younger sister he was so fond of" (Freud, 1959, p. 288).

The ecological perspective makes several points in viewing the child's pathology within a social or cultural context:

1. What is pathological is defined by the given culture (Benedict, 1934). Certain behaviors that are regarded as disturbances within our society would not be so regarded in some other so-

ciety. Psychopathology is a function of our culture's values and limits of tolerance. Hence, psychopathology could be reduced by our society being more accepting of a broader range of behaviors. Hyperactivity and learning disabilities are examples of disorders among children which have been thought to be so defined (Werry et al., 1972; Ladd, 1973; Connolly, 1971).

2. Many of the disorders of children involve problems in their learning in school. To some extent these problems may be brought about by the manner in which subjects are taught, that is, the method of education used; and by the emotional climate of the school, that is, the structure of the classroom, the rules of the principal, the warmth and discipline of the teacher, and so on. Given appropriate educational materials and procedures, individualized instruction, and an atmosphere conducive to learning, it is argued the child would learn. The fault—the psychopathology—is thus not within the child, but in the failures of the system to provide the proper means of education (Holt, 1973).
3. Since the time of Rousseau, at least, it has been recognized that a society may distress its citizenry. The problems of children—conduct disorders or juvenile delinquency, drug abuse or substance disorders—are functions of social injustices, abuses, and deprivations. Accordingly, our energies should be directed at improving our society. By so doing we would prevent the development of psychopathology and reduce the numbers of disturbed children (Coles, 1971; Goldenberg, 1977).
4. By labeling the child with a disorder; by treating the child in special facilities which emphasize the disorder, e.g., a mental hospital, a day treatment program, a classroom for emotionally disturbed children, a child guidance clinic, a mental health center; by discussing symptoms; by anticipating and condoning the child's distress, a process is set in motion that encourages and rewards the child for playing the role of a sick person. Thus the society and the mental health apparatus may actually maintain the child's psychopathology, while labeling may have additional adverse consequences (Hobbs, 1975).
5. The very erection by the society of institutions—both bricks and mortar (mental hospitals, community mental health centers, residential treatment centers) and human (juvenile courts, foster care agencies, various treatment programs—makes necessary the identification of clientele and the provision of services to them so that these resources are utilized. At the same time, questions may be raised as to the extent the identification of children for the utilization of these services is determined by their mere availability (Rhodes & Ensor, 1979).

As can be seen, the ecological or systems model incorporates a broad range of views, unified by their insistence that psychopathology is not always a matter of disturbance within the child, but instead is often a function of the child's transactions within an ever-widening network of social systems. All models recognize the validity of this assertion, and they benefit by being forcefully reminded of it. From family to school to community to society, the ecological model highlights the consequences of practices, policies, methods, and institutions. At the very least, the model rightly insists, attention should be paid to the possible influences of these variables in ascertaining how best to help a particular child. It is, also, as it has always been, a call for meaningful reforms within the society and an end to poverty and social injustices.

Normality and Abnormality

Models of psychopathology present a basis for understanding why children behave as they do, are crucial in identifying which children are in need of services, suggest means for the treatment of problems, and provide the framework for determining what constitutes normality and abnormality. Such determinations are at the heart of epidemiological studies and have practical, dollars-and-cents consequences. A society responds to a problem and allocates its resources to deal with it depending upon its urgency, which in turn is a function of how widespread the problem seems to be. Yet obviously the models do not see disturbances in the same way. Thus the orientation of an investigator is a highly significant factor in conceptualizing what problems to study, how best to study them, and whether the problems even exist!

Professionals within the mental health field recognize that there is a distinction between what they might ideally regard as normal and what they are willing to accept as normal in their general practice. Ideally, they may think of a normal person as fully-functioning, self-actualizing, creative, cooperative, altruistic, productive, sociable, autonomous, energetic, happy, purposeful, and self-satisfied. For practical purposes in their contacts with patients they may think of normality as a condition of conformity in which the person manages to cope with the problems of day-to-day living and is not overwhelmed by misery. They reconcile these two quite different conceptions by accepting that some persons may legitimately aspire and strive for the ideal of normality, while others, for valid reasons, can do little more than get by.

With children, more so than with adults, the question of normality-abnormality is complicated by the differing standards, values, and perspectives of the parties involved. Typically, when a child is brought to the attention of a professional, there are at least four points of view that must be considered:

1. What does the child think? Does the child believe a problem exists? If so, what is it? It is not unusual for a child to claim to be unaware of the existence of any problems or to present a problem that is quite different from the concerns of adults.
2. What does the referral source think? Often parents are directed to seek help for their child by a third party, such as the school, the juvenile court, or a pediatrician. It is usually necessary to evaluate the referral source's determination of abnormality and to see how it corresponds with the parents' understanding.
3. What do the parents think? Are they concerned? If so, about what? Frequently parents reject the problem of the referral source or see a quite different problem.
4. What does the examining professional think? Does the professional concur with the other judgments or see the situation quite differently?

A professional judgment of normality-abnormality, and what enters into it, is an issue we have been discussing throughout this chapter. Especially with children, that judgment must take into account normal development, which here refers to a statistical understanding, not one that is ideal or theoretical.

Statistically Normal

It is necessary to emphasize that normal can have two major and quite different meanings. It can refer to what is usual or average or common, which is what is meant by the statistical meaning of normality. And it can refer to what is ideally or theoretically regarded as healthy and desirable. Some professionals and investigators consistently speak of normal-abnormal in only one sense—generally those who advocate a behavioral model employ a statistical meaning, while those who favor a psychodynamic model make judgments from their theoretical or ideal understanding—while others shift, sometimes without warning, from one usage to the other.

The statistical determination of normality usually begins with a bit of behavior or condition, such as "takes first step without assistance," "truants from school," "has temper tantrums"; obtains samples of children of different ages; and determines the numbers of children within those samples who exhibit those behaviors. By such means it may be found that it is normal for a child to begin walking at about one year of age, that many two- to three-year-olds have temper tantrums, and that it is unusual for children of any age to truant from school.

Normal in a statistical context refers to the usual or the average age for the occurrence of behavior. Some indication of dispersion, such as a standard deviation, is frequently provided, so what is normal usually encompasses a range—children begin to walk alone from 11–15 months of age. A significant delay in evidencing a behavior would merit further inquiry.

It is in this sense that parents frequently ask, "Is it normal?" They wonder if their child is exhibiting behaviors appropriate for a child of that age, and their concern has to do with whether their child's development is progressing normally.

Normal in a statistical context also refers to what is common or frequent. An investigator may take a large number of problem behaviors or symptoms and ask teachers or parents to indicate how many are displayed by each of their children. After tabulating the data, a finding typically reported is that the normal child is reported to have two or three symptoms.

In this sense it is normal for youngsters to have problem behaviors or to experience certain kinds of fears: The infant fears falling, loud sounds, strangers, and separation from parents; in early childhood there are fears of the dark, ghosts, being injured, and losing self-control; then follow fears related to taking tests, failing, and being rejected by classmates (Mussen, Conger, & Kagan, 1979).

At this point certain issues in interpreting the statistical concept of normality should be made explicit. One, it is not the case that what is statistically normal coincides with what is desirable or ideal. Ideally, it is preferable for children not to have any symptoms. Two, what is statistically normal is very much influenced by the conditions within the society or culture. The culture may be fostering psychopathology or a disorder may be prevalent within the society. Such a determination of widespread disturbance could not be made if the statistical concept of normality were alone employed. Three, symptoms are not equal in their pathological significance. Being shy and afraid of the dark are not as portentous as setting fires and having bizarre speech. Four, by itself, the statistical concept provides useful information, but it cannot completely replace an informed judgment. Rather, it makes an essential contribution to an informed judgment. Accordingly, it is necessary to have some basis for critically evaluating behavior that is relatively independent of what happen to be central tendencies.

Ideal Normality

The most modest standards of ideal normality have started with the premise that problems and a certain degree of anxiety are to be expected as part of the human condition. However, whatever problems exist are not of sufficient severity to interfere greatly with performance in school or with the child's social adjustment. This is a somewhat negative approach; that is, it is a definition of normality by exclusion—a normal child is one who does not show the symptoms of abnormality—but it is essentially the way the medical model identifies what is normal-abnormal.

Abnormality in the medical model is characterized by a variety of behaviors, all of which suggest failure in dealing with the ordinary stresses and demands of life. A list of these failures or symptoms is compiled: problems of various kinds, such as in deciding between what is right and wrong, controlling impulses, thinking reasonably or clearly, performing intellectual tasks accurately, and recognizing reality (Grossman, 1965); exhibiting cognitive-perceptual-motor disabilities (Rubin, Simson, & Betwee, 1966); and failures in socialization, as evidenced by inattentive, nonconforming, withdrawn, aggressive, disruptive, immature, disorganized behaviors (Hewett, 1968).

Normality is indicated by the apparent absence of these problems or symptoms.

The psychiatric nomenclature, which will be discussed in some detail in the next chapter, presents a list of disorders and behaviors that are regarded as abnormal among children. Assuming the list is exhaustive, a child who cannot be categorized within the system would be judged normal. While there may be advantages to this kind of working definition, many mental health professionals would prefer to have normality defined in terms of positive characteristics, rather than by default or the absence of pathology.

Bower (1959) has argued that the major attribute of normality is a feeling of freedom about one's capacity to decide among alternatives: "To live is to make choices; when one's choices are severely limited by emotional lacks or injunctions one's behavior can be regarded as handicapped."

Abnormality would then refer to a personal feeling of being controlled, stifled, or hampered in making decisions and expressing one's individuality. Obviously both the impulsive and the inhibited child would be abnormal. The former's behavior appears driven and out of control, while the latter's appears hemmed in by doubts, fears, and feelings of inadequacy. Neither the inhibited nor the impulsive child would appear to have those attributes associated with a sense of freedom: confidence, spontaneity, flexibility, and creativity.

From a humanistic perspective, spontaneity and creativity are crucial in specifying what is ideally normal. Terms like "self-actualizing" and "fully functioning" suggest a state of better-than-average well-being: "self-actualization stresses ways by which normal [well] people can become 'weller,' that is, how dog paddlers can become Australian crawlers" (Shostrom, 1973).

Although the validity of these attributes may be debatable for adults, their relevance for children becomes increasingly remote as they are considered in relation to younger and younger children. How can one speak of an infant feeling free or a toddler being spontaneous and creative and fully functioning? Even ideal normality for children cannot be divorced from age and development.

Developmental models afford a basis for specifying what is ideally normal according to a given theory. Thus psychoanalysis suggests the child should acquire a sense of trust in people early and describes a number of characteristics to be expected

TABLE 1-1

Psychoanalytic Stages of Development

Stage	Sexual and Aggressive Expression (Freud)	Acquired Beliefs (Erikson, 1971)	Presumed Normal Psychopathology
Narcissism (Birth–3 months)	Stimulation of body surface (skin)		Pervasive developmental disorders; infantile autism
Oral (4 months–1 year)	Mouth & lips; sucking; eating; biting	Trust-suspicion	Eating disorders; conduct disorders; personality disorders
Anal (2–3 years)	Anus & buttocks; messing; moving; opposing	Self-respect, self-doubt, shame	Oppositional disorders; Enuresis & encopresis; attention deficit disorders
Phallic (4–6 years)	Penis or clitoris; love of other-sex parent; jealousy & competitiveness with same-sex parent	To do things on one's own; to be like one's parents; guilt	Anxiety disorders; psychosexual disorders
Latency (7–12 years)	Expression & control of impulses in new & varied situations; fondness toward same-sex peers	To feel capable & useful; to feel inadequate & inferior	Academic problems
Adolescence (13–18 years)	Fondness toward other-sex peers	Decisions about work & sense of accomplishment; aimlessness & drift	Identity problems
Early adult	A continuing heterosexual relationship	Intimacy with suitable companions; loneliness	
Middle adult		Life is productive and fruitful; stagnation	
Late adult		Satisfaction with one's life; despair	

given a normal sequence of growth. However, there is no consensus among professionals that this sequence should be accepted as valid.

Those professionals who subscribe to ideal conceptions of normality are apt to be more narrow in identifying who is normal than those with a statistical concept; subtle indications of disturbance are detected in relatively well-adjusted people. In evaluating studies of the incidence or prevalence of mental disorders or psychopathology it is of great importance to know the model of the investigator, since few individuals may be ideally normal and statistically significant deviations may not have clinical significance.

What is normal behavior is relative to the individual making the determination and to the person's age, culture, situation. *Normality, then, is an informed judgment concerning the age-specific effective handling of life's difficulties and challenges, the satisfactory development in feelings about oneself and others, and the modulated expression of behavior.* Such a judgment, despite its complexities, often turns out to be simple and can be readily made by parents and teachers (Kessler, 1966, p. 68). Nevertheless there are occasions—as there are bound to be in matters of judgment—when there will be uncertainty. There is nothing wrong with doubt and ambiguity so long as we seek to reduce them by the accumulation of knowledge.

REFERENCES

Ackerman, N. W. *Treating the troubled family.* New York: Basic, 1966.

Ansbacher, H. L., & Ansbacher, R. R. *The individual psychology of Alfred Adler.* New York: Basic, 1956.

Aries, P. *Centuries of childhood.* New York: Knopf, 1962.

Bandura, A. *Social learning theory.* Englewood Cliffs, NJ: Prentice-Hall, 1977.

Bandura, A. The self system in reciprocal determinism. *American Psychologist,* 1978, *33,* 344–358.

Beers, C. W. *A mind that found itself.* Garden City, NY: Doubleday, 1970.

Benedict, R. *Patterns of culture.* Boston: Houghton-Mifflin, 1934.

Blanck, G., & Blanck, R. *Ego psychology II.* New York: Columbia University Press, 1979.

Boring, E. G. *A history of experimental psychology.* New York: Appleton-Century-Crofts, 1950.

Bouchard, T. J., Jr., & McGue, M. Familial studies of intelligence. *Science,* 1981, *212,* 1055–1059.

Bower, E. M. The emotionally handicapped child and the school. *Exceptional Children,* 1959, *26,* 6–11.

Bower, E. M. *Early identification of emotionally handicapped children in school* (2d ed.). Springfield, IL: Charles C. Thomas, 1969.

Brenner, R. H. (Ed.) *Children and youth in America: A documentary history. Vol. 1, 1600–1865.* Cambridge, MA: Harvard University, 1970.

Chess, S., Thomas, A., & Birch, H. G. *Your child is a person.* New York: Viking, 1965.

Ciaccio, N. V. A test of Erikson's theory of ego epigenesis. *Developmental Psychology,* 1971, *4,* 306–311.

Coles, R. Social issues and the child psychiatrist. *Child Psychiatry and Human Development,* 1971, 2, 67–69.

Connolly, C. Social and emotional factors in learning disabilities. In H. R. Myklebust (Ed.), *Progress in learning disabilities.* Vol. II. New York: Grune & Stratton, 1971.

Cremin, L. *The transformation of the school.* New York: Alfred A. Knopf, 1961.

Despert, J. L. *The emotionally disturbed child.* Garden City, NY: Doubleday Anchor, 1970.

deVries, M. W., & Sameroff, A. J. Culture and temperament, *American Journal of Orthopsychiatry,* 1984, 54, 83–96.

Douvan, E., & Adelson, J. *The adolescent experience.* New York: John Wiley, 1966.

Ellis, A. *Humanistic psychotherapy.* New York: McGraw-Hill, 1973.

Erikson, E. H. Growth and crises of the "healthy" personality. In C. Kluckhohn, H. A. Murray, & D. M. Schneider (Eds.), *Personality in nature, society, and culture,* New York: Alfred A. Knopf, 1971.

Fancher, R. E. *Psychoanalytic psychology. The development of Freud's thoughts.* New York: W. W. Norton, 1973.

Freud, S. Analysis of a phobia in a five-year-old boy

(1909). In *Collected papers of Sigmund Freud*. Vol. 3. New York: Basic Books, 1959.

Goldenberg, H. *Abnormal psychology: A social/community approach*. Monterey, CA: Brooks/Cole, 1977.

Grossman, H. *Teaching the emotionally disturbed: A casebook*. New York: Holt, Rinehart and Winston, 1965.

Healy, W. *The individual delinquent*. Boston: Little, Brown, 1927.

Hewett, F. M. *The emotionally disturbed child in the classroom*. Boston: Allyn & Bacon, 1968.

Hobbs, N. *Issues in classification of children*. Vol. 1. San Francisco: Jossey-Bass, 1975.

Holt, J. Quackery. In A. Davids (Ed.), *Issues in abnormal child psychology*. Monterey, CA: Brooks/Cole, 1973.

Ilg, F. L., & Ames, L. B. *Child behavior*. New York: Dell, 1955.

Ilg, F. L., & Ames, L. B. *School readiness*. New York: Harper & Row, 1972.

Jarvick, L. F., Klodin, V., & Matsuyama, S. S. Human aggression and the extra Y chromosome: Fact or fantasy? *American Psychologist*, 1973, *28*, 674–682.

Jones, M. C. A laboratory study of fear: The case of Peter. *Pedagogical Seminary*, 1924, *31*, 308–315.

Kallman, F. J. *Heredity in mental health and disorder*. New York: W. W. Norton, 1953.

Kanner, L. Emotionally disturbed children: A historical review. *Child Development*, 1962, *XXXIII*, 97–102.

Kauffman, J. M. *Characteristics of children's behavior disorders*. Columbus, OH: Charles E. Merrill, 1981.

Kessler, J. W. *Psychopathology of childhood*. Englewood Cliffs, NJ: Prentice-Hall, 1966.

Kronstadt, D., Oberkalid, F., Ferb, T., & Swarz, J. P. Infant behavior and maternal adaptations in the first six months of life. In S. Chess & A. Thomas (Eds.), *Annual progress in child psychiatry and development*. New York: Brunner/Mazel, 1980.

Ladd, E. T. Pills for classroom peace? In A. Davids (Ed.), *Issues in abnormal child psychology*. Monterey, CA: Brooks/Cole, 1973.

Lahey, B. B., & Ciminero, A. R. *Maladaptive behavior: An introduction to abnormal psychology*. Glenview, IL: Scott, Foresman, 1980.

Lane, H. *The wild boy of Aveyron*. Cambridge, MA: Harvard University Press, 1976.

Lunde, A. S. Demography. *1983 Encyclopaedia Britannica Book of the Year*, 1983, 288–293.

Meichenbaum, D. *Cognitive-behavior modification: An integrative approach*. New York: Plenum, 1977.

Moos, R. H. Social ecology: Multidimensional studies of humans and human milieus. In S. Arieti (Ed.), *American handbook of psychiatry*, Vol. 6. New York: Basic Books, 1975.

Mussen, P. H., Conger, J. J., & Kagan, J. *Child development and personality* (5th ed.). New York: Harper & Row, 1979.

Potter, H. W. Schizophrenia in children. *American Journal of Psychiatry*, 1933, *12*, 1253–1270.

Premack, D. Toward empirical laws: I. Positive reinforcement. *Psychological Review*, 1959, *66*, 219–233.

Reisman, J. M. *A history of clinical psychology*. Melbourne, FL: Krieger, 1982.

Rhodes, W. C. The disturbing child. A problem of ecological management. *Exceptional Children*, 1967, *33*, 449–455.

Rhodes, W. C., & Enser, D. R. Community programming. In H. C. Quay & J. S. Werry (Eds.), *Psychopathological disorders of childhood*, (2d ed.). New York: Wiley, 1979.

Robinson, D. N. *An intellectual history of psychology*. (Rev. ed.). New York: Macmillan, 1981.

Rosen, M., Clark, G. R., & Kivitz, M. S. (Eds.). *The history of mental retardation: Collected papers* (Vol. 1). Baltimore: University Park Press, 1976.

Ross, A. O. *Psychological disorders of children*. New York: McGraw-Hill, 1980.

Rubin, E. Z., Simson, C. B., & Betwee, M. C. *Emotionally handicapped children and the elementary school*. Detroit: Wayne State University Press, 1966.

Satir, V. *Conjoint family therapy*. Palo Alto, CA: Science & Behavior Books, 1967.

Schwartz, J. C. Childhood origins of psychopathology. *American Psychologist*, 1979, *34*, 879–885.

Shostrom, E. L. Comment on a test review: The Personal Orientation Inventory. *Journal of Counseling Psychology*, 1973, *20*, 479–481.

Skinner, B. F. *About behaviorism*. New York: Alfred A. Knopf, 1974.

Szasz, T. S. The myth of mental illness, *American Psychologist*, 1960, *15*, 113–118.

Thomas, A., & Chess, S. *Temperament and development*. New York: Brunner/Mazel, 1977.

Thomas, A., Chess, S., & Birch, H. G. *Temperament and behavior disorders in children*. New York: New York University Press, 1968.

Thomas, A., Chess, S., & Birch, H. G. The origins of personality. *Scientific American*, 1970, *223*, 102–109.

Watson, J. B. What the nursery has to say about instincts. In C. Murchison (Ed.), *Psychologies of 1925*. Worcester, MA: Clark University Press, 1928.

Watson, J. B., & Raynor, R. Conditioned emotional

reactions. *Journal of Experimental Psychology*, 1920, *3*, 1–14.

Watson, R. I. *The great psychologists.* Philadelphia: J. B. Lippincott, 1963.

Weiner, I. B. *Psychological disturbance in adolescence.* New York: Wiley-Interscience, 1970.

Werry, J. S., Minde, K., Guzman, A., Weiss, G., Dogan, K., & Hoy, E. Studies on the hyperactive child. VII: Neurological status compared with neurotic and normal children. *American Journal of Orthopsychiatry*, 1972, *42*, 441–451.

Witmer, L. Clinical psychology. *Psychological Clinic*, 1907, *1*, 1–9.

Witmer, L. The treatment and cure of a case of mental and moral deficiency. *Psychological Clinic*, 1908–1909, *2*, 153–159.

Zilboorg, G., & Henry, G. W. *A history of medical psychology.* New York: W. W. Norton, 1941.

CHAPTER 2

Diagnostic Nomenclatures

John M. Reisman

Every child is different and unique, yet there are common characteristics among children. Classification is used to reduce the bewildering diversity of individuals into categories of attributes that many of them share. An early attempt to classify mental disorders was assayed by the eighteenth century physician Boissier de Sauvages, who developed a highly detailed system modeled on the botanical classification of plants. He identified four orders of psychological disturbances, twenty-three genera, and many, many species; the genus of melancholia, for example, was subdivided into fourteen species (Menninger, et al., 1963). Of course there were earlier systems of psychopathology, going back to the ancient Greeks, and much simpler systems than that of de Sauvages. Pinel's classification had only four disorders; Esquirol's had five; and the philosopher Kant noted only four disturbances—senselessness, madness, absurdity, and frenzy (Kant, 1964).

Although Kant is better known for his philosophy than for his psychiatry, the attitudes he expressed about mental illness undoubtedly influenced German psychiatrists. Kant distinguished between mental weakness (retardation and ordinary foolishness) and mental disturbances. The latter were not evidenced in children, though since Kant believed all psychological disorders were hereditary, some youngsters carried "the seed of derangement" which eventually developed into disturbances. Moreover, since he regarded all mental disorders as incurable, he was not too certain much attention needed to be directed to this area: "It is difficult to impose an orderly classification upon that which is essentially and irreparably disordered. There is also little use in occupying oneself with it; all therapeutic efforts in this direction must turn out fruitless, since the energy of the sufferer cannot contribute to them (as it would certainly do in the case of bodily ailments), and since the therapeutic goal can be reached only through the use of the sufferer's own mental resources" (Kant, 1964, p. 14).

Some of Kant's pessimism was shared by Emil Kraepelin in his highly regarded late nineteenth and early twentieth century classification of psychiatric disturbances. Mental disorders were regarded as falling into two major groups, depending upon their etiology or cause. *Exogenous disorders* were caused by external conditions, such as accidents, shocks, and poisonings, and they might be cured. *Endogenous disorders* were brought about by internal, constitutional, hereditary factors, and they were incurable (Reisman, 1982, pp. 32–33). Significantly, Kraepelin placed dementia praecox (schizophrenia) among the endogenous disorders.

For over half a century Kraepelin's system held sway in psychiatric thinking, though his nomenclature was not universally adopted. Within the United States it was not uncommon for a hospital or medical setting to develop its own departures from the traditional classification, reflecting the judgments of its staff about what additional disorders were important and how they were to be defined. The result was that communication between one setting and another was often difficult and the findings of scientific studies were frequently questioned because it was unclear if the same disorder was being diagnosed by the same criteria.

Since the end of World War II the American Psychiatric Association has worked at developing and improving the nomenclature of psychiatric disorders. Its first system, in what eventually became a series, was published in 1952 in the *Diagnostic and Statistical Manual* (*DSM*). In 1968 a second nomenclature, DSM-II, was published, and in 1980 DSM-III appeared. There is every indication that the near future holds a DSM-IV, which makes necessary some clarification of the nature of nomenclatures.

What Is a Nomenclature?

A *nomenclature* is a system of names in what purports to be a scientific classification of some group of objects or natural phenomena. The classification may be based upon knowledge of some underlying pattern or reality. For example, organic disorders of the brain or nervous system may be identified based upon an understanding of the etiologies (studies of the reasons for or causes) of these ailments, or rocks may be classified according to their chemical constituents. Such a classification is *natural,* and it indicates an ordering based upon definite information; such a system cannot be changed unless there is new information to suggest a modification, or unless deliberate violence or woeful ignorance is directed to undermine the foundation of the system.

A classification may also be *artificial,* which is to say that its names are arbitrary or merely descriptive. An artificial nomenclature is developed for purposes of communication and convenience so that people have a common understanding of what they're talking about: "A natural classification must be discovered; an artificial one is invented" (Brill, 1974, p. 1123).

This distinction immediately raises the question of whether a psychiatric nomenclature is a natural or artificial classification. While over the years the etiology of certain psychiatric disorders has been discovered, the factors responsible for many remain controversial, and so *the psychiatric nomenclature is largely artificial. It consists mainly of names given to patterns of behavior that are held to be disorders.*

Similarly, a classification system may consist of mutually exclusive categories. An exclusive system would be based upon a *class model,* and would hold that an individual either has one disorder or another; the presence of one disorder would preclude the possibility of something else in the system (Lorr, 1961). A descriptive system is based upon an effort to describe the individual adequately. It does not have mutually exclusive categories. Thus the individual might have as many disorders as are necessary to portray the individual's patterns of behavior. *The psychiatric nomenclature is a descriptive system.*

This situation is similar to that which exists in other areas of medicine. For example, an unfortunate individual may suffer from a variety of chronic and acute ailments: diabetes, convulsive disorder, strep throat, and influenza. Although some exclusivity does exist in the psychiatric nomenclature—a person can't be diagnosed as neurotic and psychotic at the same time, and there are age-defined diagnostic categories which perforce are mutually exclusive—DSM-III encourages its users to employ as many diagnostic categories as seem appropriate.

The major purpose of a psychiatric nomenclature is to present a set of clearly defined terms so that there will be some stability and uniformity in scientific discourse. This stability and agreement about the meanings of concepts should subsequently have a number of benefits: Studies investigating the same disorder will be comparable and cumulative in their findings; eventually, differential etiologies, treatments, and outcomes (prognoses) will be determined for the various disorders so that the diagnoses will have significant, practical implications for patients (Hunt, 1980); and understanding of the correlates of the disorders will be advanced, such that it will be possible to make predictions about such matters as family relationships and peer perceptions (Quay, 1979, p. 2).

However, it is not necessary that any of these benefits be realized so long as the major purpose is achieved, that there is a consensus about terms. So as to achieve this consensus, the formulators of DSM-III took a number of unusual steps.

Operational Definitions in DSM-III

In order for a classification system to be widely accepted, Brill (1974) specified that its terms should be few and simple so that they could readily be mastered, understandably defined, and comparable to those in previous and alternative nomenclatures. This last stipulation is what Reisman (1971, pp. 10–11) called *recognizability,* which is to say that insofar as possible categories and their meanings should be retained and defined in some familiar fashion.

The framers of DSM-III were mindful of the above standards and exceeded them in many instances by defining disorders operationally. For the first time many diagnoses are explicit and clear. Functional enuresis, for example, is defined as at least two involuntary voidings of urine per month by a child between five and six years of age, and at least one voiding per month by an older child that is not due to a physical disorder; schizophrenia is defined by the presence of hallucinations, delusions, and/or incoherence, with related symptoms, such as blunted affect and markedly peculiar behavior, noted over a six-month period.

Further, extensive field trials were conducted involving over 450 clinicians using the diagnostic criteria with almost 800 patients. These trials were attempts to insure that the diagnostic criteria were clinically useful and acceptable and that they led to improved reliability of DSM-III over the previous systems, DSM-I and DSM-II, and these aims, as we shall soon see, were largely achieved.

Scope of DSM-III

From 1974 and virtually until the moment of its publication, the Committee working on DSM-III strove for agreement, not only among psychiatrists, but also between psychiatrists and other disciplines within the mental health field. Representatives from the American Psychological Association were invited to submit their comments and criticisms about early drafts of the nomenclature, and to an extraordinary degree these suggestions were both seriously considered and implemented (Spitzer, Williams, & Skodol, 1980). The result is that while DSM-III has been severly criticized—in accordance with Murphy's Law: when you try to please everyone, somebody won't like it—it nevertheless represents as close to an agreed-upon system as is likely to be obtained at this time.

DSM-III's nomenclature has been deliberately made compatible with the *International Classification of Diseases* section on psychiatric disorders, although it differs in numerous ways from it. The point is that DSM-III, by virtue of the care with which it has been formulated, has been adopted by American psychiatrists and commands the attention of psychologists and psychiatrists worldwide. It is therefore an official nomenclature and it simply cannot be ignored by persons who wish to be knowledgeable in child psychopathology.

Moreover, DSM-III does not confine itself to mental disorders, but presents diagnoses for every conceivable problem that might be brought to a mental health professional. Nevertheless, one of its major achievements is that it contains a definition of *mental disorder.* Although it is recognized the term cannot be precisely defined, or defined in such a manner that it can be approved by all who subscribe to differing models of psychopathology, it is clearly an advantage to have a definition expressed so that the medical position can be made explicit and serve as a point of departure. Within DSM-III a mental disorder is defined "as a clinically significant behavioral or psychological syndrome or pattern that occurs *in* [italics added] an individual and that is typically associated with either a painful symptom (distress) or impairment in one or more important areas of functioning (disability)" (American Psychiatric Association, 1980, p. 6).

This definition specifically rejects an exclusive ecological explanation for mental disorder. There must be something internally wrong—"a behavioral, psychologic or biologic dysfunction" within the individual—and not only a problem between the person and society. If the disorder can be satisfactorily explained by societal pressures and conflicts which have not produced any impairment within the person, then the disorder is not a mental disorder. By the same token, if society judges the person's behavior as deviant but psychiatrists do not see any disability within some important area of functioning, a mental disorder does not exist.

Spitzer, Williams, and Skodol (1980) see the definition as being of special help in clarifying whether certain sexual deviations are to be regarded as mental disorders. Fetishism, exhibitionism, impotence, and frigidity are judged to represent disabilities in sexual functioning and thus are mental disorders. However, homosexuality, because of disagreements within the mental health field about whether impairment exists, is considered a mental disorder only when the homosexual is distressed by an inability to function heterosexually.

With particular relevance to children, DSM-III provides a number of diagnostic categories which are explicitly recognized as situational, social, societal, interpersonal problems. These conditions may merit the attention of mental health professionals, but they are not mental disorders.

What appears to distinguish the disorders in Table 2-1 is that either the child experiences no distress in connection with the condition and seems relatively well-adjusted, such as Borderline Intellectual Functioning, or the distress is an isolated incident or a transitory response to environmental circumstances, which when altered or removed results in equanimity. For example, the child who is unhappy and disturbed by peer rejection (Other Interpersonal Problem) immediately responds positively to acceptance by classmates.

The presence of these diagnostic categories for non-mental disorders in DSM-III emphasizes the comprehensive scope of this nomenclature. Diagnoses are provided for every conceivable disorder, including the possibility of a disorder not currently described (unspecified mental disorder) and the deferral of a diagnosis. Additional manifestations of this comprehensiveness are the presence of "atypical" and "unspecified" diagnoses scattered throughout the system and a category, adjustment disorder, which seems to occupy an intermediate position between the mental disorders and "conditions not attributable to a mental disorder."

Adjustment disorders are responses to identifiable crises and environmental

TABLE 2-1

DSM-III Categories Relevant to Children of Conditions Not Attributable to a Mental Disorder

Borderline intellectual functioning	IQ in the range of 71–84
Childhood or adolescent antisocial behavior	An isolated antisocial act
Academic problem	Difficulties in achievement in school with no apparent mental disorder
Uncomplicated bereavement	Normal depressive reaction to death of a loved one
Noncompliance with medical treatment	Refusal to cooperate for religious or reasonable reasons
Phase of life problem or other life circumstance problem	Temporary distress to some change in adjustment
Parent-child problem	An abused child or difficulties in communication with no mental disorder
Other specified family circumstances	Sibling rivalry, problem with relatives
Other interpersonal problem	Difficulties with peers, dating, teachers, and so on

TABLE 2-2

Adjustment Disorder

Adjustment disorder with depressed mood	
Adjustment disorder with anxious mood	
Adjustment disorder with mixed emotional features	
Adjustment disorder with disturbance of conduct	Several acts of truancy, vandalism, fighting, or misconduct
Adjustment disorder with mixed disturbance of emotions and conduct	
Adjustment disorder with academic inhibition	Difficulties in school after a record of adequate performance
Adjustment disorder with withdrawal	
Adjustment disorder with atypical features	

stressors; it is expected that the disorder will cease when the stressors are removed or when the person accommodates constructively to them. What distinguishes these disorders from those in Table 2-1 is that the adjustment disorder distress seems more severe or prolonged or frequent than that of the conditions. However, presumably adjustment disorders, too, are not mental disorders, since essentially they are expected to remit when circumstances change for the better (see Table 2-2).

It is important to emphasize that DSM-III in its effort to be inclusive and to provide a diagnosis for every psychological problem encompasses both mental and non-mental disorders. Its ambitious scope has alarmed some professionals, who are concerned that psychiatrists are attempting to define every problem, from baby-talk to schizophrenia, as being within their purview. However, the professed aim for DSM-III is not to stake out the professional boundaries of psychiatry, but to provide psychiatrists and professionals in the mental health field with diagnostic categories that cover every contingency (Spitzer, 1981). In accomplishing that ostensible aim there is no question of DSM-III's outstanding thoroughness.

Multiaxial System

A diagnosis according to DSM-III requires the individual to be evaluated along five independent axes. This simply means that each person is assessed in terms of five variables:

Axis I: Here are noted the mental disorders or conditions not attributable to a mental disorder appropriate to describe the individual. In general, on this axis are the diagnoses of immediate concern. For example, an adolescent boy with an IQ of 70 who smokes marijuana and bedwets daily would probably be diagnosed as functional enuresis, cannabis abuse, and mental retardation—mild on Axis I. The disorders which might be listed on Axis I are drawn from and comprise almost the entire DSM-III nomenclature (see Table 2-3).

Axis II: Only personality disorders and specific developmental disorders are listed on this axis. In general, these are chronic or longlasting disorders about which the individual may feel little concern (see Table 2-4). Since many clinicians believe the child's personality is somewhat flexible and resilient, five personality disorders are not diagnosed

TABLE 2-3

Axis I DSM-III Diagnostic Categories Relevant to Children

Category	Subtypes
I. *Disorders usually first evident in infancy, childhood, or adolescence*	
A. Mental retardation	Mild (IQ 50–70); moderate (IQ 35–49); severe (IQ 20–34); profound (IQ 19 or less); unspecified
B. Attention deficit disorder	With hyperactivity; without hyperactivity; residual
C. Conduct disorder	Undersocialized, aggressive; undersocialized, nonaggressive; socialized, aggressive; socialized, nonaggressive; atypical
D. Anxiety disorders of childhood or adolescence	Separation anxiety disorder; avoidant disorder; overanxious disorder
E. Other disorders of infancy, childhood, or adolescence	Reactive attachment disorder of infancy; schizoid disorder of childhood or adolescence; elective mutism; oppositional disorder; identity disorder
F. Eating disorders	Anorexia nervosa; bulimia; pica; rumination disorder of infancy; atypical
G. Stereotyped movement disorders	Transient tic; chronic motor tic; Tourette's disorder; atypical tic; atypical stereotyped movement
H. Other disorders with physical manifestations	Stuttering; functional enuresis; functional encopresis; sleepwalking disorder; sleep terror disorder
I. Pervasive developmental disorders	Infantile autism, full syndrome present or residual state; childhood onset pervasive developmental disorder, full syndrome present or residual state; atypical
II. Substance use disorders	Cannabis abuse; tobacco dependence; other
III. Schizophrenic disorders	Disorganized; undifferentiated; residual
IV. Affective disorders	Major depressive episode; dysthymic disorder
V. Anxiety disorders	Simple phobia
VI. Psychosexual disorders	Transexualism; gender identity disorder of childhood; atypical; ego-dystonic homosexuality
VII. Adjustment disorder	(See Table 2-2)
VIII. Conditions not attributable to a mental disorder	(See Table 2-1)
IX. Psychological factors affecting physical condition	(This condition replaces *psychosomatic* or *psychophysiologic* disorders. The physical disorder, or medical illness, is coded on Axis III.)

among children and adolescents. Although the patterns of behavior are virtually the same, on theoretical grounds before the age of eighteen years one diagnosis is given, and only after that age is a diagnosis of personality disorder made (see Table 2-5).

Axis III: On this axis are noted any physical disorders and conditions of the child. Examples: asthma, juvenile onset diabetes, nystagmus, and so on. As many are listed as are appropriate.

Axis IV: This is essentially a seven-point rating scale on which the diagnostician assesses the Severity of the Psychosocial Stressors that seemed to precipitate the disorder from 1 (none) to 7 (catastrophic, such as the deaths of two or more members of the child's family). It is assumed that the stressor will have occurred within the year prior to the onset of the disorder, and that the prognosis will be more favorable if some severe stressor can be identified rather than if the disorder occurs following mild (example: a change in school teacher) or minimal (example: vacation with family) stress.

TABLE 2-4

Axis II DSM-III Diagnostic Categories Relevant to Children

I. Personality disorders	
A. Schizotypal personality disorder	
B. Dependent personality disorder	
C. Compulsive personality disorder	
D. Narcissistic personality disorder	
E. Paranoid personality disorder	
F. Histrionic personality disorder	
G. Atypical personality disorder	
II. Specific developmental disorders	
A. Developmental reading disorder	
B. Developmental arithmetic disorder	
C. Developmental language disorder	Expressive type or receptive type
D. Developmental articulation disorder	
E. Mixed specific developmental disorder	
F. Atypical specific developmental disorder	

Axis V: This is another seven-point rating scale on which the diagnostician judges the highest level of adaptive functioning in the past year from (1) superior to (7) grossly impaired. In making this judgment the age of the individual is considered with regard to performance in social relations, work or school, and leisure activities. For a school-age child, Level 1 would be indicated by popularity with peers, excellent grades, and a constructive use of afterschool time, all accomplished with enjoyment, ease, and zest; Level 7 would be indicated by very serious deficiencies in all these areas. Presumably, the higher the level of adaptation, the more favorable the prognosis and the better the adjustment that can be expected following recovery.

This multiaxial system facilitates research and certainly provides more information than a diagnostic label. It affords impressions of both immediate and long-standing psychological problems, physical disorders, precipitating factors, and premorbid adjustment. Although it places

TABLE 2-5

Age-Determined DSM-III Diagnostic Categories

Onset Before Age 18	Onset After Age 18
Schizoid disorder of childhood or adolescence	Schizoid personality disorder
Avoidant disorder of childhood or adolescence	Avoidant personality disorder
Conduct disorder	Antisocial personality disorder
Oppositional disorder	Passive-aggressive personality disorder
Identity disorder	Borderline personality disorder
Overanxious disorder	Generalized anxiety disorder

greater demands upon diagnosticians, Spitzer, Williams, and Skodol (1980) reported clinicians favored its use.

It should be noted that DSM-III maintains the practice of regarding Mental Retardation, *ipso facto,* as a disorder. Of interest is that the World Health Organization also has a multiaxial classification but places intellectual level on an axis of its own (Rutter, Lebovoici, Eisenberg, Sneznevskij, Sadoun, Brooke, & Lin, 1969; Rutter, Shaffer, & Shepherd, 1975). This reflects a position that mental retardation is, in and of itself, no more a mental disorder than is above average intellectual functioning.

General Assumptions in DSM-III

A major assumption in DSM-III is that the validity of the different etiological models with reference to specific disorders remains to be established. While certain disorders have a definite etiology, for the great majority of problems the arguments for one theoretical position are no more compelling than they are for another. DSM-III has tried to avoid any bias toward one view over another, even going so far as to try to avoid a bias toward the medical model (Spitzer, Williams, & Skodol, 1980); though admittedly this would have been quite an accomplishment since it was written mainly by and for psychiatrists.

It is assumed that DSM-III, though a good, conscientious effort at developing a reliable and valid nomenclature, nevertheless has imperfections. Unavoidably it is dated by the limits of current knowledge. While field trials were conducted to identity problems in its use prior to its adoption, in all likelihood difficulties will emerge that were not anticipated. Moreover, despite its comprehensiveness, new syndromes may be identified. Accordingly, this classification system is seen as ever-evolving, not as a fixed statement about the existence of a certain number of definite disorders.

More explicitly, DSM-III is a classification system not necessarily of specific, clear-cut disorders, but of behavior patterns. It is not a classification of individuals, but of the behaviors that an individual may display. A person is not fully or adequately described by the diagnostic labels no matter how many are appropriately used. Moreover, it disarmingly acknowledges the lack of mutually exclusive disorders by urging that as many labels be employed as are appropriate in making the diagnosis. Although all persons with a given disorder are similar in the ways by which that disorder is defined, it must be stressed they are also quite different in many important ways. Those differences may be, and often are, of greater significance than the commonalities of the disorder.

Further, it is recognized that the boundaries that demarcate disorders in childhood from those in adulthood are artificial and contrived. Aside from the diagnostic categories which are specifically defined by age (senile dementia, for example, and see also Table 2-5), adult diagnoses may properly be assigned to children who satisfy the criteria, and disorders which originate in infancy, childhood, and adolescence may be assigned to adults when it appears those symptoms have persisted from youth. Some adult disorders which are more likely than others to be exhibited by children are noted in Categories II–VI in Table 2-3. Among the disorders of childhood that are apt to be appropriate for adults are: mental retardation; attention deficit disorder–residual; eating disorders; anorexia nervosa and bulimia; stuttering, chronic motor tic; Tourette's disorder; and residual state of infantile autism or pervasive developmental disorder.

What emerges from this flexibility is an attitude of candor about the uncertainties of this classification system. Consensus among the committee members about diagnostic categories was not always attained; in some instance a majority vote determined the issue, with the minority still strongly opposed to the ultimate decision. If ever a student of psychopathology was tempted to believe in the reality of the diagnostic categories, that temptation should be swept aside by reading the final report from the chairman and leading members of the American Psychiatric Association's Task Force on Nomenclature and Statistics (Spitzer, Williams, & Skokol, 1980) who conclude: "DSM-III represents a major investment by our profession. The real payoff, in terms of advancing the field and better understanding and care of our patients, will come from careful study in the next few years of the strengths and weaknesses of this system. This will be of great help to those brave souls given the responsibility for developing DSM-IV."

The above quotation suggests a dominant assumption in DSM-III. The individual is more important than the diagnostic categories. Justice to the individual, not to the system, is of paramount importance. If no diagnostic category is appropriate, the clinician is advised to use none, to defer a diagnosis, to offer a tentative diagnosis, or to use whatever diagnostic statement outside DSM-III seems appropriate. The uncertainties and limitations of any classification scheme are implied by these recommendations, but an attitude of freedom is also conveyed to the clinician to exercise professional judgment. DSM-III through its relatively rigorous definitions constrains and guides the diagnostic process, while through the liberality of its attitudes it conveys a becomingly modest and sophisticated appraisal of what it after all accomplishes.

Criticisms of DSM-III: Reliability

A major aim of DSM-III and its operational definitions is to increase the reliability of diagnoses. Previous research with DSM-I and II in the classification of adults and the Group for the Advancement of Psychiatry's nomenclature in the classification of children found unacceptably low reliabilities, unless judgments about broad diagnostic categories, such as psychotic, neurotic, or organic, were at issue (Beck, et al., 1962; Freeman, 1971; Sandifer, Pettus, & Quade, 1964; Schmidt & Fonda, 1956). On the face of it, the greater specificity of diagnostic criteria cannot do anything but help to increase reliabilities, particularly for disorders such as functional enuresis and encopresis, where previously there had been no age or frequency delineations. Nevertheless, the reliability of DSM-III, particularly in the diagnosis of children and adolescents, is still a matter for investigation.

The field trials assessing the reliability of DSM-III had pairs of experienced clinicians interview 281 patients. At times two clinicians interviewed the same patient independently. In some cases the interviews were conducted jointly by the two clinicians. Agreement was higher under the latter set of circumstances than under the former, was higher than had been found for DSM-I and II, but was still only moderate. The reported coefficient of agreement was .78 for diagnoses on Axis I and .61 for diagnoses on Axis II (Spitzer, Forman, & Nee, 1979). More disconcerting is the fact that agreement was counted when the clinicians agreed upon the general class of disorder, (for example, affective), even though they might have disagreed upon the specific diagnosis. It is the decision having to do with the specific diagnosis that is often the issue in clinical practice. Agreements on Axes IV and V were at similar levels, .62 and .80, respectively (Spitzer & Forman, 1979). And remember the field trials were conducted only with adult patients!

With regard to children, a study conducted by Cantwell, Mattison, Russell, and Will (1979) provides some enlightenment. These investigators selected twenty-four case histories of child and adolescent patients who presented a variety of diagnoses and diagnostic issues. After agreeing among themselves about the DSM-II and III diagnoses that should be assigned ("the expected diagnosis"), they submitted the case histories to twenty child psychiatrists for their diagnostic judgments. They were interested in how much agreement there would be among their judges (interrater agreement) and how often the judges' diagnoses would agree with those of the investigators.

Unavoidably the study was conducted with an early draft of DSM-III, which differed in certain respects from the final version and which meant that the judges had little familiarity with the nomenclature. Although the judges were given an opportunity to familiarize themselves with the system, they did not have the benefit of a training program. Such a program has appeared to result in higher reliabilities than is found otherwise (Webb, et al., 1981). Further, judgments were based on case material, not patient interviews, and the judges differed considerably among themselves in their experience in child psychiatry; eight were faculty members in psychiatry, but the remainder were students, of whom six were in their first year of training with children.

Considering the above problems and the fact that judges were required to agree on the specific diagnosis, it is not too surprising that interrater agreement averaged 57 percent for DSM-II and 54 percent for Axis I of DSM-III. More informative than these averages were the agreements on particular disorders: 100 percent for infantile autism, 85 percent for mental retardation, 75 percent for attention deficit disorders and specific developmental disorders, but only 35 percent for organic brain syndromes. There also seemed to be difficulties in diagnosing depression, schizophrenia, and anxiety disorders, again, perhaps because the judges were working with a new system.

The investigators found that the great majority of the judges preferred DSM-III to DSM-II. They also found that the multiaxial system led to more attention being given to the possibility of Axis II disorders so that they were more often noted under DSM-III than they were under DSM-II. The same was true for non-mental medical disorders on Axis III. Their general conclusion was that the DSM-III diagnosis was more clinically useful and that there were no difficulties with the system of any significant nature.

Strober, Green and Carlson (1981) investigated interrater agreement on Axis I in the diagnosis of hospitalized adolescents. In this study there were only two judges, Strober and Green, both experienced clinicians who had some familiarity with DSM-III. Although Strober is a clinical psychologist and Green is a psychiatrist, profession need not be a significant variable in the use of this nomenclature

(Morey, 1980). The procedure they followed was such as to maximize reliability. In addition to their close collaborative relationship, their diagnostic judgments were based on joint interviews with each of ninety-five patients and readings of all available case history information. Under these circumstances, disagreements would tend to point to diagnostic categories that were not clearly defined.

Overall, there was a moderate degree of agreement between Strober and Green; the coefficient of concordance (K) was .74. But there was also considerable variation. Agreement was high in the diagnosis of eating disorders (.94) and schizophrenia (.82), but was low for anxiety disorders. Since the investigators were working with the 1977 draft of DSM-III, which was being revised until virtually the moment of its publication in 1980, it is possible that some sources of vagueness and confusion in the nomenclature were subsequently reduced.

These two studies demonstrate that a high degree of agreement can be expected with the use of DSM-III in the diagnosis of certain disorders—attention deficit with hyperactivity, mental retardation, pervasive developmental disorders, eating disorders—but not in the diagnosis of others—organic brain syndromes and anxiety disorders. Low reliability seems to occur when a child exhibits a disorder that is infrequently seen or rarely considered. High reliability is associated with disorders that are defined by easily verified behaviors. The very thoroughness of DSM-III in providing diagnostic categories for almost any contingency cannot help but act to reduce reliability when agreements are compared for specific disorders rather than general classes of disorder because as the number of diagnostic options increase so too do the possibilities for disagreement.

Criticisms of DSM-III: Validity

Ordinarily in discussions of the validity of a psychiatric nomenclature it is reasonable to note that a diagnostic category may be reliable (i.e., people can agree on the diagnosis) even when it may not be valid (i.e., the category may not define a mental disorder or it may be heterogeneous and consist of two or more disorders). This criticism does not seem to faze those who developed DSM-III since they did not regard the diagnostic categories as necessarily descriptive of mental disorders or as mutually exclusive; the system allows for conditions not attributable to a mental disorder and for multiple diagnoses. Such a sophisticated attitude is quite disarming, and would be appropriate if everyone were well-informed about DSM-III. However, assuming that not everyone is knowledgeable, it is important to be alert to the hazards and confusions that can result.

The probability is high that if someone sends a child to a psychiatrist and the psychiatrist diagnoses a disorder, it will be assumed that the child has a psychiatric disorder. A "psychiatric disorder" carries a number of implications, none of which is very positive or favorable: disease, mental illness, instability, craziness, and unpredictability, to mention a few. Yet the assumption that a psychiatric diagnosis under DSM-III means a mental disorder is, as we have seen, not valid. According to DSM-III, all that a psychiatric diagnosis means is that the child has some problem, which may or may not be a mental disorder. But it is highly unlikely that the public will be aware of this distinction. Nor is this the entire story.

Certain conditions in DSM-III have

been specified as *not* due to a mental disorder. This would lead one to assume that all the remaining conditions not so specified are due to mental disorder or disabilities within the person. Many of those problems are not regarded as mental disorders by many professionals and a sizable part of the general population, but as problems associated with a lack of adequate training or ineffective educational practices and procedures, such as stuttering; functional enuresis and encopresis; developmental articulation, reading, or arithmetic disorders; and pica. Behavioral professionals, of course, would argue that improper training is involved in far more disorders than the few just mentioned (Ross, 1980; Schwartz & Johnson, 1981).

Therefore, the extent to which DSM-III is a classification of mental disorders, even when it says it is, is questionable. It has been estimated that according to the criteria of this system about 80 percent of all the criminals in this country are now able to be diagnosed as antisocial personality disorder (Frances, 1980); in contrast, according to DSM-II criteria only 25 to 33 percent of inmates received that diagnosis (Goldenberg, 1977, p. 565). Hence it would not be valid to interpret a significant increase in the numbers of criminals diagnosed as antisocial personality disorder as indicative of a dramatic increase in the incidence of this disorder.

Prevalence refers to the number of cases in a given population at a given time who have a particular condition. Estimates of children who are emotionally disturbed have ranged from 2 to 20 percent (Kauffman, 1981, pp. 22–23; Weiner, 1970, pp. 50–52). President Carter's Commission on Mental Health estimated about 20 percent of school-age children have psychological problems for which they might need professional help. These estimates were based upon diagnoses when DSM-II was in effect. What will be the anticipated impact of DSM-III?

It was intended that DSM-III be a comprehensive system and this very comprehensiveness will probably act to inflate prevalence of mental disorder figures. Two new disorders alone, avoidant disorder and oppositional disorder, will enable children who are shy and disobedient to be diagnosed as having psychiatric disorders and bring a sizable number of youngsters into the realm of what is regarded as the mentally disturbed. Garmezy (1978) has vigorously objected to the overinclusiveness of DSM-III. In particular he has questioned the inclusion of specific developmental disorders within the nomenclature, contending that these problems are neither diagnosed nor treated by psychiatrists and that psychiatry has no special expertise in these areas: "The entire taxonomy has been made vulnerable by an overreaching effort by the creators of the children's section to bring under psychiatry's wing deficits and disabilities that are not mental disorders" (Garmezy, 1978, p. 4).

Although the committee which developed DSM-III acted with a refreshing candor and humility in recognizing the limits of knowledge about etiology and the questionable validity of the system, the result is a heterogeneous, mixed-bag classification system. They have thrown together mental disorders and disorders that are not mental disorders, in some cases making clear which are which, but in most instances merely assuming that when the etiology is unknown, the problem is a mental disorder. It is a system of rocks and fruits. It is definitely an artificial system. It is also a system of unknown and dubious validity.

In the years to come the validity of DSM-III should be investigated and the findings of this research should be incorporated in DSM-IV. Questions, however, have been raised about the validity of a number of specific categories where diagnostic criteria depart markedly from previous understandings of the disorders or where labels have been significantly changed (Frances, 1980; Goldstein, 1983; Hyler & Spitzer, 1978; Lyskowskil & Tsuang, 1980; Rieder, 1979; Spitzer & Endicott, 1979). With particular relevance to children are the concepts of "early infantile autism" and the "borderline child."

The disorder early infantile autism was identified by Leo Kanner in 1943 and named by him in 1944. The major symptom of the disorder, the one which gave the syndrome its name and identifying characteristic, was the profound inability of these children to relate themselves to people "*from the beginning of life*" (italics added; Kanner, 1943). Although the syndrome was immediately recognized by clinicians and grew to be the subject of an extensive literature (Rimland, 1964; Rutter, 1971; Schopler & Reichler, 1976; Lovaas, 1977; Morgan, 1981), early infantile autism did not find its way into the psychiatric nomenclature until DSM-III.

Somewhat surprisingly, DSM-III criteria for infantile autism differ from Kanner's by specifying that the symptoms be present prior to the child's attainment of thirty months of age. Note that Kanner specified the disorder must be evidenced virtually from birth. He took pains to mention the parents must report the child never evidenced normal responsiveness to social stimulation. Such a determination is, of necessity, dependent upon case history material, whose reliability is often suspect. Accordingly, the less stringent criterion for onset in DSM-III should make for greater reliability in diagnosing this disorder. However, what is its effect on validity?

From a psychodynamic point of view the child who *never* has evidenced an interest in others represents a quite different problem from the child who has developed normally for a time and who then shows signs of an autistic disorder. The former suggests an early fixation in development or an inherent or early acquired incapacity to make and emotionally invest in relationships. The latter suggests a regression in development due to some psychological conflict or trauma.

Clinically, this distinction has been recognized and has been thought to have meaningful implications for treatment. Des Lauriers and Carlson (1969), among others (Rimland, 1964; Schopler & Reichler, 1976), have postulated an organic problem among children who exhibit the Kanner syndrome and have advocated they be helped by means of pleasant, intrusive, physical stimulations, such as tickling. Mahler (1952) and Bettelheim (1967) have addressed themselves to what has been termed "secondary autism," or "symbiotic psychosis," in which a discernable period of apparently normal development during infancy is followed by the symptom picture of autism; here a treatment involving psychotherapy has been advocated.

The DSM-III criteria obliterate the clinical distinction between early infantile autism (primary autism) and secondary autism, or symbiotic psychosis. Since an ultimate aim of a psychiatric nomenclature is to evolve into mutually exclusive categories of known etiology, it is difficult to see how this aim has been furthered by what has happened in the diagnosis of infantile autism.

Similarly, the concept of the borderline child was a clinically recognized disorder which was not previously acknowledged in the official nomenclature. As understood, the borderline child referred to a youngster who maintains an uneven, precarious balance between a somewhat marginal adjustment and emotional outbursts so extreme that contact with reality is temporarily lost. Relatively unprovoked temper tantrums, a low tolerance for frustration, and poor peer relationships characterize these children, who are evidently not unknown to clinicians (Ekstein & Wallerstein, 1954; Marcus, 1963).

The diagnostic category of borderline personality disorder in DSM-III has symptoms that differ in several respects from those of the borderline child and in any event is an age-specified diagnosis, that is, professionals are urged to reserve the diagnosis of this disorder for those who are eighteen years old or older. The homogeneity of this adult category has already been questioned (Lyskowskil & Tsuang, 1980), but the concern raised here is that a term which was widely used by professionals working with children has been appropriated by DSM-III and redefined so that it no longer has the meaning previously understood. This redefinition cannot help but cause confusion.

Adding to this problem is the suggestion within DSM-III that those considering the diagnosis of "borderline child," which does not exist in the nomenclature, consider the diagnosis of schizotypal personality disorder, which does. While there are similarities between the symptom pictures of the two disorders, it is conceivable that a child who would be thought to be borderline would not meet the diagnostic criteria stipulated by DSM-III for schizotypal personality disorder.

In sum, DSM-III is highly vulnerable to criticism on the gounds of its validity. While it appears to make for greater reliability in diagnosis, the validity of some of the diagnostic categories is suspect. These conclusions make it necessary to be cautious in conducting and evaluating research bearing upon a number of the disorders identified by DSM-III: "For research purposes the current diagnostic schema is only a preliminary classification and should be regarded as tentative in the same sense that the first interpretations of the data of any experiment are tentative" (Zubin, 1977–78, p. 6).

Criticisms of DSM-III: Doctrinaire

DSM-III has endeavored to be atheoretical and has left moot the issues of etiology whenever factors responsible for a disorder are controversial. Therefore it has been criticized by advocates of one or another model of psychopathology for neglecting proper attention to behavioral (Schwartz & Johnson, 1981), psychodynamic (Francis & Cooper, 1981; Karasu & Skodol, 1980), and systems or ecological (McLemore & Benjamin, 1979; McReynolds, 1979) explanations. To the extent that research determines the significance of behavioral, psychodynamic, and ecological variables in the etiologies of disorders, these criticisms will have validity, but at present it is difficult to say. Thus far, the impressive research of behaviorists has been addressed to the maintenance and modification of behavior, not etiology.

DSM-III has also been criticized for being based on the medical model, despite its disclaimers to the contrary. The fact is that DSM-III is the official nomenclature of the American Psychiatric Association and thus cannot help but connote a medical responsibility for its disorders. It seems about as reasonable to criticize DSM-III for being based on a medical model as it would be to criticize Anna

Freud's (1965) description of children according to developmental lines for being based on a psychodynamic model or to object to Ross's (1980) classification of childhood disorders for being based on a behavioral model.

Alternative Classification Systems

Although DSM-III is the prevalent nomenclature in use in the United States, there are other classification systems in use elsewhere, such as the International Classification of Diseases or the systems employed within foreign countries. Thus what might be called identity disorder in this country is apt to be known as philosophical intoxication in the Soviet Union (Rollins, 1972). Rather than present these more or less similar medical model systems, it may be more instructive to consider the classifications proposed by American proponents of psychodynamic and behavioral models so that their merits can be assessed.

Psychodynamic. The psychosexual-psychosocial theory of development discussed in Chapter 1 can be considered a form of classification. Behaviors of the child would be examined to determine whether the child evidences undue fixations in the oral, anal, phallic, or other, stages and how these particular fixations are manifested. Since a fairly comprehensive theory of personality is involved, knowing that a child is fixated at one or another stage immediately suggests corresponding conflicts, ways of dealing with them (defenses), and treatment strategies (See Table 2-6).

An eight-year-old boy, for example, who ordinarily is constipated except for the day or two each week he soils his pants, assuming there is no physical basis for these symptoms and his parents have endeavored to toilet train him, would be regarded as exhibiting a disorder within the anal stage of development. There would be interest in determining whether the problem represents a fixation—a continuation of anal concerns—or a regression—a retreat to the problems of anality because the conflicts of a subsequent stage are more threatening and disruptive. Anal conflicts suggest this boy is probably concerned with issues of autonomy, which would indicate difficulties with authority about matters of who exercises control, problems in the open expression of hostility and self-assertiveness, a lack of certainty about what it is he really does want, and the use of isolation as a defense. Treatment would be directed toward making these problems more available to conscious expression and control, both for the boy and his parents.

Anna Freud (1965) has recommended that a diagnostic description be ordered along a number of different lines or where the child is performing on each of several different progressive stages of development. The exact number and the kinds of developmental lines were not specified by her, but presumably there would be as many as our knowledge indicated would be appropriate for a meaningful description. In addition to Freud's psychosexual and Eriksen's psychosocial stages, there might be lines for intellectual, moral, and peer relationship development. To illustrate: Relations with peers would progress from indifference to other children, to recognition of their presence, to regarding peers as competitors, to occasional interaction when the peer is of some use, to seeing peers as helpers and playmates, to the exchanging of confidences with peers

TABLE 2-6

A Psychoanalytic Scheme of Defenses and Defensive Characteristics

Stage	Defense Mechanisms	Personality Characteristics
Narcissism	Denial: fantasy hallucinations Repression	Withdrawn, schizoid, autistic Impulse-ridden, sociopathic
Oral (trust—mistrust)	Introjection Projection	Passive, dependent, gullible Suspicious, paranoid Demanding, critical, unappreciative
Anal (autonomy—shame, doubt)	Isolation Undoing Displacement Reaction Formation Intellectualization Reversal of Affect	*Obsessive-compulsive:* Thrift, uncertainty, attention to details, neatness, orderliness, stubbornness, opposition to authority, negativism
Phallic (initiative—guilt)	Repression Identification Counterphobic	*Hysteric:* Fearful, anxiety-ridden, naive, dramatic, emotional, intuitive, disorganized, self-indulgent, dissociative
Latency (industry—inferiority)	Rationalization	*Competitiveness:* Feelings of superiority in relation to peers
Early gential (identity—confusion)	Asceticism Intellectualization Sublimation	Search for meaning, values, sexual identity, roles, vocation, purpose

Note: As a defense, regression can occur at any stage following the first. Early defenses may occur from time to time at later stages; what is significant is the persistent use of a defense and its frequency, to the extent that the person is characterized by its use.

and seeing them as persons with feelings of their own, to close relationships with peers of the same and other sex, to intimate relations with a peer of the other sex. Research would be important to establish the sequences of stages in the developmental lines, the age range for each stage, and their correctness (see, for example, Selman and Jaquette, 1978).

An elaborate diagnostic scheme based upon Anna Freud's recommendation and drawing upon Mahler, Pine, and Bergman (1975) and Piaget (1969) has been presented by Greenspan (1981; Greenspan & Lourie, 1981). Specifically criticizing DSM-III because it is "unsystematic" and "lacks a cohesive developmental focus that encompasses developmental lines," Greenspan (1981, p. 12) goes on to offer a highly detailed system for describing children up to ten years of age. His system consists of developmental lines for: physical and neurological growth; mood or emotional tone; capacity for human relations, affects displayed by the child and means of coping with anxiety; how the child uses available space and materials; and the child's communication of themes and problems. The validity of these lines seems open. Physical and neurological growth, for example, appears soundly based upon the large body of empirical research in child development. However, other lines, such as the child's communication of themes and problems, are on less secure foundations and in need of much research to establish their validity.

Statistical. A common strategy in a statistical determination of diagnostic groupings is to take a number of symptoms or problems—e.g., shy, steals, withdrawn, wets bed, overactive—ask judges, often parents or teachers, to rate children, usually those who are being considered for professional help, as to which of these problems they have; and employ a statistical technique, factor analysis, to determine which problems are intercorrelated, that is, clustered together into syndromes, and how many clusterings or factors are needed to account for the results. Presumably the reliability and validity of a classification system would be enhanced if the large number of diagnostic groupings could be reduced to a few empirically verified categories. Moreover, this procedure demonstrates which symptoms do seem to cluster together into observable patterns of disorder.

Peterson (1961) found that two factors could account for many of the difficulties of elementary school children. One factor, *personality problems*, referred to children who were shy, anxious, fearful, self-conscious, easily embarrassed, socially withdrawn, and inadequate. The second factor, *conduct problems*, related to children who fought, were noisy and boisterous, restless, disruptive, attention-seeking, and disobedient. Subsequent research has tended to confirm these two factors.

Achenbach (1966) had raters go over the case material of 600 boys and girls, four to sixteen years of age, referred to a child psychiatry unit of a university hospital, deciding which of ninety-one problems and complaints they seemed to exhibit. The major principle factor that emerged from an analysis of the data was labelled *internalizing-externalizing.* The problems subsumed at the two poles of this factor, "problems within the self" at one end and "conflict with the environment" at the other, indicate its correspondence to Peterson's "personality problems-conduct problems." Of interest was that among girls internalizers were twice as frequent as externalizers, while the reverse was true among boys.

A second principal factor in Achenbach's study was called "severe and diffuse psychopathology," which consisted of items involving bizarre behaviors, delusions, hallucinations, and extreme aggressiveness. Since this second factor is an independent dimension, it indicates that severity of pathology can be in either internalizing or externalizing directions.

The problem with factor analytic research and these broad dimensions is that although they provide a general idea of the child's problem, they are not specific enough to be clinically useful. Given a child who is an externalizer or an internalizer provides less information about the nature of the child's difficulties than does a DSM-III diagnosis. Although the reduction of diagnostic categories is desirable, it is not the sole consideration. After all, if simplification were the only aim, it would be sensible to adopt a single category classification system that recognized all psychopathologies as merely different forms of deficiencies in learning or training. This criticism of nomenclatures derived from factor analyses seems to have been accepted in more recent presentations of empirical efforts.

After surveying the literature on empirical forms of classification, Achenbach and Edelbrock (1978) suggested there are broad-band and narrow-band factors. One broad-band factor is *undercontrolled* and *overcontrolled,* which corresponds to the externalizing-internalizing dimension. A second is *pathological detachment,* which is similar to the factor of severe and diffuse psychopathology. A third is *learning problems,* which consists of failures to achieve at an expected grade level in one or more academic areas. As broad-band factors these dimensions could be relevant in any narrow-band factor or syndrome.

Achenbach and Edelbrock identified the following fourteen narrow-band syndromes or specific disorders: (1) aggressive; (2) delinquent; (3) hyperactive; (4) schizoid; (5) anxious; (6) depressed; (7) somatic complaints; (8) social withdrawal; (9) academic disability; (10) immature; (11) obsessive-compulsive; (12) sexual problems; (13) sleep problems; and (14) uncommunicative.

Similarly, Quay (1979) suggested that a survey of the research literature, much of it the same as that reviewed by Achenbach and Edelbrock, indicated the presence of five patterns of disorder: (1) *conduct disorder,* which involves verbal and physical aggression, as well as poor social relationships with both children and adults; (2) *anxiety-withdrawal,* a pattern of anxious and/or withdrawn behaviors; (3) *immaturity,* consisting of short attention span, daydreaming, poor coordination, passivity, and inattentiveness; (4) *socialized-aggressive disorder,* which refers to delinquent activities perpetrated by members of gangs who have some loyalty and friendliness to one another; and (5) *psychosis,* which has to do with social unresponsiveness and avoidance or hypersensitivity to stimulation.

Certainly five or even fourteen disorders are far fewer than the number of syndromes found in DSM-III for the diagnosis of children, so that these efforts do suggest directions for simplication and enhanced reliability. Nevertheless, it must be reiterated that in clinical practice economy in diagnostic categories is seldom a major consideration, and in fact it is usually no consideration at all. A clinician is rarely striving to describe the problems of patients in the least number of categories, but is most often trying to do justice to the syndromes or behavior patterns that each individual patient presents.

Accordingly, clinicians may be particularly interested in those very clusters of behaviors that are exceedingly rare. In these instances, statistically it may be very difficult, if not impossible, to isolate the clinically observed syndrome. Early infantile autism and anorexia nervosa are not readily apparent from a statistical analysis of data. Nevertheless, these disorders do occur, their syndromes are distinctive, and they have definite prognostic and treatment implications that are not conveyed by any of the statistically-derived narrow-band syndromes.

Moreover, the analysis and interpretation of statistical results are by no stretch of the imagination straightforward and unequivocal. Low to moderate, though statistically significant, correlations are often ambiguous in their implications. In discussing the findings of a number of factor analytic studies, Quay was led to the conclusion that: "Considering all of the data, the evidence for the independence of hyperactivity as independent from conduct disorder is dubious at best" (Quay, 1979, p. 23).

Certainly the number of studies evaluated by Quay which failed to find a hyperactivity factor exceeded the number of studies which did. But a moderate, or even a very high, correlation between variables has never meant they are necessarily identical or equivalent, as witness the relationship in childhood between height and weight. The reality is that in clinical settings individual children are observed to exhibit independent patterns of behavior which may cluster together as a common factor. Some children diagnosed as hyperactive do not fight and hit, which is a leading component of conduct disorder. This brings us to the following critical point.

Although some factor analytic groupings appear to be relatively homogeneous, others do not. Instead, they represent an aggregate of problems which statistically may cluster together but which occur in isolation often enough to necessitate their separate consideration when working with individual children.

In the final analysis, what information do we have knowing that a child has a sleep problem or a conduct disorder? Given the former diagnosis, would we not be better informed if we knew the sleep problem was insomnia or nightmares; given the latter diagnosis, would it not be more helpful to learn the specific nature of the conduct disorder, whether it be stealing or defiance of authority?

Statistics is, after all, only a tool, a means for the ordering and evaluation of data. In its use the exceptional, the individual case, is often ignored in pointing the way toward the general trend. It directs attention to uniformities and generalizations, and these are meaningful and helpful in furthering understanding and in making informed judgments. Nevertheless, in clinical interactions it is the individual child who is present and who is at issue. This individual child is like no other, despite similarities among the members of those abstractions known as factors or diagnostic categories. It seems that an aim of DSM-III, insofar as it is possible, is to recognize diversity through its multiaxial approach, its large number of clinically based diagnostic groupings, and its open-ended nature. (If none of its diagnostic categories seems appropriate, the creative clinician is advised to insert an original description.) It should frankly be recognized that in its objective of encompassing uniqueness, DSM-III is openly at variance with the goal of a statistical or empirical classification, and that the choice of system involves the question of values.

General Criticisms of Classifications

No matter what classification system is used, the fact that a person is classified has certain negative consequences. The label or diagnostic category calls attention to itself and to the class characteristics which have been assigned to it. As a result the uniqueness of the individual, the differences of this situation from any other, may be minimized or lost. Even worse, the assets and strengths of a child, or a child's family, may be so ignored or distorted that they fail to be utilized.

What is one to make of the bit of information that the prognosis for children diagnosed as infantile autism is not very favorable (Kanner, 1971) when dealing with a child who exhibits that disorder? Will this information assist, hinder, or have no effect upon treatment efforts? To the extent that the label and its correlates discourage or hinder treatment and the expectations of improvement, it can be argued that this knowledge has been a disservice to this child.

The negative consequences of labeling are particularly strong in the field of psychopathology. In spite of many years of publicity about mental health, and though improvements in attitudes have occurred, it is still true that psychological disturbances occasion more negative feelings than do physical ailments. Franklin D. Roosevelt, though crippled from the effects of polio, was nominated and elected president four times; in contrast a later candidate for the vice presidency was compelled to withdraw, due, in large part, to his having undergone treatment for depression, although the therapy had been successful in alleviating the symptoms and he appeared in all respects to be functioning effectively.

Psychiatric diagnoses and terms have often assumed pejorative characteristics. As the public and children become familiar with a label, it often ceases to be used in a sensitive, detached, nonevaluative manner and is employed to ridicule, insult, and deprecate the person. "Feebleminded," "moron," "imbecile," "disturbed," "retard," "mentally ill": the terms are not in and of themselves the issue but the attitudes and values elicited by them are. These attitudes and values associate a persistent stigma with the behaviors of mental illness, a wish to isolate and extrude the mentally ill person from society, and fears about the irrationality and unpredictability of those afflicted.

To label a child mentally retarded or emotionally disturbed can have immediate and far-ranging effects upon the child's education, social relationships, and life. Many of these effects may be intended to be helpful and constructive through the identification of children for treatment programs, special educational classes, and tutoring. But at the same time it must be recognized that even a beneficial and appropriate service can have adverse effects by segregating the child from peers and by oversensitizing the child and others to the existence of problems.

In a study by Langer and Abelson (1974) a group of psychoanalytically oriented clinical psychologists was shown a videotaped interview of a young man discussing his job history. Half these psychologists were told the man was a "job applicant"; half were told he was a "patient." The analytic clinicians who thought the man was an applicant described him as: "attractive and conventional looking," "candid and innovative," "straightforward," "upstanding," "middle class," and "fairly open." Those who thought he was a patient described him as: "tight, defensive," "passive," "considerable hostility," and "despondent." As an applicant, the man was rated as significantly better in psychological adjustment than when he was identified as a patient.

Similarly Critchley (1979) found adverse effects of labels when ninety nursing students observed films of three normal children. When a child was identified as schizophrenic or obsessive compulsive, the youngster was judged significantly more disturbed than when labeled normal.

While it is not especially distressing that a person who is given a pathological label is regarded as more disturbed than one who is not—if we label one bottle of clear, colorless liquid "vodka" and another "poison," we would hardly be surprised at the different reactions these labels evoke—it is disconcerting that professionals make quite different personality judgments about the same behaviors. Evidently labeling biases are quite pervasive, though in the general population they may be ill-founded in fears about the mentally ill, while among professionals they may be associated with stereotypes involved in theoretical orientations.

Hobbs (1975) has detailed the many harmful consequences of labels when applied to children. Yet he has also recognized that the classification of children serves many useful purposes in organizing research, facilitating communication, grouping children with certain meaningful characteristics in common for treatment and help, and in providing a means for rallying parents and pressure groups for the enactment of suitable legislation and programs.

As we have tried to emphasize, it is not the label that is in itself harmful, but the feelings and behaviors aroused by the label, which in turn would seem to depend upon the behaviors and personality attributes associated with the label. Classifying and labeling are significant steps in scientifically ordering observations and data. A diagnostic nomenclature can be empirically and clinically useful. Its terms are best employed when it is remembered they are merely convenient devices for identifying presumably significant commonalities among individuals rather than being encompassing descriptions of the individual children.

REFERENCES

Achenbach, T. M. The classification of children's psychiatric symptoms: A factor-analytic study. *Psychological Monographs,* 1966, *80* (6, Whole No. 615).

Achenbach, T. M., & Edelbrock, C. S. The classification of child psychopathology: A review and analysis of empirical efforts. *Psychological Bulletin,* 1978, *85,* 1275–1301.

American Psychiatric Association. *Diagnostic and statistical manual of mental disorders* (3d Ed.). Washington, D. C.: American Psychiatric Association, 1980.

Beck, A. T., Ward, C. H., Mendelson, M., Molk, J. E., & Erbaugh, J. K. Reliability of psychiatric diagnoses. Two: A study of consistency of clinical judgments and ratings. *American Journal of Psychiatry,* 1962, *119,* 351–357.

Bettelheim, B. *The empty fortress.* New York: Free Press, 1967.

Brill, H. Classification and nomenclature of psychiatric conditions. In S. Arieti (Ed.), *American handbook of psychiatry.* Vol. I. New York: Basic, 1974.

Cantwell, D. P., Mattison, R., Russell, A. T., & Will, L. A comparison of DSM-II and DSM-III in the diagnosis of childhood psychiatric disorders. *Archives of General Psychiatry,* 1979, *36,* 1208–1228.

Critchley, D. L. The adverse influence of psychiatric diagnostic labels on the observation of child behavior. *American Journal of Orthopsychiatry,* 1979, *49,* 157–160.

Des Lauriers, A. M., & Carlson, C. F. *Your child is asleep.* Homewood, IL: Dorsey, 1969.

Ekstein, R., & Wallerstein, J. Observations on the psychology of borderline and psychotic children. *Psychoanalytic Study of the Child,* 1954, *9,* 344–369.

Frances, A. The DSM-III personality disorders section: A commentary. *American Journal of Psychiatry,* 1980, *137,* 1050–1054.

Francis, A., & Cooper, A. M. Descriptive and dynamic psychiatry: A perspective on *DSM-III. American Journal of Psychiatry,* 1981, *138,* 1198-1202.

Freeman, M. A reliability study of psychiatric diagnosis in childhood and adolescence. *Journal of Child Psychology and Psychiatry,* 1971, *12,* 43–54.

Freud, A. *Normality and pathology in childhood.* New York: International Universities Press, 1965.

Garmezy, N. DSM-III: Never mind the psychologists; is it good for the children? *The Clinical Psychologist,* 1978, *31*(3,4), 1, 4–6.

Goldenberg, H. *Abnormal psychology: A social/community approach.* Monterey, CA: Brooks/Cole, 1977.

Goldstein, W. N. DSM-III and the diagnosis of schizophrenia. *American Journal of Psychotherapy,* 1983, *XXXVII,* 168–181.

Greenspan, S. I. *The clinical interview of the child.* New York: McGraw-Hill, 1981.

Greenspan, S., & Lourie, R. S. Developmental structuralist approach to the classification of adaptive and pathologic personality organizations: Infancy and early childhood. *American Journal of Psychiatry,* 1981, *138,* 725–735.

Hobbs, N. *The future of children: Categories, labels, and their consequences.* San Francisco: Jossey-Bass, 1975.

Hunt, W. A. History and classification. In A. E. Kazdin, A. S. Bellack, & M. Harsov (Eds.), *New perspectives in abnormal psychology.* New York: Oxford University Press, 1980.

Hyler, S. E., & Spitzer, R. L. Hysteria split asunder. *American Journal of Psychiatry*, 1978, *135*, 1500–1504.

Kanner, L. Autistic disturbances of affective contact. *Nervous Child*, 1943, *2*, 217–250.

Kanner, L. Early infantile autism. *Journal of Pediatrics*, 1944, *25*, 211-217.

Kanner, L. Follow-up study of eleven autistic children originally reported in 1943. *Journal of Autism and Childhood Schizophrenia*, 1971, *1*, 119–145.

Kant, I. *The classification of mental disorders*. Doylestown, PA: The Doylestown Foundation, 1964.

Karasu, T. B., & Skodol, A. E. VIth Axis for DSM-III: Psychodynamic evaluation. *American Journal of Psychiatry*, 1980, *137*, 607–610.

Kauffman, J. M. *Characteristics of children's behavior disorders*. Columbus: Merrill, 1981.

Langer, E. J., & Abelson, R. P. A patient by any other name . . . : Clinician group differences in labeling bias. *Journal of Consulting and Clinical Psychology*, 1974, *42*, 4–9.

Lorr, M. Classification of the behavior disorders. In P. R. Farnsworth, O. McNemar, & Q. McNemar (Eds.), *Annual review of psychology*. Palo Alto: Annual Reviews, 1961.

Lovaas, O. I. *The autistic child: Language development through behavior modification*. New York: Irvington, 1977.

Lyskowskil, J. C., & Tsuang, M. I. Precaution in treating DSM-III Borderline Personality Disorder. *American Journal of Psychiatry*, 1980, *137*, 110–111.

Mahler, M. S. On child psychosis and schizophrenia: Autistic and symbiotic infantile psychosis. *Psychoanalytic Study of the Child*, 1952, *7*, 286-305.

Mahler, M. S., Pine, F., & Bergman, A. *The psychological birth of the human infant, symbiosis and individuation*. New York: Basic, 1975.

Marcus, J. Borderline states in childhood. *Journal of Child Psychology and Psychiatry*, 1963, *4*, 207–218.

McLemore, C. W., & Benjamin, L. S. Whatever happened to interpersonal diagnosis? A psychosocial alternative to DSM-III. *American Psychologist*, 1979, *34*, 17–34.

McReynolds, W. T. DSM-III and the future of applied social science. *Professional Psychology*, 1979, *34*, 17–34.

Menninger, K. A., Mayman, M., & Pruyser, P. *The vital balance*. New York: Viking Press, 1963.

Morey, L. C. Differences between psychologists and psychiatrists in the use of DSM-III. *American Journal of Psychiatry*, 1980, *137*, 1123–1124.

Morgan, S. B. *The unreachable child*. Memphis: Memphis State University Press, 1981.

Peterson, D. R. Behavior problems of middle childhood. *Journal of Consulting Psychology*, 1961, *25*, 205–209.

Piaget, J. *The psychology of the child*. New York: Basic Books, 1969.

Quay, H. C. Classification. In H. C. Quay & J. S. Werry (Eds.), *Psychopathological disorders of childhood*. New York: Wiley, 1979.

Reisman, J. M. *Toward the integration of psychotherapy*. New York: Wiley-Interscience, 1971.

Reisman, J. M. *A history of clinical psychology*. Melbourne, FL: Krieger, 1982.

Rieder, R. O. Borderline schizophrenia: Evidence of its validity. *Schizophrenia Bulletin*, 1979, *5*, 39–46.

Rimland, B. *Infantile autism*. New York: Appleton-Century-Crofts, 1964.

Rollins, N. *Child psychiatry in the Soviet Union*. Cambridge, MA: Harvard University Press, 1972.

Ross, A. O. *Psychological disorders of children*. New York: McGraw-Hill, 1980.

Rutter, M. *Infantile autism: Concepts, characteristics, and treatment*. London: Churchill Livingston, 1971.

Rutter, M., Lebovici, S. Eisenberg, L., Sneznevskij, A. V., Sadoun, R., Brook, E., & Lin, T. Y. A triaxial classification of mental disorder in childhood. *Journal of Child Psychology and Psychiatry*, 1969, *10*, 41–61.

Rutter, M., Shaffer, D., & Shepherd, M. *A multi-axial classification of child psychiatric disorders*. Geneva: World Health Organization, 1975.

Sandifer, M. G., Pettus, C., & Quade, D. A study of psychiatric diagnosis. *Journal of Nervous and Mental Disease*, 1964, *139*, 350–356.

Schmidt, H. O., & Fonda, C. The reliability of psychiatric diagnosis: A new look. *Journal of Abnormal and Social Psychology*, 1956, *52*, 262–267.

Schopler, E., & Reichler, R. J. *Psychopathology and child development*. New York: Plenum, 1976.

Schwartz, S., & Johnson, J. H. *Psychopathology of childhood*. New York: Pergamon, 1981.

Selman, R. L., & Jaquette, D. Stability and oscillation in interpersonal awareness: A clinical-developmental analysis. In H. E. Howe, Jr. (Ed.) *Nebraska symposium on motivation 1977*. Lincoln, Neb.: U. Nebraska Press, 1978.

Spitzer, R. Nomedical myths and the DSM-III. *APA Monitor*, 1981, *12* (Oct.), 3, 33.

Spitzer, R. L., & Endicott, J. Justification for separating schizotypal and borderline personality disorders. *Schizophrenia Bulletin*, 1979, *5*, 95–100.

Spitzer, R. L., & Forman, J. B. W. DSM-III field

trials: II. Initial experience with the multiaxial system. *American Journal of Psychiatry,* 1979, *136,* 818–820.

Spitzer, R. L., Forman, J. B. W., & Nee J. DSM-III field trials: I. Initial interrater diagnostic reliability. *American Journal of Psychiatry,* 1979, *136,* 815–817.

Spitzer, R. L., Williams, J. B. W., & Skodol, A. E. DSM-III: The major achievements and an overview. *American Journal of Psychiatry,* 1980, *137,* 151–164.

Strober, M., Green, J., & Carlson, G. Reliability of psychiatric diagnosis in hospitalized adolescents: Interrater agreement using DSM-III. *Archives of General Psychiatry,* 1981, *38,* 141–145.

Webb, L. J., Gold, R. S., Johnstone, E. E., & Dielamente, C. C. Accuracy of *DSM-III* diagnoses following a training program. *American Journal of Psychiatry,* 1981, *138,* 376-378.

Weiner, I. B. *Psychological disturbance in adolescence.* New York: Wiley-Interscience, 1970.

Zubin, J. But is it good for science? *The Clinical Psychologist,* 1977–78, *31*(2), 1, 5–7.

CHAPTER 3

Epidemiology and Outcome

Sheldon Cotler

Parents, teachers, and mental health professionals are continually making judgments about the suitability and acceptability of children's behavior. These judgments are frequently value-laden because they are often based on a person's own normative standard of conduct. Children are evaluated by comparison with other children and then labeled as deviant if their behavior is not within the evaluator's range of acceptability. The criterion for deviance is usually quantitative instead of qualitative, e.g., it is the degree or extent of aggression or shyness that is salient, not the mere existence of these behaviors. In other words, all children exhibit many qualities of behavior, but when certain behaviors are judged unusual in terms of intensity, frequency, or duration, the behavior and the child are likely to be classified as deviant.

Labeling a child as deviant and then intervening to change that child's behavior involves ethical as well as professional considerations. Children are dependent upon adult caretakers and consequently are at the mercy of adult judgments about them. We must understand that the very process of labeling children's behavior as deviant may have damaging implications for their self-images, and prejudice how they are viewed by others. Care is also needed in prescribing and applying interventions designed to bring children's behaviors within normative standards. Mental health professionals are often accused of being agents of the society empowered to preserve the status quo by utilizing their resources as a way to achieve "social control"(Hurvetz, 1973; Gross, 1978), so it must be determined whether the child or the situation is more in need of intervention.

In considering treatment interventions,

the questions are: Who should be treated? What should be treated? and What should the goals of treatment be? The identification of "problem children" and the application of treatment methodologies imply that there are general standards of conduct that apply to everyone. But is the child being changed to conform to the psychologist's standards, or to the parent's standards, or to the teacher's standards?

Given the diversity of opinions about the causes of human behavior, let us adopt a definition of adjustment that is generally compatible with different theoretical orientations. Based on Knopf's (1979) ideas, adjustment can be related to efficient intellectual and cognitive operations, reasonable expressions of emotions, and satisfying interpersonal relationships. Children need to be able to approach their worlds openly and spontaneously and fulfill their needs in a positive social manner without interfering with the rights of other people. Ideally, behavior should be motivated by the desire to seek new experiences and not by the wish to avoid difficult or threatening circumstances. Intellectually curious, emotionally expressive, and friendly children will neither see themselves nor be seen by others as being disruptive and unhappy.

In this chapter we shall examine how many children are considered disturbed—the occurrence or the epidemiology of disordered behavior. The relative efficacy of psychotherapeutic treatment of children and adolescents will then be addressed to see what light these results shed on the prognosis or outcome of disorders. Even though the literature primarily focuses on the individual child as a source of concern, we will also look at social institutions and social standards and their influences upon diagnosis and outcome.

Epidemiology

Basically, in epidemiology questions are asked about how disorders are distributed in the population with respect to age, sex, socio-cultural factors, and place of residence. There is a distinction drawn in the literature between the *prevalence* of a disorder, which is essentially the number of those exhibiting the disorder in a given population in a given time, and the *incidence* of a disorder, which consists of the number of new, identified cases that occur in a given population in a specified period. An important consideration is that the prevalence of a disorder does not necessarily indicate the need to provide professional services (Graham, 1979). Since prevalence is an enumerative event, only the presence of a given handicap is identified, and no determination is made about whether the disorder is sufficiently debilitating to require professional intervention. In making that determination we must be cognizant of population base rates before reaching any conclusions. For examples, the average "normal" child in Achenbach's study had between eight and twenty-eight problems. A survey, using the Louisville Behavior Checklist with 500 parents of children seven to twelve years of age, determined that the average child reportedly manifested between eleven and thirteen problem behaviors (Miller et al., 1971). Some common problems may be transitory or are to be expected of children of a certain age.

A reported prevalence of disorders is often related more to who is doing the classifying and labeling and the accessibility of mental health resources in the community than to the actual frequency of the disordered behavior. A type of behavior may be diagnosed as serious by some professionals and considered normal by others. Also, availability of services affects prevalence. For example, some prosperous school systems in suburban Chicago identify as many as 10 percent to 20 percent of their students as learning disabled or educationally handicapped. Those school districts that can financially afford to treat deviance have established an extensive network of special education classrooms and ample personnel to serve children with special needs. With such resources available, school personnel are encouraged to select children and refer them for that help. Other school districts, which have limited resources, less personnel to assess and identify children with "special" educational needs, and relatively few classrooms to serve these children, typically identify a smaller number—3 to 5 percent—of their children as requiring special educational services. This illustrates that the availability of professional resources substantially affects how prevalence data are determined and interpreted.

Studies of prevalence also vary with respect to: (1) the ages of the children; (2) the source of the report, whether parents, teachers, mental health workers or the children themselves; and (3) the nature of the sample, either clinic or non-clinic. This section will conclude with a discussion of studies representative of each of the above areas.

In studies of preschool children, teachers and mental health workers have identified as many as 20 percent of these children as exhibiting signs of deviant behavior. Richman, Stevenson, and Graham's (1975) epidemiological study of 705 "normal" three-year-olds indicated that 15 percent had mild and 6 percent had moderate to severe behavior problems, with no clear-cut differences between the sexes. A study of 462 Headstart children identified 31.6 percent who had psychological problems severe enough to require professional attention (Anderson, 1983).

These data are generally confirmed in a study of behavior disorders among 588 two- to five-year-old children in a daycare setting (Crowther, Bond, & Reff (1981). They administered the ninety-item Vermont Behavior Checklist to the children's teachers. Their data indicated that 20 percent of two- to four-year-old males had high activity levels and another 20 percent of all two- and three-year olds were classified as inattentive. The teachers rated the misbehavior of two- and three-year-olds as more severe than older children. The acting-out or inattentive behavior of all groups of children gradually decreased as they approached year five. Sex differences were found in the study and consisted of boys being more likely to be classified by their teachers as deviant if they frequently engaged in externalizing behaviors, such as destructive and aggressive activities. On the other hand, girls were more likely to be seen as deviant if they were shy, withdrawn and spoke in a soft voice. It is interesting that the teachers apparently responded to quantitative extremes in stereotyped boy and girl behaviors in making their judgments about deviance.

An attempt to understand the large proportion of reported behavior disorders among preschool age children found that among three-year-olds, behavior problems and expressive language delays were substantially correlated (Richman, Stevenson, & Graham, 1975). Thirty-nine percent of the children with problems had expressive language delays, but only 14 percent of children in the total population had language delays. Also, at a one year follow-up of behavior problem preschoolers, two-thirds of the language-delayed children remained disordered, while only one-half of the children without language delays were still classified as disordered. These data suggest that mediating developmental factors may be associated with the base rate of preschool children's behavior disorders. While cause and effect cannot be established, it seems logical that children who have difficulty expressing themselves would be more likely to experience frustrations with peers and adults and consequently react with disordered behavior.

Another study of disordered behavior of young children (Lahey et al., 1980) found preschool teachers rated first-born sons as significantly more disturbed than later born males or females. First-born males were rated as having more behavior problems and being more anxious, hostile and hyperactive. First-born males also had higher referral rates to mental health centers. Again this relationship is correlational in nature and it is not known whether first-born males simply receive more attention and concern or whether they have unique developmental experiences which interfere with their social adjustment.

In the preceding and subsequent studies teachers were often relied upon to identify children who have behavior disorders. Researchers like Zax and Cowen (1967), Glidewell, Domke, and Kantor (1963), and Achenbach and Edelbrock (1984) see teachers as playing a leading role in the early identification of behavior problems. Teachers usually have a much wider range of experience with children and can compare them more reliably than parents. In addition, the classroom is a more standardized situation than the home in which to evaluate children's behavior and conduct.

Other researchers (Green et al., 1980) examined the validity of teacher evaluations of ninety-five third grade children who had an average age of 9.5 years. Teachers classified each child in their class as normal, conduct disorder, or withdrawn. The teacher judgments were compared with sociometric ratings, behavior observations by trained observers, and independent evaluations of each child's academic performance. Children with conduct disorders reacted more negatively and inappropriately with peers and had lower achievement test scores. The sociometric data were consistent with teacher impressions and showed that conduct disorder children were liked less by their classmates. The children judged normal by teachers were accepted more, rejected less, and liked more by their peers than those children rated deviant. While the withdrawn children did not seem deviant to outside raters, the academic and sociometric evaluations of these children showed they were less liked by their peers and did more poorly in school. It was concluded from this study that teachers can reliably identify disturbed children in their classrooms and that teacher descriptions are in concert with evaluations of social and academic performance by peers and outside experts.

The social adjustment of over 2,500 five- to fifteen-year-old children in public and private schools in Ontario, Canada, was evaluated (McDermott, 1980). Approximately 25 percent of the sample were mildly to severely maladjusted. Of this 25 percent, 60 percent showed multiple symptoms of maladjusted behavior. McDermott used a social adjustment index to survey the children and was able to classify them into several types of distinctive disorders, ranging from lack of assertiveness and initiative, to depression and withdrawal, to hostility. He concluded that behavioral maladjustment is more than just an "under- vs. over-reaction," and that it also consists of specific syndromes of behaviors.

What is remarkable about these studies is the amazingly high prevalence of disordered behaviors in normal, presumably typical samples of young children. A survey of the epidemiology of children's disorders reviews earlier studies which also indicate that between 10 percent and 20 percent of normal children demonstrate some degree of disordered behavior (Graham, 1979). This range is reported consistently, with the percentages becoming somewhat higher during teenage years, particularly for boys. It does not seem to matter if prevalence data are derived from parents, teachers, or mental health professionals. It is consistently estimated that about 7 percent of the child population have moderate to severe behavior problems, while another 15 percent have mild behavior problems. These prevalence data are roughly equal for boys and girls, even though the number of boys referred for mental health services outnumber girls by about two or three to one.

In comparison to samples of normal children, a study of a cross-section of children receiving medical care (Jacobson et al., 1980) indicates that few of these children are likely to receive a psychiatric diagnosis. The investigators studied the prevalence of children's disorders at four comprehensive health care facilities on the East Coast. They were interested in determining the percentages of children under eighteen getting general medical care who also received a psychiatric diagnosis. They found that one health care agency identified 8.2 percent of the children as requiring psychiatric services, while three other agencies had rates between 2.2 to 3.6 percent. In addition, diagnosed disturbances among boys were one and one-half times higher than among girls, a ratio somewhat lower than usually found in the general population. Most of these children received relatively mild diagnoses; they were either classified as behavior disordered or reacting maladaptively to situational demands. Severe psychiatric diagnoses were attributed to less than 4 percent of disordered children. Overall, the study concluded that 3 to 10 percent of the children seen in general medical outpatient clinics are diagnosed as having some form of mental disturbance. The rates are higher in clinics serving urban and suburban children, as opposed to clinics serving rural children, a finding consistent with other studies. Another important result was that children with psychiatric diagnoses utilized all medical services two to four times as often as children who did not receive a psychiatric diagnosis. It is logical that children and their parents who are experiencing behavioral disruption might seek professional services, including medical services, much more frequently than untroubled children and families. These data suggest that the early identification and treatment of problem children may be cost-effective in that such children and families may ultimately require less medical care than otherwise.

Adolescents are much more likely to be hospitalized or incarcerated for aberrant behavior than younger children. It is ironic that there is less tolerance for deviance among adolescents, even though our culture expects them to assert themselves and abandon their dependent status. Moreover, our society fosters dependence-independence conflicts by uncertain economic conditions and by extending the period of adolescence into the twenties. Yet the prevalence of psychological disorders among adolescents is not appreciably different from other age groups in our population (Graham, 1979; Edelbrock & Achenbach, 1980).

Adolescents themselves confirm that they are functioning fairly comfortably in society. In a unique study, adolescents were asked to provide self-reports of their levels of personal satisfaction and adjustment (Offer, Ostrov, & Howard, 1981). Using questionnaire data from over 20,000 students, the authors concluded that about 20 percent of the adolescents felt troubled, a figure congruent with the prevalence data derived from parents, teachers, and mental health professionals. On the positive side, 80 percent of the adolescents surveyed felt secure with friends and family, relatively non-anxious, and optimistic about their families.

A problem-oriented classification of adolescent disorders (Weiner, 1980) was based on an extensive survey of 1,334 twelve- to eighteen-year-old adolescents registered for mental health services in Monroe County (Rochester, New York). Approximately 95 percent of all psychiatric contacts in the community were identified in this register. While more severely disordered adolescents are overrepresented in this sample, the data are nevertheless informative. The percentages of disturbed adolescents in each of six descriptive categories were: schizophrenia, 8.5; neurosis, 13.3; personality disorder, 31.4; situational disorder, 27.1; suicide attempt, 2.8; and other 16.9.

Weiner reclassified DSM-II diagnoses into six categories that he thought were particularly salient to the adolescent population: schizophrenia, depression, suicide, problems of school achievement, problems of school attendance, and delinquency (including personality disorders). With respect to schizophrenia, he reported that roughly 2 percent of the child/adolescent psychiatric population is considered schizophrenic, but 25 to 30 percent of adolescents admitted to psychiatric hospitals are so classified. Males, it should be noted, are more often hospitalized with psychotic disorders, while female hospitalizations tend to be due to psychophysiological conditions (Beitchman & Dielman, 1982).

Weiner's data show that 6 to 8 percent of adolescents seen in clinics and offices have symptoms that appear schizophrenic. The prognosis for adolescent onset of schizophrenia is unfavorable. It is estimated that half the hospitalized adolescents with schizophrenia show little or no progress over several years of treatment.

Although less than 10 percent of children and adolescents in psychiatric treatment were diagnosed depressed, half these patients showed significant depressive symptoms. Many normal adolescents do have occasional feelings of sadness or worthlessness (Offer, Ostrov, & Howard, 1981). Depression as a symptom is often expressed by fatigue, hypochondriacal complaints, and difficulty concentrating and completing one's work. Moreover, depression prominently affects a wide range of adolescent behaviors and plays a significant role in adolescent suicide. It is estimated that approximately one out of every thousand adolescents in the United States attempts suicide. Six percent of the known suicides each year are adolescent suicides. In addition, adolescents receiving mental health services frequently report suicide ideation and suicide gestures, with the figure going as high as 50 percent in some clinical settings.

Historically, delinquent behavior has been separated from other kinds of disturbances in adolescence because delinquency is a legally defined category and is not a specific psychiatric diagnosis. For instance, society tends to apply different standards to adolescents than to adults—age restrictions on driving, drinking, and so on—that inflate delinquency figures.

While many adolescents are likely to

demonstrate "externalizing" behaviors and act out toward society, the true prevalence of these behaviors is difficult to ascertain. Many rule violations go undiscovered or unreported by parents, school authorities, or law enforcement officers. Lower-class children are probably overrepresented as delinquents because their parents are less able to provide compensation or restitution for damages and so they are more apt to be brought to court.

Correlates of "externalizing" behaviors among adolescents include low socioeconomic status, low intelligence, low school achievement, and poor family background. One study by (Moffitt et al., 1981) attempted to establish a relationship between socioeconomic status (SES), intellectual ability, and delinquent behavior. The authors discovered that IQ and school achievement were more directly related to delinquent activity than was SES. They concluded, at least on a tentative basis, that adolescents with lower verbal abilities are relatively less able to cope with academic and social demands and consequently are more likely to act out against society.

It is obvious that school performance is also likely to be affected by external stressors in the lives of children and adolescents. Weiner (1980) reported that approximately 25 percent of all adolescents underachieve in school, with an extraordinary 50 percent of the children who are receiving mental health services classified as underachievers. School achievement and attendance may likely be the most obvious and frequent casualties of stress. Since children have a record of performance in school, drops in achievement, which are potentially symptomatic of psychological difficulties in a child's life, are often used by mental health professionals as a gauge of behavioral deterioration.

A study in Norway examined the effects of parental influence on children's aggression (Olweus, 1980). Olweus studied seventy-six twelve- to fourteen-year-old and fifty-one fifteen- to seventeen-year-old boys and their parents. Peer ratings and parental interviews were the primary sources of data. He concluded that children's temperament was related to subsequent aggression. Mothers' permissiveness for aggression and both parents' use of power assertive methods of discipline with their children resulted in relatively more aggressive behavior. Boys with aggressive temperaments affected their mothers' attitudes, in that the mothers would either become permissive about the aggression or would become punitive and negativistic toward their sons—both reactions contributing to increased aggressive behavior on the part of the adolescent boys. It was assumed that if the mothers reacted in a more balanced and positive way toward their aggressive sons, subsequent aggressive behavior would be minimized. Finally, Olweus found that fathers had much less influence on their sons' aggressive behavior than did mothers.

The effects of family influences on disordered behavior is a favorite topic in the psychopathology literature, but the findings are not always supportive of troubled family systems. In an extensive review published in 1975, Jacob examined the interaction patterns in disturbed and nondisturbed families. He concluded from his review of nonschizophrenic disturbed and normal families that there were very few differences in their interaction patterns. There were no reliable distinguishing characteristics in communication clarity, dominance, sex of children, and nature of conflict between them. Families who have a child or adolescent identified as deviant do not necessarily have interactional styles that are different from families whose children are normal.

In order to understand the correlates of

children's disorders better, psychologists have examined the influence of the family's social and economic status (Dohrenwend & Dohrenwend, 1974; Heitler, 1976; Lorion, 1978). It is frequently suggested that children from lower SES backgrounds tend to be diagnosed as having more severe disorders than middle-class children because the poor are less likely to receive high quality mental health services early in their lives when problems often begin. The fact that there is a higher prevalence of psychopathology among lower class children has also been explained in terms of poorer health services, poor nutrition (Birch & Gussow, 1970), the lack of preventive medical and psychological services, and poorer educational and recreational resources.

Many social and cultural factors interact to bring about the prevalence of mental disorders among lower-class people (King, 1978). Families of poverty are continually confronted with fulfilling basic needs in the face of economic deprivation, crowding, and threats of physical violence. To these factors add the absence of intimacy and the frequent disruptions of family life, all of which contribute to the stress upon lower SES children and their families.

In addition to the lower-class having greater stress, there is also the probability of a "downward drift"(Dohrenwend & Dohrenwend, 1974)—that is, people who are more disturbed or who have more difficulty functioning in society are more likely to end up in lower class status. This downward drift is another variable which seems to account for some amount of class differences.

Lorion (1978) noted low-income status generally contraindicates psychotherapeutic services being provided. Even when lower SES patients are accepted into psychotherapy, they tend to be seen by less experienced therapists. Also therapists' expectations about improvement in their patients is a significant determinant of outcome of treatment, and it is a common misconception that lower-class patients cannot benefit from psychotherapeutic intervention. Consequently, it may be difficult to find professionals who are eager or willing to offer their services to lower-class children. For example, it has been suggested (Goldstein, Heller, & Sechrest, 1966) that people from lower-class backgrounds require more direct action-oriented interventions that have practical and immediate significance for their day-to-day lives as opposed to more traditional psychotherapies. However, when low SES families are, in fact, treated in psychotherapy, their outcome data are similar to those of other classes (Lorion, 1978).

At any rate, there is little question that the availability of mental health resources is much less in lower-class communities and prevalence of school failures, judged conduct disorders, delinquency, and institutionalization (either prison or mental hospitals) is greater in lower-class children. Given these higher frequencies, professionals question the applicability of the criteria for making diagnostic judgments about lower SES children and their families. Standards of behavior differ between subcultures and middle-class values and standards may not be valid when imposed on groups of people who are responding to very different sets of circumstances. Mental health planners need to acknowledge that social and environmental factors restrict what children can be expected to achieve.

In addition, what may be dysfunctional or even nonadjustive in one group of children may be socially adaptive in another. For example, children in threatening, dangerous environments would be expected to learn to be vigilant and suspicious of other people. In those circumstances cooperation and sharing materials and feelings may actually increase a child's vulnerability to exploitation. On the other hand, these same behaviors may be viewed as hostile and components of a personality disorder when they occur in a truly benign situation. The task of mental health professionals is twofold: to help children and families function in society at large and yet to recognize adjustments that are compatible with subcultural standards and realities.

The final epidemiological issue to be considered is whether the occurrence of disorders in childhood is predictive of maladjustment in adult life. Kohlberg, LaCrosse, and Picks (1972) developed an elaborate system to distinguish long-lasting behaviors from transient or situational behaviors. They classified childrens' problem behaviors into three main categories: (1) *developmental-adaptational traits,* which were viewed as problem behaviors that decline with age and consist of lying, speech problems, enuresis, and phobias; (2) *temperamental traits,* which are not age-related, include behaviors such as activity level, intelligence, shyness, and irritability; and (3) *phase specific reactions to developmental crises,* which take place at two principal times in childhood: five to seven and ten to thirteen—when beginning school and puberty.

The above classification identified a few childhood factors predictive of adult adjustment. Intellectual ability was found to be the temperamental trait which is the best predictor of later adjustment. Also, traits like shyness and reserve are likely to continue throughout childhood and into adulthood (Robins, 1972). Antisocial behavior in childhood is an excellent predictor of similar types of problem behavior in adulthood, as are poor schoolwork, challenging teachers' authority, and unpopularity with classmates. Finally, children's biological (including genetic) predispositions to schizophrenia are significantly associated with later disturbance in adulthood.

However, there are many childhood disorders that do not seem predictive of later adjustment. Drawing heavily from the Berkeley growth studies (a longitudinal investigation of development from infancy through adulthood), Robins concluded that most children's problems are age-specific and transitory. Kohlberg points out that children's emotional reactions, like anxiety and fears, do not predict later adjustment. Shyness and dependency are also poor indicators of adult behavior. Finally, and counter to prevailing belief, both Kohlberg and Robins suggest there is little support for the notion that maternal deprivation and psychological trauma in early childhood are related to disturbance later on. Robins does say that physical abuse is an exception and portends later behavior disturbance.

Given the preceding findings, Kohlberg characterized children's problem behaviors as either long-lasting or transitory. Certain troublesome behaviors are likely to be maintained because they are trait-related or are a function of critical experiential or biological determinants. Other behaviors are characteristic of a certain age (e.g., fear of the dark) or are situationally induced, and both these types decline in importance as the child grows older. Kohlberg plays down the effects of early stresses on the grounds that they seem unrelated to the later occurrence of disordered behavior. This may or may not be a valid conclusion, depending on whether children are able to overcome threatening and stressful events without damage to their feelings of self-efficacy and whether the effects of the stressors may not be evidenced in less obvious adult problems. Nevertheless, most children do gow up to be productive citizens, despite the tremendous economic, social, and experiential differences among families in contemporary American society. In the next section we will evaluate the attempts that have been made to psychotherapeutically intervene with deviant children.

Evaluating the Treatment of Children, Adolescents and Families

Levitt's 1957 review of the child treatment literature set the tone in evaluating child therapy for the next twenty-five years. He originally reviewed thirty-five studies of psychotherapy with children, some of which dated back to the 1930s. Eighteen studies reported results at the close of treatment, seventeen at follow-up (typically one to two years after treatment was completed), and five studies reported measures for both times. By averaging the outcomes at the conclusion of treatment, Levitt reported that only 34.5 percent of the children receiving psychotherapy showed "much improvement," 32.5% showed "partial improvement," and the balance (33%) showed "no improvement." The outcome data are more favorable at follow-up, when 78 percent of the treated children were reported as improved or partially improved approximately one year after treatment. This latter finding is confirmed in a literature review (Wright, Moelis, and Pollack, 1976), which indicated that treated children show continued growth and improvement after their psychotherapy ended.

At first glance those outcome data seem favorable and support the efficacy of psychotherapeutic intervention with children. However, science demands that treated children be compared with a "control group" of children who do not receive any treatment. Levitt used as a control group children and families who were "defectors" from treatment; that is, people who terminated treatment before the therapist thought they were ready to leave. He determined that 72.5 percent of the defectors actually showed improvement, even though they did not begin or complete their prescribed psychotherapy. Levitt's results were almost identical to Eysenck's (1952) controversial findings about adult psychotherapy—approximately two-thirds of adult patients show improvement, a rate no greater than that found for "untreated controls." The studies cited by both Levitt and Eysenck have since been widely criticized on methodological grounds, and both men are accused of drawing erroneous conclusions from their data. For example, their control groups had many inadequacies; the nature of the patient samples was poorly specified and ranged from "neurotic" to "psychotic"; and treatment conditions, therapist variables, and outcome standards were often not taken into account.

Yet the preceding studies are representative of the type of research that has led to substantial concern about whether psychotherapy with children and adolescents is effective. In 1971, Levitt presented the argument that child psychotherapy has been based on two questionable hypotheses. He discussed the "continuity" hypothesis that essentially states that untreated children who are emotionally disturbed will ultimately become emotionally disturbed adults. The second hypothesis, the "intervention" hypothesis, suggests that psychotherapeutic treatment will reduce the incidence of future adult problems. Levitt maintained that the research on the effects of child therapy has not supported either of these hypotheses. Kohlberg, LaCrosse, and Ricks (1972) reached the same conclusion, while conceding that the hypotheses made sense logically and conceptually.

These unfavorable conclusions about child psychotherapy have been justly criticized. Heinecke and Strassman (1975) claimed that often the functions and objectives of child psychotherapy have not been specified. Barrett, Hampe, and Miller (1971) identified four conditions that need to be satisfied in order to validly assess child therapy: (1) the children and their disorders must be carefully selected to control for age, intelligence, type of onset, and severity of disorder; (2) the therapist and his or her personality must be seen as active ingredients in the therapy process; (3) a comprehensive assessment of intervention techniques and the impact of these techniques must be examined; and (4) there needs to be a way of measuring outcome that consists of reliable indices of change. Serious consideration of the preceding elements in constructing and assessing psychotherapeutic interventions with children results in a formidable task but to do less invites equivocal findings and much confusion.

Progress in evaluating child psychotherapy also requires that researchers become sensitized to three additional methodological issues. First is the selection or *sampling* of the "target" children. How and why were these children selected for treatment? Children do not simply walk into their local mental health center, nor do they telephone a child psychologist for an appointment. An adult representative of society, typically a parent or a teacher, brings a child in for treatment because he or she believes the child is violating normative standards of behavior. The children who are presented for treatment for the majority of disorders are only a percentage of the total population of children who show similar deviations (Shepherd, Oppenheim, and Mitchell, 1966). In the sampling process, the nature of the child patient sample must be specified and distinguished from others in similar environments who are not involved in psychotherapy.

Second is the consideration of *specificity*, which relates to both the reliable description of the child and his disorder and to the nature of the treatment intervention. Kiesler (1966) talks about the "uniformity myths" that have been carelessly attributed to the problems being treated, to the child, and to therapist populations. For example, all phobias are not alike, and yet in the literature they are discussed as though they were identical; and clinicians certainly do not treat all children alike, though most outcome studies do not discriminate among the kinds of psychotherapy offered. There are also inevitable differences between therapists, and yet the specific contributions of the individual therapists to treatment outcome are usually not assessed.

Moreover, psychotherapeutic intervention is not equally effective or ineffective. A study (Cotler et al., 1982) at a community mental health center indicates that short-term outpatient treatment of children is relatively more successful with children classified as anxious or neurotic than with children who seem character disordered. The data indicate that approximately 70 percent of lower middle class and lower-class children who were judged to be anxious and fearful improved in short-term psychotherapy, while only about 50 percent of children who had antisocial problems improved.

Third is the establishment of *criteria for change* and the identification of goals for treatment; these are particularly perplexing problems with children. Adults in treatment are often able to articulate their concerns and have some ideas about what they expect from therapy, but children typically do not. Frequently the child's problem is not the exclusive concern in treatment. In Levitt's literature review, only in 10 percent of the studies cited was the child the sole focus of treatment, while in 40 percent of the studies the mother was the only member of the family seen for treatment. Adams (1975) feels that children have been short-changed in psychotherapy and really have not been a major focus of attention with respect the development and application of intervention techniques. Adams points out that many children receive indirect services through parents or schools and that their own needs and concerns are not highly valued. At any rate, the criteria for change should include not only the "target" child, but also the other significant people in the child's life who were involved in the treatment intervention.

To summarize, there are many methodological issues that affect how we evaluate children's treatment: appropriate sampling of both children and therapists; being able to specifically describe the children, their disorders, and the nature of the interventions; and establishing reasonable criteria for change. Many of these issues are also relevant to control groups. The dependency of children and adolescents adds to the complexity of providing and evaluating helping services because, among other variables, parents are often included in the treatment process.

Behavior Therapy and Children

The social learning approach toward child therapy (Ross, 1980; Mischel, 1968; and Bandura, 1977) places more emphasis on the measurement of disordered behavior, the determination of conditions associated with its occurrence, and individualization of therapeutic interventions than do dynamic therapies. Rather than depending solely on other people's judgments about behavior, the behavior therapist assesses the functional value of a given behavior in a given situational context (Mischel, 1973). The emphasis of treatment is to enhance the efficacy of the child's behavior in the natural environment (Bandura, 1977). The social learning orientation promotes a narrowing of the definitions of children's problems, explicitly formulating treatment goals, and pursuing outcomes that can be characterized in behavioral terms.

In Ross' (1980) review of behavior therapy with children, he divides children's problems into behavior deficits and behavior excesses. The working assumption in designing treatment interventions is that children have learned disordered or "bad" behaviors that result in relatively little positive reinforcement and/or have not learned appropriate "good" behaviors that produce desirable and rewarding consequences. The characterization of a behavior deficit suggests that certain skills need to be taught to, and practiced by, the children.

For example, among the deficits that Ross identifies are deficits in social skills, academic skills, language skills, attending behavior, sphincter control, appropriate gender behavior, and knowing which social norms to follow. Behavior excesses may consist of certain behavioral reactions that need to be reduced or relearned in order for the child to have rewarding experiences. Here Ross includes excessive avoidance behaviors, such as phobias, overeating, and self-injurious behavior, and aggressive or disruptive behavior.

Within the parameters of a social learning conceptualization, the task of the behavior therapist becomes one of a teacher helping a child to acquire specific kinds of skills that are going to facilitate functioning in specific situations, resulting in personal and social satisfactions. At the same time, the child is helped to extinguish other behaviors that are dysfunctional and result in social punishment and a lack of personal accomplishment.

It is difficult to compare the outcomes of behavior therapy with children to the treatment studies summarized by Levitt (1971). Behavioral research is most frequently done with small groups, often consists of case studies, and is generally not subject to traditional statistical analyses. The evidence for therapeutic efficacy is consequently presented in terms of changes in the specific target behaviors of individual children. The success of an intervention is not presented in all-or-none terms, but is represented by progressive changes in behavior, e.g., reducing "out-of-seat behavior" of a given child in school from 50 percent of the time to 10 percent. To their credit, behavior therapists try to compare the behavior of the target child with the base-rate, normative child from the same situation. For example, the average child in a specific third grade classroom may be "out of seat" only 15 percent of the time.

Returning to methodological considerations for behavior therapists, sampling consists of identifying specific kinds of disorders; there is relatively little interest in the qualities of the children aside from the target symptom or behavior. Accordingly, the criteria for change are primarily behavioral and do not consist of reorganizing personality functioning; the specificity of the intervention is quite distinct, with the purpose limited to certain behaviors in given situations; and the goals of treatment and measure of outcome are directly linked to how the problem is defined in terms of measurable behavioral events. It should be obvious that behavioral interventions are not always comparable to psychodynamic treatments either in terms of conceptualizing children's problems or with respect to how therapy is defined and evaluated. The different orientations of behavior therapists provide useful alternative approaches to the treatment of children's problems. Given the above considerations, it is not too surprising that considerable success has been reported.

Adolescents and Psychotherapy

The data derived from outcome studies of psychotherapy with adolescents closely parallel the findings in the children's literature. Tramontana (1980) reviewed eighteen clinical and fifteen experimental studies of psychotherapy outcome with adolescents covering a ten-year period, 1967–1977, and reported a 75 percent median rate of positive outcomes for treated adolescents, compared with a 39 percent median rate of positive outcomes for adolescents not receiving treatment. These improvement statistics are not appreciably different from the improvement rates of treated adults or children reported earlier, but the improvement rate for the untreated controls is much lower than what is usually used. Tramontana concluded that adolescent problems may be acute, and therefore adolescents may show less improvement on their own than if seen in treatment. In addition, Tramontana noted that many of the untreated adolescents in the research studies were classified as delinquents and the rate of improvement of delinquents, treated or untreated, tends to be relatively low compared with other samples of disordered adolescents.

The treatment literature with adolescents has the same problems as the child treatment literature with respect to specifying the types of children, the nature of the problems, and the type of interventions used. Psychotherapy with adolescents lacks any specific character of its own; techniques are borrowed from child and adult treatment and there do not seem to be differential prescriptive interventions suitable for different kinds of adolescent disturbance. In the clinical studies of adolescents, group therapy is a common mode of treatment, with delinquents and hospitalized (seriously disturbed and psychotic) adolescents overrepresented relative to other adolescent disorders. Studies of treatment with younger children usually sample the less disturbed, most of whom are being treated in outpatient centers.

One of the infrequent examples of an impressive clinical research study of psychotherapy with adolescents was done by Shore and Massimo (1969, 1973). They conducted a comprehensive, vocationally oriented psychotherapy program with boys who were primarily character disordered or delinquent. These adolescents were provided with vocational and personal counseling by social service workers and helped to find jobs. Their comprehensive approach toward adolescent disturbance consisted of attending to school, family, and work relationships, and not just to the personality of the adolescent. Rather than permitting adolescents to continue in roles which perpetuate a sense of "negative identity" (Erikson, 1963), it is much more sensible to train adolescents to function effectively in the mainstream of society. Shore and Massimo reported success even ten years after psychotherapy and demonstrated that treated teen-agers showed better adjustment at work and in school and had fewer legal problems than untreated controls.

Families and Psychotherapy

Today, with an emphasis on prevention and a heightened awareness of social influences, there is tremendous interest in trying to involve a system in working with young people—this may include the extended family, as well as the school and community agencies. Including the family in treatment was a natural evolutionary step in psychotherapeutic practice. In family therapy there is typically a target child or adolescent who is originally referred as the person with the "problem," but treatment is performed in a family context. It is assumed that the child's disorder is actually symptomatic of a family disturbance. Family therapy then consists of working with all or some of the members of the family simultaneously, with the general goal of improving family functioning so that everybody's needs are expressed and met, including those of the target child's.

Developments in evaluating the effects of family therapy have proceeded quite slowly. Family therapy is routinely practiced by a variety of mental health practitioners, and consequently there are many different languages used to talk about its processes and objectives. As might be expected, family therapy is also combined with other types of treatment, resulting in difficulties in its assessment as a distinct therapeutic intervention. The evaluation issue is further complicated because the unit of treatment is the family system and researchers have developed neither the descriptive nomenclature nor sufficient technological expertise to reliably measure changes in systems. Given the previous discussion on the difficulty in evaluating changes in an individual child's behavior, specifying goals and measuring simultaneous changes in the behavior of several people in a family become extraordinarily complicated tasks.

In evaluating the effectiveness of family therapy, DeWitt (1978) determined the research was disappointing in both quantity and quality. He surveyed thirty-one studies of family therapy and found only eight methodologically adequate. Most studies did not have satisfactory control groups, random selections of subjects, adequate posttest follow-up measures, and appropriate statistical analyses. Nevertheless, the impression was that success rates of family therapy interventions are comparable to those reported for the treatment of individual children; two-thirds of identified child patients appear to improve. In fact, a comprehensive review chapter (Gurman & Kniskern, 1978) noted that "every study to date that has compared family therapy with other types of treatment has shown family therapy to be equal or superior" (p. 835).

While Jacob (1975) does not dispute the above percentages, he judged the outcome data from his review of 57 family therapy studies to be inconclusive because of their serious methodological difficulties.

Like all therapists, family therapists work with heterogeneous groups of people and problems. Accordingly, care must be taken to specify what is being done and with whom. For example, family therapy can be a particularly successful treatment for psychosomatic problems and is an alternative to psychiatric hospitalization (Wells & Duzen, 1978).

One approach to family therapy, developed by Minuchen (1974), is generally referred to as *structured family therapy*. This is a directive system of therapy, which includes encouraging parents to take charge of their children and establish specific rules that must be followed by all members of the family. Children who were experiencing serious physical problems, such as anorexia and heroin addiction, as well as asthmatics and diabetics, were treated and obtained a remarkable 91 percent rate of improvement at follow-up, which was several months after the conclusion of therapy (Minuchen, et al., 1975).

Langsley and Kaplan (1968) described using family therapy as a crisis intervention technique with very disturbed adolescents and their parents; this proved to be much more effective than hospitalization and individual treatment. Hundreds of adolescents and their parents were studied and outcome was evaluated by examining both length of treatment or hospitalization and the rate of recidivism after the completion of therapy. Family therapy was a superior treatment, as measured by the maintenance of adolescents in their community and their ability to resume normal social activities. Including parents in the treatment of adolescents in crisis proved to be efficacious, since they were able to change and serve as resources for their children.

A particular series of studies on family therapy with delinquent adolescents is impressive because the investigators developed a conceptual basis for their work, which they called *functional family therapy* (Alexander & Parsons, 1982). The family treatment is systematic and sequential, and an evaluation system is tied directly to their intervention. The studies began when Alexander (1973) identified differences between disturbed and normal families with respect to their communication process. There were more defensive communications in delinquent families and delinquent children expressed higher rates of system disintegrating communications (defensive communications including arguing and making excuses) than system integrating communications (supportive communications, such as listening and showing concern).

Parsons and Alexander performed a therapy outcome study using social learning principles and Alexander's notions about defensive and supportive communications: "Using the concept of reciprocity, the program was aimed at systematically extinguishing maladaptive interaction patterns. Based on the matching to sample philosophy, the goal was to modify the interactions of deviant families so that they would approximate those patterns characteristic of 'normal' or adjusted families found in prior research" (1973, p. 196). The therapy program involved differentiating rules from requests; establishing a token economy system so that there would be specific contingencies associated with appropriate behaviors; and finally, a social reinforcement system used to improve communication patterns. The members of the family were taught to communicate more appropriately by learning how to "interrupt for clarification," to find out more information about topics or people, and to offer positive feedback to other family members.

The data from these studies indicated that not only were the researchers able to modify communication patterns in the families, but that these modifications were directly associated with reductions in deviant behavior of the target adolescent. Alexander and Parsons (1973) compared their family treatment approach with either no-treatment groups or groups of children treated by other kinds of therapy. They reported that recidivism (as measured by referrals to juvenile court and problems with law enforcement authorities) was much less among those families who were treated with their functional approach toward family therapy. Moreover, those children who showed the lowest recidivism rates seemed to learn the most in the family therapy sessions, as measured by changes in communication patterns between the children and their parents.

A subsequent study (Alexander et al., 1976) examined the role of relationship factors in the treatment of families of delinquents. It was previously determined that family therapists who apply the techniques of structured family therapy produce results consistent with the objectives of their treatment. Relationship factors also significantly contributed to positive outcome; that is, it was not only the application of specific interventions that contributed to positive outcomes, but also the style in which therapists related to families that affected the results of the intervention. Apparently even in well specified treatments the personal qualities of the therapist influenced the treatment equation.

Perceptions of Children's Behavior

Judgments about the appropriateness of children's behaviors are usually based on the perceptions of adult caretakers. Achenbach and Edelbrock (1978) point out that parents are the psychologist's most important source of information about the nature of children's disorders. It is generally conceded that parents can be very reliable reporters. In a study of phobic children (Hempe et al, 1973) parents were very effective at assessing and documenting their children's phobic behaviors. As a matter of fact, in this case, reports proved to be just as valid as the information provided by experienced clinicians.

One study (O'Leary, Turkowitz, & Taffel, 1973) showed that parents and therapists had a 77 percent concordance rate in evaluation of children's improvement in outpatient psychotherapy. Another one (Glidewell, Domke, & Kantor, 1963) compared teachers' and parents' evaluations of children who were referred to a mental health clinic. They determined that there was a positive relationship between the number of symptoms reported by the child's mother and the degree of maladjustment reported by his teacher. Seventy-four percent of the mothers are cited as agreeing with teachers' ratings of their children's symptomatology.

A study of parent perceptions of schizophrenic children (Leim, 1974) shows that parents can be depended upon to interact with their disturbed children reliably and objectively. Leim compared the interactions of parents with schizophrenic children to parents with normal children. Both sets of parents responded to their own children and to other people's children. Essentially, the parents of schizophrenic children did not show any distortions in perception and did not act any differently toward their sons and other people's sons than did the parents of normal children.

Leim also concluded that parents of schizophrenic young male adults were as able to understand their sons' verbal expressions and associations as well as the parents of normal children listening to the same schizophrenic communications. Both sets of parents became confused by interacting with the young schizophrenics, and neither group of parents was particularly effective at influencing the behavior of the schizophrenic sons. The Leim study is an excellent demonstration that parents' perceptions and behavior can be stable and consistent, whether they are reacting with their own children or someone else's children.

While there tends to be high agreement among parents', teachers', and clinicians' ratings of children's behavior, it must be remembered that behavior is situation-specific (Mischel, 1973). One can only expect a moderate degree of overlap in conduct at home, conduct in school, conduct with peers, and conduct in the clinicians's office. Mitchell and Shepherd (1966) noted that one-half of the pupils characterized as having several problems at home were reported trouble-free by their teachers. Conversely, one-third of the children who were free of symptoms at home had at least one significant problem at school. Several sources of information have to be considered in order to distinguish those situations where behavior is acceptable from those where it is not. It follows that treatment interventions frequently need to be designed to enable children to function successfully in specific situations.

A distinction should be drawn between ratings of children receiving clinical treatment and ratings of children in the general population. Agreement among parents, teachers, and clinicians tends to be much higher for children who need professional assistance and engage in treatment than for normal children. A mutual consensus about the existence of a problem no doubt affects the amount of agreement about problem definition.

When there is a broad sampling of a cross-section of "normal" children, there is less agreement, with parents showing more concern about deviant behavior than teachers. Touliatos and Lindholm (1981) obtained ratings from mothers, fathers, and teachers on 1000 white, elementary school children in grades kindergarten through eighth. They used the Quay and Peterson Behavioral Problem Checklist (1979) in order to assess children's problems. The correlations between parental ratings and teacher ratings were in the low to moderate range, suggesting that the two groups of observers were seeing or reacting to different behaviors. Parents reported a greater amount of disordered behavior in their children, with both mothers and fathers reporting more conduct and personality problems than teachers. Social class was related only to conduct problems, with fewer conduct problems being attributed to children higher in SES status.

Three important questions can help us understand better the influence of parents' reactions to their children's behaviors (Rogers, Forehand, & Griest, 1981): (1) How do parents perceive their children and how do they make judgments about whether their children's behaviors are either deviant or nondeviant? (2) How do parents actually behave toward their children? (3) What is the personal adjustment level of the parents? The answers to these questions should help determine how the behaviors of clinic children and their families differ from behaviors of nonclinic children and their families.

By definition, parents of clinic children tend to see their children as more deviant and less compliant. Studies suggest that parents of clinic children give more commands or orders, are more likely to use coercive techniques, and generally respond more critically to their children that do nonclinic parents (Rogers et al., 1981). If parents are going to take their children to a mental health center, these parents are going to be distressed about their children's conduct and perhaps respond more punitively and negatively to their children. In fact, boys in treatment do show a lower percentage of compliance to parental demands and are perceived as engaging in a higher percentage of socially undesirable behavior by both parents and teachers than nonclinic children.

Finally, the perceptions of others are influenced by their frame of reference, their needs, and their level of adjustment. The same mothers who rate their children as more deviant are themselves rated by clinic personnel as more anxious and depressed and showing more personal and marital adjustment problems than nonclinic mothers (Rogers et al., 1981). It is very tempting to conclude that children and parents, and perhaps teachers as well, are influenced in their judgments by their levels of adjustment and that their perceptions of the child's behavior is affected by how they see themselves.

For example, children may be brought to a mental health professional because the parents have personal and marital adjustment problems and are projecting those problems onto their children. Also, if a parent has difficulty relating intimately with his or her spouse, the "blame" may be attributed to a demanding, dependent child who "insists" on sleeping in the parents' bed. In addition, parents may perceive themselves as deviant and noncompliant and feel unable to respond to their children's needs. Therefore, they exaggerate the child's problem and seek outside help so that they can develop their own skills to become more effective parents.

There is often some combination of the above factors (Bell, 1968). Certain children and certain parents, because of mutual adjustment problems and differences in temperament and orientation, have difficulty functioning together and end up perceiving each other's behavior as intolerable. Interpersonal influence is seldom unidirectional, with arrows just going from parent to child. Clearly, children can affect adult behavior, and Bell discussed instances of a "poor fit" between certain children and their parents. For example, a placid, easy-going child may frustrate energetic and competitive parents. Likewise, children who are active and seek much stimulation can cause stress and frustration for parents who operate at low-keyed levels. Parents of children who are "incompatible" are likely to make judgments about their children's behavior that result in the children being labeled as deviant and behavior disordered.

Children's Perceptions

An area that has been long neglected in terms of understanding the development of children's disorders and the treatment of those disorders is that of how children themselves perceive deviant behaviors. If behavior change is influenced by expectancy effects (Wilkins, 1979), children's expectations probably play a role in what they derive from treatment.

A first step is to determine how and if children are aware of psychological problems. Dollinger, Thelen, and Walsh (1980) conducted an open-ended survey with over 1,000 fifth- through twelfth-grade children to determine what roles children ascribed to clinical psychologists. They asked the question (p. 192): "Clinical psychologists help people with problems. What kinds of problems do you think they help people with? (Try to name at least three.)" The most frequently cited problem was family problems, with marital problems, mental health problems, interpersonal problems, and emotional problems following in that order. Types of problems were coded as internal to the person, such as thoughts and feelings; external, which included environmental factors such as drugs or alcohol; and social, which referred to problems involving other people. There were sex differences, with boys seeing problems as more internally mediated while girls made more social attributions to account for personal difficulties.

A companion study (Dollinger & Thelen, 1978) interviewed children about what they thought about psychologists. Girls were more likely to perceive psychologists as helping agents than were boys, while boys were more likely to see psychologists as people who study or do research. However, for the most part, children conceive of psychologists as primarily therapeutic agents. With age, children know more about the functions of psychologists and generally have more positive attitudes about them.

Roberts, Beidleman, and Wurtele (1981) found that children had very different perceptions of medical versus psychological disorders. Children saw medical disorders as being resolved through the use of medication and self-help, such as, "take aspirin, stay home, and take care of your cold." Psychological disorders, on the other hand, were seen as much more enduring and requiring some change in life circumstances. Interestingly, the fifth- and sixth-grade children in this study did not spontaneously identify mental health professionals as primary resources for children with psychological disorders. Lay professionals and salient people in their lives (teachers, parents, ministers, etc.) were seen as the primary providers of psychological help.

Maas, Marecek, and Travers (1978) addressed two major questions: what do children believe causes deviant behavior and what do they believe happens to enable children to change their behavior? After studying sixty children from grades two through six, they concluded that younger children saw internal factors (qualities intrinsic to the child) as the predominant causes of disordered behavior, while older children saw social and environmental factors as the main contributors to behavior disorders. In a manner consistent with their perceptions, younger children saw behavior change taking place through the child using internal resources, while older children were more likely to associate behavior change with changes in external social conditions, combined with some internal effort. Finally, children who acted out against society were seen as enjoying and wanting to act out. Children who were anxious, self-punitive, or socially withdrawn were perceived as behaving that way because of compelling inner forces which they were unable to control.

In open-ended interviews with first- through eleventh-grade boys and girls, the children were asked to characterize the behavior of deviant peer group members (Cole & Pennington, 1976). Younger children had great difficulty in making judgments of deviance. Seven and eight-year-olds were unable to place behavior in a normative context and, while they were able to talk about same or different, they were unable to characterize behavior in terms of group norms. Children in middle school years (ages nine through thirteen) were able to make normative comparisons and, in a manner consistent with Piaget's developmental findings, directly associated deviance with the violation of concrete social codes and rules. For adolescents in their mid-teens, judgments about deviance were normatively based, with the definition of the deviance related to the violation of social and group norms. Seventeen-year-olds relied on their own individual social judgments in order to make deviance attributions they were the only group to classify disorders apart from normative standards and to attribute behaviors to the unique personal characteristics of children and adolescents. The norms invoked by adolescents were more likely to be rooted in specific situations, compared with younger children, who based their attributions on generalized rights and wrongs independent of situational factors.

Questionnaires and rating scales determined how parents and children accounted for the success or failure of children's behavior (Compas et al., 1980). The researchers evaluated sixty-five elementary school children who were identified by either schools, professionals, or their parents as having learning or behavior problems. They found that the parents of these children made more internal than external attributions for the children's problems than did the children themselves. The children on the whole tended to see their problems as more externally mediated than did their parents. With respect to success experiences the picture changed, with both parents and children attributing the reasons for success to internal factors (things about the child and his/her personality) rather than to external social factors. For children, learning problems were seen as being mediated more by internal factors and conduct problems mediated by external factors. It is not surprising that children accepted more personal responsibility for success than for problems or failures. Parents, on the other hand, had a position that favored internal explanations for both success and failure in either learning or conduct situations. This finding is consistent with the attribution literature in the sense that outside observers (in this case parents) make more internal attributions, while the actors themselves are more likely to attribute their behaviors, particularly their unsuccessful behaviors, to external factors.

A review of the child perception literature suggests that children differ from adults with respect to ideas about: (1) the development of psychological disorders,

(2) what factors account for changes in behavior, and (3) the roles of professional helpers. Further clarification of the preceding issues will assist in understanding children and involving them in decisions that affect them directly.

Adolescents' Perceptions

Offer, Ostrov, and Howard (1981) presented detailed descriptions of adolescents' self-perceptions. Adolescents were asked to complete the Offer Self-Image Questionnaire, which provided information about how they felt about themselves. Data were gathered from four groups: 1970s normals, 1960s normals, adolescents from other cultures, and deviant adolescents. The deviant adolescents were classified as delinquent, psychiatrically disturbed, or physically ill. It was assumed that both younger adolescents (thirteen- to fifteen-year-olds) and older adolescents (sixteen- to eighteen-year-olds) could reliably evaluate their own feelings and emotions and systematically report their observations about themselves. The investigators examined the psychological self, the social self, the sexual self, the familial self, and the coping self of the respondents.

The *psychological self* was equated with emotionality, control over impulses, and perceptions of body image. Normal adolescents tended to see themselves as enjoying their lives, being happy with school most of the time, not feeling inferior, and seeing themselves as being treated fairly. They also described themselves as relaxed most of the time (90 percent), but anxious some of the time (50 percent). The only sex difference worthy of note was that girls were more conscious of, and more negative about, their bodies and reported themselves to be somewhat sadder and lonelier than boys.

In contrast to normal children, physically ill teen-agers had more negative emotions about themselves and their body image, and reported feeling unattractive and inferior. Delinquents described themselves as being sadder and more lonely, feeling that they got less out of life; they seemed more worried about their health than normals. Interestingly, the delinquents did not see themselves as having any more problems controlling their aggression than did normals. The psychiatrically disturbed adolescents presented themselves as having relatively good impulse control, but they reported problems with mood and body image.

With respect to their *social self*, normal teen-agers tended to be career oriented, had a strong work ethic, and enjoyed social activities in the company of others. Girls reported more traditional moral standards and more positive attitudes toward careers, while boys reported themselves to be more independent and more often saw themselves to be in a leadership position. There were no differences in social self between normal and physically ill children. Juvenile delinquents tended to report being less social, and 33 percent said they preferred to be alone, as compared with 20 percent of normal adolescents who felt the same way. Psychiatrically disturbed adolescents reported difficulties with relationships with the same and opposite sexes and reported feeling more vulnerable and insecure in the presence of others than did the other groups of adolescents.

With respect to the *sexual self*, most normal teen-agers reported being unafraid of their own sexuality, and positively valued changes in their own body. Boys tended to be more open than girls about sexuality and thought more about sex. There were age differences among girls, with the older girls (sixteen- to eighteen-year-olds) thinking about sex more and enjoying sexual experiences more than the younger girls (thirteen- to fifteen-year-olds). Older teenagers in general tended to be more confident about their physical appearance than younger teenagers. The physically ill children reported poorer self images, did not think as often about sex, and saw themselves as lagging in sexual experiences. There were no reliable differences between the reports of delinquents, psychiatrically disturbed adolescents, and normal adolescents with respect to sexual interests or activities.

Normal teen-agers reported relatively few major problems with respect to their *familial self* in terms of relationships with parents. The notion of a "generation gap" was generally discounted, with normal adolescents feeling close to their parents and seeing their parents as proud of them. The physically ill children felt even closer to their parents than the normal ones, saw themselves as a greater source of pride to their parents, and saw their roles as children as more important to their parents in the future than did normals. On the other hand, juvenile delinquents had more negative feelings toward their parents, did not see their parents as being satisfied with them, and frequently believed their parents were ashamed of them. Psychiatrically disturbed adolescents were similar to delinquents in feeling more distant from the parents—only 60 percent of both groups felt their parents were satisfied with them, as compared to 90 percent of normal adolescents.

Normal adolescents saw themselves coping with their lives with confidence and relatively little fear. They were hopeful about the future, and even if they failed, they felt they could learn from that experience. Approximately 20 percent of the normal children felt some emotional emptiness and saw life as a series of problems, with relatively little hope to make significant changes in those problem areas. The younger adolescent females saw themselves as more disturbed and less able to cope successfully than the other three groups. Younger girls more often felt experiences of shame, and felt they were criticized more often by their relatives and even by their peers. Physically ill children saw themselves as socially more vulnerable and more self-conscious and uncertain about their ability to cope with day-to-day circumstances. Finally, juvenile delinquents and psychiatrically disturbed adolescents saw their lives as consisting of endless problems; they reported confusion, tended to be more ashamed of their behavior, and saw their academic performances as being more problematic.

Looking at their data as a whole, Offer, Ostrov, and Howard saw girls as having more negative feelings about themselves than boys, and being more concerned about their bodies. On the other hand, girls tended to be more positive about their interpersonal relationships. Except as previously mentioned, there were no dramatic age or cross-cultural differences, and surprisingly there were no consistent differences between the adolescents of the 1960s and the 1970s. There were very significant differences with respect to the negative attitudes of juvenile delinquents and psychiatrically disturbed children toward their family relationships. In addition, these same adolescents were clearly more unhappy with their lives. Physically ill children did distinguish themselves in terms of their feelings of vulnerability and their concerns about body image, and yet they claimed a sense of optimism about the future and a feeling of closeness to their families.

The general findings of these investigators indicate that most American teenagers basically perceive themselves as confident, happy and self-satisfied individuals. Their data are in opposition to the turmoil theory of adolescence, which assumes that the adolescent period is generally and normally one of considerable distress, mood swings, and rebellion. They see adolescence as a period in which there are some crises, but no major disruptions for most adolescents. The findings that 50 percent of adolescents report occasional periods of anxiety does not distinguish them from adults. With the national divorce rate currently over 40 percent, it is sobering that 20 percent of normal adolescents report significant disruptions in family relationships. It would seem that the effectiveness of the adolescents' coping strategies are certainly no worse than other age groups

The issues raised in this section consider the relationships among children's and adolescents' perceptions of their own behavior and parents', teachers', and clinicians' perceptions of these same behaviors. The concordance rates among adult observers tends to be quite high, with parents and teachers usually proving to be reliable reporters of children's behavior. However, there is little doubt that there are distortions and that greater effort is needed to understand how children perceive their own conduct. In determining what is abnormal behavior, not only must the situation in which the behavior is taking place and the usual social expectations be considered, but also the observer who is reporting the behavior. If we are to respect the rights of the children and adolescents we serve and actually accommodate our efforts to their needs, we must broaden the source of data about deviant and normative functioning to include the very children we are serving.

REFERENCES

Achenbach, T. M., & Edelbrock, C. S. (1984) Psychopathology of childhood. In M. R. Rosenzweig & L. W. Porter, (Eds.), *Annual review of psychology,* Vol. 35. Palo Alto, CA: Annual Reviews, Inc.

Adams, P. L. Children and para-services of the community mental health centers. *Journal of the American Academy of Child Psychiatry,* 1975, *14*(1), 18–31.

Alexander, J. F. Defensive and supportive communications in normal and deviant families. *Journal of Consulting and Clinical Psychology,* 1973, *40*(2), 223–231.

Alexander, J. F., Barton, C., Schiavo, R. S., & Parsons, B. V. Systems-behavioral intervention with families of delinquents: Therapist characteristics, family behavior, and outcome. *Journal of Consulting and Clinical Psychology,* 1976, *44*(4), 656–664.

Alexander, J., & Parsons, B. V. Short-term behavioral interventions with delinquent families: Impact on family process and recidivism. *Journal of Abnormal Psychology,* 1973, *81*(3), 219–225.

Alexander, J., & Parsons, B. V. *Functional family therapy.* Monterey, CA: Brooks/Cole, 1982.

Anderson, D. R. Prevalence of behavioral and emotional disturbance and specific problem types in a sample of disadvantaged preschool-aged children. *Journal of Clinical Child Psychology,* 1983, *12*(2), 130–136.

Bandura, A. *Social learning theory.* Englewood Cliffs, NJ: Prentice-Hall, 1977.

Barrett, C. L., Hampe, E., & Miller, L. Research on psychotherapy with children. In A. E. Bergin and S. L. Garfield (Eds.), *Handbook of psychotherapy and behavior change.* New York: Wiley, 1971.

Beitchman, J., & Dielman, T. Predicting hospitalization in child psychiatry: The influence of diagnosis and demographic variables. *Journal of Clinical Child Psychology,* 1982 *11*(2), 116–122.

Bell, R. Q. A reinterpretation of the direction of effects in studies of socialization. *Psychological Review*, 1968, *75*, 81–95.

Birch, H. G., & Gussow, J. D. *Disadvantaged children: Health, nutrition, and school failure.* New York: Harcourt, Brace, 1970.

Cole, J. D., & Pennington, B. D. Children's perceptions of deviance and disorder. *Child Development*, 1976, *47*, 407–413.

Compas, B. E., Friedland-Bandes, R., Bastien, R., & Adelman, H. S. Parent and child causal attributions related to the child's clinical problem. *Journal of Abnormal Child Psychology*, 1981, 9(3), 389–397.

Colter, S., Jason, L. A., Middelberg, C., Ribordy, S. C., Dinello, F. A., & Frey, M. J. Issues in introducing program evaluation in a community mental health center. In G. L. Judy (Ed.), *Successful innovations in child guidance: Unique management techniques and services for children and their families.* Springfield, IL: Charles C. Thomas, 1982.

Crowther, J. H., Bond, L. A., & Reff, J. E. The incidence, prevalence and severity of behavior disorders among preschool-aged children in day care. *Journal of Abnormal Child Psychology*, 1981, 9:*1*, 23–42.

DeWitt, C. N. The effectiveness of family therapy. *Archives of General Psychiatry*, 1978, *35*, 549–561.

Dohrenwend, B. S., & Dohrenwend, B. P. Overview and prospects for research on stressful life events. In Dohrenwend, B. S. and Dohrenwend, B. P. (Eds.), *Stressful life events: Their nature and effects.* New York: Wiley, 1974.

Dollinger, S. J., & Thelen, M. H. Children's perceptions of psychology. *Professional Psychology*, 1978, *9*, 117–126.

Dollinger, S. J., Thelen, M. H., & Walsh, M. L. Children's conceptions of psychological problems. *Journal of Consulting and Clinical Psychology*, 1980, Fall, 191–194.

Edelbrock, C., & Achenbach, T. M. A typology of child behavior profile patterns: Distribution and correlates for disturbed children aged 6–16. *Journal of Abnormal Child Psychology*, 1980, *8*(4), 441–470.

Erikson, E. H. *Identity, youth and crisis.* New York: Norton, 1968.

Eysenck, H. J. The effects of psychotherapy: An evaluation. *Journal of Consulting Psychology*, 1952, *16*, 319–324.

Glidewell, J. C., Domke, H. R., & Kantor, M. B. Screening in schools for behavior disorders: Use of mothers' reports of symptoms. *Journal of Educational Research*, 1963, *56*, 508–515.

Goldstein, A. P., Heller, K., & Sechrest, L. B. *Psychotherapy and the psychology of behavior change.* New York: John Wiley, 1966.

Graham, P. Epidemiological studies. In H. C. Quay and J. S. Werry (Eds.), *Psychopathological disorders of childhood* (2nd ed.). New York: John Wiley, 1979.

Green, K., Beck, S., Forehand, R., & Vosk, B. Validity of teacher nominations of child behavior problems. *Journal of Abnormal Child Psychology*, 1980, *8*(3,) 397–404.

Gross, M. L. *The psychological society.* New York: Simon & Schuster, 1978.

Gurman, A. S., & Kniskern, D. P. Research on marital and family therapy: Progress, perspective and prospect. In A. E. Bergin and S. L. Garfield (Eds.), *Handbook of psychotherapy and behavior change.* New York: John Wiley, 1971.

Hempe, E., Noble, A., Miller, L. C., & Barrett, C. L. Phobic children one and two years posttreatment. *Journal of Abnormal Psychology* 1973, *82*(3), 446–453.

Heinicke, C. M., & Strassmann, L. H. Toward more effective research on child psychotherapy. *Journal of American Academy of Child Psychiatry*, 1975, *15*, 561–588.

Heitler, J. B. Preparatory techniques in initiating expressive psychotherapy with lower-class, unsophisticated patients. *Psychological Bulletin*, 1976, *83*, 339–352.

Hurvitz, N. Psychotherapy as a means of social control. *Journal of Consulting and Clinical Psychology*, 1973, 40(2), 232–239.

Jacob, T. Family interaction in disturbed and normal families: A methodological and substantive review. *Psychological Bulletin*, 1975, *82*, 33–65.

Jacobson, A. N., Goldberg, I. D., Burns, B. J., Hoper, E. N., Hankin, J. R., & Hewitt, K. Diagnosed mental disorder in children and use of health services in four organized health care settings. *American Journal of Psychiatry*, 1980, *137*(15).

Kiesler, D. J. Some myths of psychotherapy research and the search for a paradigm. *Psychological Bulletin*, 1966, *65*, 110–136.

King, L. M. Social and cultural influences on psychopathology. *Annual Review of Psychology*, 1978 *29*, 405–433.

Knopf, I. J. *Childhood psychopathology: A developmental approach.* Englewood Cliffs NJ: Prentice Hall, 1979.

Kohlberg, L., LaCross, J., & Ricks, D. The predictability of adult mental health from childhood behavior. In B. B. Wolman, *Manual of child psychopathology.* New York: McGraw-Hill, 1972.

Lahey, B. B., Hammer, D., Crumrine, P. L., & Forehand, R. L. Birth order and sex interactions in child behavior problems. *Developmental Psychology,* 1980, *16*(6), 608–615.

Langsley, D. G., & Kaplan, D. M. *The treatment of families in crises.* New York: Grune and Stratton, 1968.

Leim, J. H. Effects of verbal communications of parents and children: A comparison of normal and schizophrenic families. *Journal of Consulting and Clinical Psychology,* 1974, *42*(3), 438–450.

Levitt, E. E. The results of psychotherapy with children: An evaluation. *Journal of Consulting Psychology,* 1957, *21,* 189–196.

Levitt, E. E. Research on psychotherapy with children. In A. E. Bergin and S. L. Garfield (Eds.), *Handbook of psychotherapy and behavior change.* New York: Wiley, 1971.

Lorion, R. P. Research on psychotherapy and behavior change with the disadvantaged. In A. E. Bergin and S. L. Garfield (Eds.), *Handbook of psychotherapy and behavior change.* New York: Wiley, 1978.

Maas, E., Marecek, J., & Travers, J. R. Children's conceptions of disordered behavior. *Child Development,* 1978, *49,* 146–154.

McDermott, P. Prevalence and constituency of behavioral disturbance taxonomies in the regular school population. *Journal of Abnormal Child Psychology,* 1980, *8*(4), 523–536.

Miller, L. C., Hampe, E., Barrett, C. L., & Noble, H. Children's deviant behavior within the general population. *Journal of Consulting and Clinical Psychology,* 1971, *37,* 16–22.

Minuchin, S. *Families and family therapy.* Cambridge, MA: Harvard University, 1974.

Minuchin, S., Baker, L., Rosman, B., Liebman, R., Milman, L., & Todd, T. A. conceptual model of psychosomatic illness in children. *Archives of General Psychiatry,* 1975, *32,* 1031–1038.

Mischel, W. *Personality and assessment.* New York: Wiley, 1968.

Mischel, W. Toward a cognitive social learning reconceptualization of personality. *Psychological Review,* 1973, *80,* 252–283.

Mitchell, S., & Shepherd, M. A comparative study of children's behavior problems at home and at school. *British Journal of Educational Psychology,* 1966, *36,* 248–254.

Moffitt, T. E., Gabrielle, W. F., Mednick, S. A., & Schulsinger, F. Socioeconomic status, IQ and delinquency. *Journal of Abnormal Psychology,* 1981, *90*(12), 152–156.

Offer, D., Ostrov, E., & Howard, K. I. *The adolescent: A psychological self-portrait.* New York: Basic Books, 1981.

O'Leary, K. D., Turkowitz, H., & Taffel, S. J. Parent and therapist evaluation of behavior therapy in a child psychological clinic. *Journal of Consulting and Clinical Psychology,* 1973, *41,* 279–283.

Olweus, D. Familial and temperamental determinants of aggressive behavior in adolescent boys: A causal analysis. *Developmental Psychology,* 1980, *16*(6), 644–660.

Parsons, B. V., & Alexander, J. F. Short-term family intervention: A therapy outcome study. *Journal of Consulting and Clinical Psychology,* 1973, *41*(2), 195–201.

Quay, H. C., & Peterson, D. R. *Manual for the behavior problem checklist, 1979.* Available from D. R. Peterson, 39 North Fifth, Highland Park, NJ 08904.

Richman, N., Stevenson, J., & Graham, P. Prevalence of behavior problems in 3-year-old children: Preliminary findings. *Journal of Child Psychology and Psychiatry,* 1975, *16,* 272–287.

Roberts, M. C., Beidleman, W. B., & Wurtele, S. K. Children's perceptions of medical and psychological disorders in their peers. *Journal of Clinical Child Psychology,* 1981, *10,* 76–78.

Robins, L. N. Follow-up studies of behavior disorders in children. In H. C. Quay and J. S. Werry (Eds.), *Psychopathological disorders of childhood.* New York: J. Wiley, 1972.

Rogers, T. R., Forehand, R., & Griest, D. L. The conduct disordered child: An analysis of family problems. *Clinical Psychology Review,* 1981 *1,* 139–147.

Ross, A. O. *Psychological disorders of children: A behavioral approach to theory, research and therapy.* (2nd ed.). New York: McGraw-Hill, 1980.

Shepherd, M., Oppenheim, A. N., & Mitchell, S. Childhood behavior disorders and the child-guidance clinic. *Journal of Child Psychology and Psychiatry,* 1966, *7,* 39–52.

Shore, M., & Massimo, J. Five years later: A follow-up study of comprehensive vocationally oriented psychotherapy. *American Journal of Orthopsychiatry,* 1969, *39,* 769–773.

Shore, M., & Massimo, J. After ten years: A follow-up study of comprehensive vocationally oriented psychotherapy. *American Journal of Orthopsychiatry,* 1973, *43,* 128–132.

Touliatos, J., & Lindholm, B. W. Congruence of parents' and teachers' ratings of children's behavior problems. *Journal of Abnormal Child Psychology*, 1981, 9(3), 347–354.

Tramontana, M. G. Critical review of research on psychotherapy with adolescents: 1967–1977. *Psychological Bulletin*, 1980, *88*(2), 429–450.

Weiner, I. B. Psychopathology in adolescence. In J. Adelson (Ed.), *Handbook of adolescent psychology*. New York: Wiley, 1980.

Wells, R. A., & Duzen, A. E. The results of family therapy revisited: the nonbehavioral methods. *Family Processes*, 1978, *17*, 251–274.

Wilkins, W. Expectancies in therapy research: Discriminating among heterogeneous nonspecifics. *Journal of Consulting and Clinical Psychology*, 1979, *47*(5), 837–845.

Wright, D. M., Moelis, I., & Pollack, L. J. The outcome of individual child psychotherapy: Increments at follow-up. *Journal of Child Psychology and Psychiatry*, 1976, *17*, 275–285.

Zax, M., & Cowen, E. L. Early identification and prevention of emotional disturbance in a public school. In E. L. Cowen, E. A. Gardner, and M. Zax (Eds.), *Emergent approaches to mental health problems*. New York: Appleton-Century-Crofts, 1967.

PART II

DISORDERS

Introduction

The eleven chapters in Part II have been arranged in basically a developmental sequence, according to when in the life span the disorder is first apt to be diagnosed. Thus Chapter 4, on "Mental Retardation" leads off, since severe forms of retardation can be diagnosed and, in cases such as phenylketonuria, prevented early in infancy. However this developmental scheme is only approximate because many of the chapters, including "Mental Retardation," cover the appearance of their disorders in infancy, childhood, and adolescence. Reactive attachment disorder of infancy appears in Chapter 9, where it is appropriately discussed among the depressive disorders. Nevertheless, there is a developmental progression, with the last two chapters giving attention to problems of adolescence.

DSM-III has no categories for juvenile delinquency, suicide, and psychophysiologic (psychosomatic) disorders. These omissions were deliberate and are reasonable. Delinquency, a legal term which varies in meaning from place to place and year to year, receives consideration under conduct disorders in Chapter 13 and substance use disorders in Chapter 14. Suicide is associated with depression, and so is discussed in Chapter 9. Psychophysiologic conditions are handled in DSM-III by specifying the medical disorder in question on Axis III and noting on Axis I that there are psychological factors affecting the physical condition, if indeed that is the case. Obesity is *not* a psychiatric disorder, but as a medical condition which has attracted the efforts of many psychologists, it is in Chapter 8, "Eating and Elimination Disorders."

Although the authors of these chapters try to be balanced in their presentations of etiology and treatment, they do have biases which it may be helpful to make explicit. Some are behavioral (as in Chapters 5, 6, and 8); some are psychodynamic (as in Chapters 10, 13, and 14); and some have a beguilingly practical, commonsensical orientation (as in Chapters 7 and 12). All try to be mindful of other points of view. Moreover, all share the same goal: to provide you with a comprehensive understanding of psychopathology in infancy, childhood, and adolescence and to communicate why it is so interesting, complex, and worthy of serious study.

CHAPTER 4

Mental Retardation

Penelope H. Brooks and Pamela Doxsey West

Mental retardation has been recorded in all known civilizations. In the ancient Greek city-state of Sparta, infants with obvious physical or mental handicaps were slain. In Rome and subsequently in much of Europe, the dull were often kept for the entertainment of wealthy citizens. In medieval times, Christian leaders believed the mentally retarded were "possessed" by the devil and often inflicted severe punishment in an attempt at exorcism (Baumeister, 1970).

Treatment for the mentally retarded was unheard of until the early 1800s when Jean Itard attempted to educate the feral boy Victor (see Chapter 1). Although he was only minimally successful, his work was continued by his student, Dr. Edouard Seguin. Seguin helped to establish several schools for the mentally retarded, and in 1876 was selected as the first president of the Association of Medical Officers of American Institutions for Idiotic and Feeble-minded Persons, now called the American Association on Mental Deficiency (AAMD) (Baumeister, 1970).

This research was supported by National Institute of Child Health and Human Development Grants HD-07226 and HD-15052 to George Peabody College of Vanderbilt University.

Defining Mental Retardation

Following the work of Itard and Seguin, definitions of mental retardation evolved. Unfortunately, no single definition of mental retardation has proven to be universally acceptable or useful. One reason for this lies in the difficulty inherent in defining the underlying concepts involved in mental retardation, such as intelligence and socially acceptable or adaptive behavior. In addition, a definition may serve a number of functions and hence may change, depending on what it is attempting to do.

For example, one function of a definition of mental retardation might be to specify severity of deficit in intellectual performance and be based on IQ scores. A second function might be to specify severity of deficit in social behavior and be based on an adaptive behavior scale. However, any good definition should facilitate communication and determine a course of action (Baumeister & Muma, 1975). Therefore, definitions of retardation must be specific enough to convey information, but may vary depending upon the treatment plan. If mental retardation is viewed as a genetic problem, for example, the treatment plan may involve genetic counseling, whereas if it is viewed as a learning problem, treatment would involve education. In addition, definitions may vary depending upon one's theoretical orientation, e.g., whether the "deficit" is viewed as existing within the person or within society's expectation of what is "normal."

Historically, mentally retarded persons have been defined as persons with a low intelligence. This has typically been determined by a score significantly below the mean on a test such as the Stanford-Binet Intelligence Scale (Terman & Merrill, 1973) or the Wechsler Intelligence Scale for Children–Revised (WISC–R) (Wechsler, 1974). Implicitly this definition conveys the deficit as existing within the person.

Although a definition based on scores on intelligence tests is somewhat circular (i.e., one has low intelligence because of a low IQ; one has a low IQ because of low intelligence), it has the advantage of being fairly simple, easily communicated, and reasonably predictive of behaviors, such as school success. It also provides a well-defined standardization group with which to make comparisons.

According to the Stanford-Binet intelligence classification system, persons with IQs between 30 and 59 are mentally defective, and persons with IQs between 60 and 79 are borderline defective. A similar psychometric classification, based on the Wechsler Adult Intelligence Scale, was devised by Wechsler in 1955.

These psychometric approaches have been incorporated into an "official" definition of mental retardation adopted by the American Association on Mental Deficiency and recognized by DSM-III. The latest definition, written in 1983, states that: "Mental retardation refers to significantly subaverage general intellectual functioning existing concurrently with deficits in adaptive behavior and manifested during the developmental period" (Grossman, 1983, p. 1). Each of the major concepts included in the definition—significantly subaverage, general intellectual functioning, adaptive behavior, and developmental period—will be discussed further.

Significantly Subaverage

An individual's score on an intelligence test is meaningful relative to the norms established on the standardization sample. A standardization sample is a group of people of varying abilities to whom a test is originally administered. All other administrations of the test can then be compared to this standardization sample. The standard deviation (SD) refers to the degree to which an individual score deviates or varies from the standard mean (i.e., the average score of the standardization sample). It is with the use of the standard deviation concept that we refer to a score being *significantly* above or below the average or mean. All IQ scores are *normally* distributed around the mean. In other words, there are an equal number of scores above and below the mean; most scores cluster around the mean; and there are fewer and fewer scores as they get farther away from the mean.

A significantly subaverage IQ is necessary in order to classify a person as mentally retarded. An IQ of less than 70 has become the popular cut-off indicative of mental retardation. These scores correspond to two standard deviations below the mean score obtained on the Stanford-Binet and Wechsler scales. The mean score on both the Stanford-Binet and Wechsler scales is 100 points and the standard deviation at each age is 15 points on the Wechsler and 16 points on the Stanford-Binet. Theoretically, 2.28 percent of the population achieve IQ scores of more than two standard deviations below the mean, and 2.28% achieve IQ scores of more than two standard deviations above the mean. Sixty-eight percent achieve IQ scores within one standard deviation of the mean. See Figure 4-1 for the theoretical distribution of intelligence quotients.

Intelligence tests, such as the Stanford-Binet and the Wechsler Scales, were developed through a process of identifying questions and problems that seem to tap areas we commonly associate with intelligence (e.g., memory, vocabulary, similarities) and that discriminate between different ages and abilities. In other words, items are selected for a test if they discriminate between individuals and if individuals' performance on those items is normally distributed around a particular age. An intelligence test on which performance was not normally distributed would not be acceptable because it is *believed* that intelligence is normally distributed within the population. Thus, if intelligence is normally distributed within the population, then scores must be normally distributed on intelligence tests.

General Intellectual Functioning

DSM-III specifies intellectual functioning be measured by an assessment with an individually administered intelligence test developed for that purpose. The most respected tests include the Stanford-Binet Intelligence Scale (1972 version) and the three Wechsler scales: The Wechsler Preschool and Primary Scale of Intelligence (WPPSI), the Wechsler Intelligence Scale

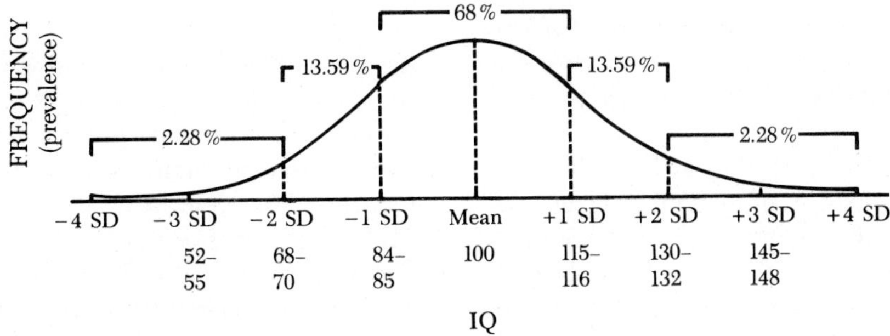

Figure 4-1

for Children–Revised (WISC–R), and the Wechsler Adult Intelligence Scale–Revised (WAIS–R). These tests require trained examiners and at least forty-five minutes to administer. A great deal of care has gone into the revisions and standardizations of these tests. For example, the 1974 standardization sample for the WISC–R consisted of 2,200 children aged six-and-one-half to sixteen-and-one-half years. In addition, variables such as sex, race (white-nonwhite), geographic region, occupation of head of household, and urban-rural residence were included at each age level tested, creating a more diverse standardization sample than included on the original WISC. The importance of a representative standardization sample becomes evident when one attempts to select a test for a particular child. Clearly it would be difficult to compare a rural black child with the all-white standardization sample of the Stanford-Binet since inadequate performance may be due to differential experiences.

Assessment in Infancy. The assessment of intellectual development can begin in infancy. Early assessment has become a popular area due to the belief that developmental problems may be remediated through early intervention. Early detection of mental retardation is difficult, however, unless there is an observable syndrome present which is commonly associated with mental retardation, such as Down syndrome. Assessment is typically done with infants who are considered at risk for mental retardation because of socioeconomic or medical reasons.

Commonly used infant intelligence or developmental tests include the Bayley Scales of Infant Development (Bayley, 1969), and the Infant Intelligence Scale (Cattell, 1940). These tests yield a DQ (developmental quotient) rather than an IQ. Although the means and standard deviations on these tests are the same as on intelligence tests (mean = 100; standard deviation = 15), infant tests measure the rate of development rather than an abstract concept such as intelligence. Infant tests usually include behavioral items, such as stacking blocks; motor items, such as sitting; social items, such as smiling; and verbal items, such as babbling. A DQ provides the age at which infants normally perform a set of behaviors. For example, an infant with a DQ of ten months behaves, on average, like a typical ten month old.

Infant assessment is critical to intervention because it provides a means to detect developmental delays and measures progress. Nevertheless, infant tests are not highly predictive of subsequent IQ (Golden & Brins, 1976; Haviland, 1976; Honzik, 1976; McCall, 1979). Generally, the younger the infant, and the larger the duration between test administrations, the lower the correlation. Although predictions may begin by six months of age for specific behaviors, they are not reliable until after twenty-four months. Prediction is best in the case of very low scoring infants since these infants do tend to continue to be assessed as mentally retarded through childhood and adulthood (Honzik, 1976).

There are several possible explanations for the low predictability of IQ from infancy. Infant tests may not tap those behaviors which correlate highly with subsequent IQ; for example, visual or perceptual activity may correlate more highly with IQ than motor activity (Zelazo, 1979; Kearsley & Zelazo, 1975). There also may be a qualitative change from infancy to childhood in which new intellectual abilities emerge and result in a reduced relationship between performance in one age and the other (Kagan,

Kearsley, & Zelazo, 1978). Other explanations include: the possibility that prenatal maturational effects must wear off before infants can be differentiated from one another; the *rate* of development during infancy should not correlate with subsequent intelligence, as exemplified by school performance, except in the case of an extremely delayed infant; and infants with a mild delay can have this effect inflated on a DQ, when chronological ages are so small.

Nevertheless, infant tests do allow us to identify infants with serious delays. It is not actually possible, however, to definitively diagnose mental retardation until the child is old enough to be given both an IQ test and an adaptive behavior scale, some time after twenty-four to thirty months of age.

Adaptive Behavior

Adaptive behavior refers to a person's ability to get along in the mainstream culture and to perform everyday activities, such as bathing, dressing, eating, socializing, shopping, etc. The construct of adaptive behavior assumes no underlying competence but measures what a person does. This notion is unlike intelligence, which has a connotation of underlying intellectual potential. Intelligence supposedly refers to what a person is capable of doing, not necessarily what they actually do. Adaptive behavior is not concerned with whether individuals know how to brush their teeth; it is concerned with *whether* they brush their teeth.

Because adaptive behavior is about an individual's typical behavior, it is not measured in the same way as intelligence. Instead of a formalized testing situation, the measurement of adaptive behavior relies on informants who answer questions about what an individual does.

How a person behaves in everyday activity is certainly subject to cultural determinants. Anger, for example, is considered a normal display in some cultures but not others. Any definition of adaptive behavior must take into account an individual's culture reference group. Similarly, some behaviors are appropriate for younger children, but not adults, e.g., temper tantrums. The AAMD definition of adaptive behavior includes such qualifications: "Adaptive behavior is defined as the effectiveness or degree with which an individual meets the standards of personal independence and social responsibility expected for age and cultural group" (Grossman, 1977, p. 11).

In all, there are more than 100 adaptive behavior scales currently in use, some more rigorously developed than others. These scales differ along several dimensions (Meyers, Nihira, & Zetlin, 1979), such as whether adaptive behavior is considered a unitary trait yielding a single test score, a product of many traits, or a product of separable but related domains. Further, each of these scales may be embedded within either an assessment system or a programming system. Most multidomain scales have at least some of the following components (Meyers, Nihira, & Zetlin, 1979): (a) daily living activities (self-help skills, vocational activities, and domestic activities); (b) cognitive, social, perceptual-motor, and self-direction aspects; and (c) role performance activities (community citizens, family, etc.).

The area of adaptive behavior measurement is currently going through the throes of scale construction, reliability and validity studies, revision, and arguments over appropriate use of instruments. Meyers, Nihira, and Zetlin (1979) predict that the flurry of activities around scale development and the proliferation of tests will soon subside, leaving us with some reasonably sound, useful scales. They claim that what is left to be measured, in the realm of adaptive behavior, is social intelligence and motivation. Until these constructs are measured and worked into the definition of adaptive behavior there are still gaps in or limits to the adequacy of our measure.

Developmental Period

The developmental period refers to the first eighteen years of life. A person whose limited skills appear prior to eighteen will be classified as mentally retarded. Someone whose limitations appear after eighteen will be classified as brain damaged, aphasic, or by some other label. Part of the rationale for the cut-off at eighteen years is related to the view that mental retardation is a developmental phenomenon, i.e., that it is delayed or halted development, regardless of the cause. Someone who sustains injury or disease after age eighteen will theoretically have developed his or her intellectual capabilities completely. Damage then is to a fully developed individual, not someone in the process of developing.

It is true that the cutoff at age eighteen is an arbitrary one. There may be very little difference in someone who was neurologically impaired as a result of a motorcycle accident at seventeen and a half and one who was similarly injured at eighteen and a half. Yet the seventeen-and-a-half-year old would be classified and treated as mentally retarded while the older person would probably be treated as mentally ill or brain damaged. This arbitrariness would exist for any age which would be designated as a cutoff. While the developmental age criterion in the definition certainly makes theoretical sense, in actual practice there may be little difference in the treatment programs for the two individuals.

Classification Systems

A classification system may have a great impact on an individual's everyday life. Depending on how one is classified within the mental retardation system, one may be institutionalized, receive free services (such as day care, medical, dental, and psychological screening), qualify for supplemental income, be placed in special education classes, or be allowed to participate or try to participate in the mainstream culture. Classification typically has both positive and negative consequences. That is, one may benefit from a society's resources as a result of being classified, but one may also be burdened with a socially degrading label. A retarded individual may be under the jurisdiction of state departments of corrections, education, mental health, or mental retardation, depending on what is considered the primary diagnosis, That is, depending on whether the primary concern involves an educational problem, a psychiatric condition, a legal or criminal offense, or simply mental retardation. In many cases these different departments treat people quite differently depending on their service philosophy and budget. The nature of the prevailing classification system can determine the allocation of hundreds of millions of dollars within a state or national budget.

Any classification system that has such serious personal and political consequences is going to be controversial. Because there is no single classification system that will satisfy the needs of all the people who are involved in serving the retarded, there are at least four major systems used to classify mentally retarded individuals.

Intellectual Performance

The most frequently used classification system was proposed by the American Association on Mental Deficiency in 1983 (Grossman, 1983). This system categorizes individuals on the basis of their level of intellectual functioning as measured by intelligence tests. In other words, it is a classification based on a person's behavior on an intelligence test. According to this system there are four levels of retardation:

Subtypes of Mental Retardation	IQ Levels
Mild mental retardation	50–55 to 70
Moderate mental retardation	35–40 to 50–55
Severe mental retardation	20–25 to 35–40
Profound mental retardation	Below 20 or 25

There have been a number of changes in this classification system over the years. The most momentous was the elimination of a fifth category, "borderline" mental retardation, in 1973. This category, reserved for individuals who performed between one and two standard deviations below the mean on intelligence tests, was eliminated because these individuals seemed to be able to adapt well within society. It is sometimes said that in 1973, 25 million mentally retarded people were cured.

Adaptive Behavior

Individuals may also be classified according to a behavioral system involving their adaptive behavior. Unlike intellectual performance, adaptive behavior does not have a long history of test development and measurement. However, since the 1973 AAMD definition has stipulated that deficient adaptive behavior be part of the criteria, several tests of adaptive behavior have been developed.

Although adaptive behavior and intelligence test performance are related, the American Association on Mental Deficiency prefers to use both systems, and designates someone as retarded only if he or she is low on both kinds of behavior. Figure 4-2 shows the relationship between the two types of behavior that result in mental retardation.

What kinds of adaptive behaviors might be expected from mentally retarded individuals at each level of retardation? In order to answer this question, we will examine a few levels of retardation with respect to behavior capabilities.

Adaptive Behavior in Severe Retardation. Carrie is nine years old and a victim of a relatively rare disorder (Cornelia de Lange syndrome) which left her at serious risk for retardation. Although she has been in intervention programs since infancy, her physical growth is quite delayed. She tries to eat but requires a great deal of help. She is not toilet trained but

Intellectual Functioning

Adaptive Behavior	RETARDED	NOT RETARDED
Retarded	RETARDED	Not classified as Retarded
Not Retarded	Not classified as Retarded	Not classified as Retarded

Figure 4-2

will sometimes indicate that her pants are wet and will help with the bathroom activities. She can undress but not dress herself. Her communication is limited to a few words and clicks with her tongue and she can point to things she wants. Although she recognizes familiar faces and is wary of strangers, she is generally unresponsive to the environment or to social interaction. Originally her unresponsiveness led teachers to believe she was deaf, but that did not turn out to be the case. Carrie would be classified as profoundly mentally retarded.

Adaptive Behavior and Moderate Retardation. Most adults with Down syndrome are found to be moderately retarded. This means that they can feed, dress, and prepare simple foods. People who are moderately retarded are usually capable of grooming themselves well, reading a few words and sentences, and carrying on a reasonable conversation. These people may also compete well in most games and sports, such as in the Special Olympics. They seem to have trouble with more complex tasks, like adding and subtracting, although making change for a dollar is typically within their capability. Moderately retarded individuals are often good candidates for sheltered workshops because they like the income, can attend to a task for fifteen to twenty minutes, and are often willing to assume responsibility

Educational Classification System

A third system of classification is based on the educability of retarded individuals and is, therefore, used frequently by schools to classify people for educational purposes. The term *educable* or EMR is roughly equivalent to mild retardation; *trainable* (TMR) refers to moderate retardation; and *custodial* refers to severe and profound retardation. The educational categories are based largely on observed behavior bolstered by scores from an individual intelligence test. Some states, such as California, have mandated that intelligence test scores may not be the only criterion used for placement because of their cultural bias. Others have argued against a behavioral criterion because of the potential for culture bias (Mercer, 1970), i.e., problem children are more likely to be a member of a minority group and are also more likely to be placed in a special education placement because of that behavior. The solution to the problem of cultural orientation and educational placement is not an easy one.

Some (Mercer & Lewis, 1978) have proposed that a battery of tests be used with each test normed or standardized on the particular group to be tested. Thus, there would be a special set of tests based on each cultural tradition, such as Mexican-Americans. The tests would differentiate between individuals *within* that cultural identity. Only those who performed poorly on the culture-specific tests would be assigned a special education placement. Unfortunately, there is no guarantee that the remaining individuals would do well in the regular classroom, because they do not always behave in ways consistent with the dominant culture. Mercer (1970) would argue that this is not a retardation issue but an educational one, that is, the problem is *not* that these children are *unable* to perform appropriately, but that they have *not* been *taught* to do so.

Another solution is to employ behavioral classification systems. Here the focus is on behavior rather than etiology. All that matters is what the individual can and cannot do; not whether the disorder is caused by Down syndrome or meningitis. There are some very good reasons, however, for wanting to know the causes of mental retardation and, therefore, when possible, for classifying retarded individuals according to the cause of their retardation.

Medical Classification System

A medical classification system is under development to allow classification according to biological bases of retardation. Such a classification facilitates research and encourages policy decisions to be made regarding efficient use of funds for further study and treatment. Thus far there are ten categories in this system.

Infection and Intoxication. This category encompasses a large set of maternal problems. Some infections of pregnancy which are common and have been identified as damaging to the unborn child are syphilis, rubella, and toxoplasmosis. Others, especially viruses, may affect the embryo without having noticeable or serious effects on the mother. One of these, cytomegalovirus, is a virus which only affects the salivary glands of the mother but causes the fetus to suffer a permanently destructive inflammation of the brain and surrounding tissue.

Maternal infections are believed to be a significant cause of mental retardation. About 80 percent of the residents of mental retardation facilities, who are known to be retarded because of infections, were subjected to maternal infections prenatally (Menolascino & Egger, 1978; Yannet, 1950). The maternal infection category is a conglomerate of a number of different kinds of disease. Rubella and cytomegalic inclusion disease are caused by viruses, syphilis is caused by bacteria, and toxoplasmosis is caused by a parasite. Many maternal infections do not cause mental retardation either because the infectious agent does not cross the placental barrier (viral hepatitis) or because it has no damaging effect on the fetal brain (e.g., malaria).

Infective agents work by damaging the brain at a critical time in its development. The severity of the damage depends on a number of factors. Among the most important of these are the health and nutritional status of the fetus and timing of infection in the course of fetal development.

The infection which we know most about is rubella (also known as German measles or three-day measles). Mental retardation is not the most frequent handicap resulting from maternal rubella; rubella is more likely to produce other abnormalities such as eye cataracts, deafness, and heart defects. Not all infants born to mothers who have had rubella during pregnancy are noticeably affected. About 15 to 20 percent of the infants whose mothers contracted the virus during the first trimester will exhibit some malformations. Retardation tends to occur when the infection appears between the sixteenth and twenty-fourth weeks of pregnancy (Menolascino & Egger, 1978). A disastrous epidemic in 1963–64 produced 50,000 stillbirths and abortions and 20,000 affected babies. Prevention is encouraged and implemented by vaccinating school-age children because they are the ones who are not immune and who transmit it to susceptible pregnant mothers.

Intoxication includes drugs and poisons, whether they are ingested by the mother or produced by her own body. Any agent which produces defects in the fetus before birth is called a *teratogen.* According to Menolascino and Egger (1978), there are many teratogenic agents. The most common drugs known to be teratogens are:

1. Endocrine substances, such as the sex hormones and those produced by the adrenal glands, and hypoglycemia drugs that lower the blood sugar, such as those used in the treatment of diabetes.
2. Specific drugs that interrupt the metabolism of a group of compounds in the body, such as antipurines, antipyrimidines, and antiglutamines.
3. Alkylating agents, or drugs that selectively destroy human cells, such as nitrogen mustard.
4. Antibiotics.
5. A miscellaneous group of drugs such as hallucinogens, azo dyes, and thalidomide.

Not all of these are suspected of causing mental retardation. Some, like thalidomide and streptomyicin, have very specific action sites, i.e., developing limbs and the auditory nerve, respectively.

Much depends on the timing of the drug intake, fitting the general rule "the earlier, the worse." During the first two weeks of pregnancy, the fetus is probably not vulnerable to teratogenic agents because the embryo has not been firmly implanted and established. However, from two to ten weeks of pregnancy, the fetus is particularly vulnerable to teratogens because its organs, such as brains, heart, liver, etc., are being formed. After three months, the fetus is susceptible in different ways, that is, either or both the rate and course of the growth and development of these organs may be affected. The central nervous system may be particularly susceptible during myelinization (from seven months of pregnancy to shortly after birth) when nerve fibers are being enclosed by a protective sheath. Any disruption of the myelinization process causes serious and long-lasting effects.

Not a great deal is known about the ability of specific drugs to cause defects in the fetus because of the difficulty in conducting well-designed research on humans. Further, it is not always possible to generalize research from animals to humans. A case in point is the catastrophe caused by the drug thalidomide, which was once sold as a tranquilizer. This drug caused defects in laboratory animals, but only when it was given in doses several times as large as the recommended human dosage, and only in certain strains of rabbits, mice, and rats. When taken by pregnant women, however, the recommended human dosage caused serious defects in the fetus.

The best data that we have on human beings are retrospective information, that is, information obtained from the mother after her defective baby is born. The problem with retrospectively gathered data is that the mothers may not remember accurately or may remember selectively. In fact, mothers of babies with defects are much more likely to remember drugs, illness, and emotions, during pregnancy, than mothers of normal babies (Menolascino & Egger, 1978). Ideal data would be obtained from prospective studies in which thousands of women would be followed prior to and during pregnancy. Careful records of all drugs and food consumed would be made and pregnancy outcomes would be related to these records. Such studies, as advantageous as they are, are rare because of the enormous expense and time involved.

Trauma or Physical Agent. Cases within this category involve brain injury due to trauma or physical agents. Included are prenatal injuries, such as radiation exposure during pregnancy; mechanical injuries at birth due to labor complications; prenatal, perinatal, and postnatal hypoxia resulting from a prolonged period of oxygen reduction; and postnatal injuries such as a fractured skull followed by a significant change in development (Grossman, 1983). This category is nonspecific in terms of both the timing and the agent involved. Trauma may occur prenatally, perinatally or postnatally and can be caused by a number of physical agents, such as radiation, oxygen deprivation, or forceps. Mental retardation is a result of permanent damage to some portion of the brain, irrespective of the particular external agent involved. Two agents commonly associated with prenatal injury are radiation and prenatal anoxia.

Prenatal exposure to *radiation* may result from a number of sources, including natural radiation, X-ray examinations and treatments, and fallout from atomic explosions. The amount of background or natural radiation varies in different locations. There is no evidence, however, that natural radiation causes mental retardation, even in areas in which large quantities of radiation are produced. For example, no increase in genetic damage has been reported in Travancore, India, where the natural radioactivity of the soil produces background ten times greater than average (Cooper & Cooper, 1966). Exposure to higher doses of radiation appears to have more serious consequences. Therapeutic and diagnostic exposure to radiation has been linked to mental retardation. However, very little can be said with absolute certainty because doses producing deformities in laboratory animals are generally higher than those used in typical X-ray examinations. Furthermore, women seeking medical attention early in pregnancy are often already experiencing complications that may cause developmental problems in their infants so it is difficult to disentangle the singular effect of the radiation (Menolascino & Egger). In any event, it is generally recommended that women avoid exposure to X-rays during pregnancy, particularly between two to six weeks after conception.

The therapeutic use of radiation in pregnant women, such as in the treatment of cancer, has been linked to serious developmental problems. Murphy (1929) was the first to show a relationship between radiation exposure during pregnancy and subsequent development problems. In this study, the effects on infants born to 625 pregnant women receiving therapeutic pelvic radiation was examined; 30 percent of these infants had some kind of malformation, most commonly, microcephaly. Jones and Neill (1944) also reported mental retardation in 20 percent of the infants whose mothers had undergone radiation treatment for pelvic cancer before the fifth month of fetal development. Treatment of pelvic cancer typically involves 150 rads daily for weeks. Because gene mutations may occur following exposure to only five rads (Neel, 1962), therapeutic abortions are often recommended to women repeatedly exposed to more than 10 rads. Limitation of head growth and mental retardations are the primary effects of radiation exposure (Miller, 1956). Overall, the amount of damage following exposure to any form of radiation depends on the dosage (rads) and the phase of development (with the most severe effects occurring before 15 weeks gestational age).

The most dramatic effects of radiation exposure during prenatal development were seen in the survivors of Nagasaki and Hiroshima. Approximately 50 percent of the children of women pregnant during the Nagasaki explosion died prenatally or as infants, and approximately 25 percent were subsequently classified as mentally retarded (Yamazaki, Wright, & Wright, 1954). Twenty percent of the surviving children of pregnant women who were within 2,000 meters of the center of the Hiroshima explosion had head circumferences significantly below average. Approximately half of these children were classified as mentally retarded, and most of these were between one and fifteen weeks gestational age at the time of exposure (Yamazaki, 1966).

No detectable genetic damage has been found in the first generation survivors of these explosions. There remains the possibility, however, that a mutation will affect a subsequent generation through a recessive trait. Gene changing effects of radiation have been demonstrated in fruit flies and mice, and this effect may hold true for humans as well (Menolascino & Egger, 1978).

The only treatment approach available to deal with the effects of prenatal exposure to radiation is prevention. It is typically recommended that pregnant women avoid X-rays, and consider therapeutic abortions if they have been exposed to massive amounts of radiation.

Prenatal anoxia, or oxygen deprivation, also produces defects in human and animal fetuses (Blattner, 1958; Ingalls, 1956; Menolascino & Egger, 1978). Oxygen deprivation causes serious problems perinatally and postnatally as well. Perinatal anoxia may be due to a number of factors, such as premature placental separation or knotted cords. The view that oxygen deprivation at birth causes permanent damage in human infants is controversial (Robinson & Robinson, 1976). There seems to be no doubt, however, that anoxia at birth *can* cause persistent damage in animals, depending on the length of deprivation. In one study (Sechzer, Faro, & Windle, 1973) signs of brain damage were observed in rhesus monkeys deprived of oxygen for up to seven minutes at birth. Temporary signs of brain damage were observed in monkeys deprived for eight to eleven and a half minutes. Monkeys deprived of oxygen for twelve to seventeen minutes manifested more extensive brain lesions and deficits which persisted over time.

The effects of perinatal anoxia on the cognitive development of children are not clear, but seem to relate to impaired cognitive functioning. In one study, preschoolers, who were full-term but hypoxic (deficient in oxygen reaching the tissues) at birth, performed significantly less well than preschoolers born with no complications on tests of cognitive and perceptual functioning (Graham, et al., 1963). More recent evidence suggests that anoxia alone does not necessarily result in mental retardation, but that the probability of mental retardation is increased twelve times in infancy and 6 times at age 7 over nonanoxia groups (Broman, 1979). Thus, newborns with clinical signs of anoxia are at risk for less than normal cognitive development. Furthermore, the risk for serious cognitive deficits or mental retardation are even greater when other signs indicative of central nervous system impairment are also present.

Mental retardation can be caused postnatally by anoxia or injury. Postnatal anoxia may result from severe anemia, shock, poisoning, convulsions and other conditions, such as atrophy, hemiatrophy and porencephaly. Postnatal injury may be caused by severe trauma, such as a fractured skull or prolonged unconsciousness. Mental retardation is attributed to the trauma if the event is followed by a marked change in development. The incidence of mental retardation due to all postnatal causes is small, however. Yannet (1950) estimated that 6 out of 1,729 residents in one training school were mentally retarded because of postnatal physical causes. Postnatal factors may play a more significant role among mildly retarded individuals who may not be institutionalized.

The three most common causes of head injury are automobile accidents, falls, and child abuse (Robinson & Robinson, 1976). Although relatively little is known about the effects of head injury, there is some evidence that the effects of trauma may be better compensated in younger children than in adults or older children, possibly because the organization of certain functions is more plastic at an early age (Teuber, 1970).

Overall, whether injury is caused prenatally, perinatally, or postnatally, the consequences of damage depend on the timing (e.g., two to six weeks gestation age), the severity (e.g., length of oxygen deprivation or severity of physical blow), the location of damage, and the extent of brain tissue involved.

The ambiguities within this category are due to a number of factors. For one thing, it is impossible to do the controlled research on humans necessary to answer the many questions raised. For example, we do not want to expose infants to radiation prenatally because of the possibility of producing effects, and yet, without systematic exposure of various gestational ages to various levels of radiation, it is impossible to make clear predictions. Another problem confusing diagnosis in this area is the fact that the causal agent is commonly inferred as such only when developmental problems emerge that cannot be otherwise explained.

Disorders of Metabolism or Nutrition. A large number of genetically determined chemical disorders may also cause mental retardation. Many have rather unfamiliar names: neuronal liped storage disease, ganglioside storage diseases, galactosemia, hypoglysemia, nucleotide disorders, Wilson's disease, ideopathic hypercalcemia, and so on. There are several hundred known varieties due to metabolic errors. They can be classified into four kinds of disorders: protein, carbohydrate, and lipid metabolism disorders and connective tissue disorders (Menolascino & Egger, 1978). A dramatic breakthrough in the prevention and cure of one such form of mental retardation occurred following a series of events which began in 1934.

A concerned Norwegian mother of two retarded children noted that both her children emitted an unpleasant, musty odor, especially in their urine. She went to several doctors with her observations and finally found one who was interested. Only five months later A. Følling, an Oslo physician, completed a paper describing ten retarded patients, who were found to excrete phenylpyruvic acid in their urine (Følling, 1934). Subsequently, the genetic mechanism for this disorder was identified by Jervis (1939, 1947) as an autosomal recessive disorder in which phenylalanine is accumulated as a result of an inability to oxidize it into tyrosine. This disorder became known as phenylketonuria (PKU).

The treatment of PKU is a special dietary regimen in which phenylalanine is almost eliminated. The diet is unpleasant to eat and difficult to accommodate; however, it prevents severe retardation if it is implemented while a child is very young. Although research has indicated that there is always some loss of intellectual ability (Berman & Ford, 1970), untreated children seldom develop any communication skills and many cannot be toilet trained. If not bedridden and completely helpless, untreated children typically have serious behavior disorders, ranging from shy, anxious, and restless behavior to extreme irritability with recurring destructive and noisy episodes. Identification of PKU has become simple and routine. An inexpensive screening test and follow-up evaluation have been developed (Guthrie & Susi, 1963) to identify victims soon after birth, enabling caretakers to implement preventive measures immediately (Menolascino & Egger, 1978; Robinson & Robinson, 1976).

The development of an appropriate treatment diet was plagued with difficulties. Occasionally, infants had high phenylalanine blood levels without having phenylketonuria. The restricted dietary regimen given to these infants was fatal (Robinson & Robinson, 1976). Furthermore, it was originally thought that treatment could be terminated when the major phases of brain growth were completed. Investigators have found, however, that school performance was significantly impaired, long after the brain was fully developed, when serum phenylalanine levels were allowed to rise above a certain level (20 mg/100ml) (Berry & Sutherland, cited by Berry et al., 1977). When girls who have been victims of PKU grow up and have children, those children have a very high incidence of mental retardation, congenital abnormalities, and episodes of psychotic behavior (U.S. Dept. of Health and Human Services, 1982).

The exact biochemical mechanism whereby PKU takes its toll is unknown. The primary damage is to the liver, causing it to produce a deficiency of phenylalanine hydroxylase enzyme (Robinson & Robinson, 1976). The lack of this enzyme results in the accumulation in the brain of phenylalanine, which in turn, is thought to interfere with amino acid transport. A dietary supplement of amino acids (valine, isoleucine and leucine) has been found to decrease brain phenylalanine levels, increase amino acid concentrations in the brain of animals, and reduce behavioral deficits in both animals and humans (Berry et al., 1977).

The incidence of PKU is quite low, occurring in only 1 in 8,000–10,000 live births. Fewer than 1 percent of residents of institutions are affected. Despite the rareness of the disease it has been extensively studied for several reasons:

1. It was the first inborn metabolic error identified as causing mental retardation. As such it was seen as the beginning of a series of such discoveries that would eventually whittle away at the problem of mental retardation.
2. It was seen as a possible model for the discovery, treatment, and detection of other metabolic errors.
3. Its treatability gave people, especially parents, hope that mental retardation could be prevented, if not cured.
4. The success story and the attention surrounding it were responsible for policy changes which concentrated on biomedical research on inborn errors of metabolism (Menolascino & Egger, 1978).

Gross Brain Disease. Several disorders, probably associated with dominant autosomal heredity mechanisms, produce malformations of the brain and skin. The two most prominent of these are tuberous sclerosis and neurofibromatosis.

The first, *tuberous sclerosis,* is a rare congenital disorder (1 per 150,000 births; Dawson, 1954) in which tumorous growths appear on organs of the body, especially the brain and skin. These growths produce seizures and retardation when they appear in the brain. The combination of skin tumors (sebaceous adenoma), mental retardation, and the seizures act as a set of symptoms which are predictve of tuberous sclerosis. Mental retardation does not always result from the disease but is quite likely because of the damage and blockage caused by the tumors. Lagos and Gomez (1967) reported a prevalence of mental retardation in 62 percent of tuberous sclerosis (out of 71) patients.

Developmentally, the seizures usually appear between twelve and eighteen months, followed by skin lesions which appear between two and six years (sometimes in adolescence). The mental retardation will appear even later, if at all. This gradual onset of symptoms, combined with the delay between onsets, make diagnosis difficult. There is no cure for tuberous sclerosis, although genetic counseling is recommended if cases have appeared previously in a family. Seizure control is important to prevent oxygen deprivation to the brain, a possible cause of some mental retardation. There is no treatment for the skin lesions (Menolascino & Egger, 1978).

Neurofibromatosis is similar to tuberous sclerosis in that it is probably inherited and appears as multiple benign fibrous tumors in the brain and skin. The types of lesions and tumors and the frequency of seizures and mental retardation differ, however. The disorder is also known as von Recklinghausen disease and was featured in a recent novel and movie, *The Elephant Man*. Its estimated prevalence is 1 in 2,000 in the general population and approximately 8.5 percent of the mentally retarded suffer from neurofibromatosis. Among the victims of neurofibromatosis, about 50 percent will prove to be retarded. The mental retardation is probably caused by pressure from intracranial tumors or faulty brain development. The tumors vary in composition—connective tissues of thin fibrous bands (neurofibromas)—and can develop anywhere, but seem to have an affinity for neural tissue. The onset of neurofibramatosis can occur from birth to age fifty; the presence of six or more cafe-au-lait or brown pigmented spots on an individual is considered definitive by some diagnosticians (Menolascino & Egger, 1978).

There is no known cure for neurofibromatosis. Tumors that create pressure on important structures or that are horribly disfiguring or that become malignant may be surgically removed.

Unknown Prenatal Causes. Conditions for which no definite etiological cause can be determined, but which exist at or prior to birth, make up the fifth category. Anencephaly, Cornelia de Lange syndrome, microcephaly and hydrocephaly are only a few of the syndromes known to exist at birth and yet have no definite etiology.

Anencephaly is a type of cerebral malformation in which a portion of the brain and skull are absent, due to a defect in the closure of the neural tube. The overall incidence of anencephaly is between .5 and 4.0 per 1,000 births and is four times more prevalent in females than in males. There is also a 10-percent risk of recurrence, i.e., of having a second child with a neural tube closure defect following the birth of an anencephalic infant. Interestingly, although there is no known etiology, there is a definite seasonal variation, with a peak in the winter months (Menolascino & Egger, 1978).

Clinically, anencephalic children are often missing skull bones on the top, sides, or front of their heads and generally have grotesque facial features. Because of the severity of this condition, these children rarely live longer than a week. Although there is no cure, genetic counseling may decrease the recurrence of the birth of an anencephalic child.

Cornelia de Lange syndrome and microcephaly are two craniofacial anomalies of unknown etiology. Infants born with Cornelia de Lange syndrome are generally less than 5½ pounds at birth and remain physically retarded. They typically have an abnormal growth of hair on their eyebrows and eyelashes, forehead, upper lip, back and forearms. Their heads are often small and short and they may have deformed limbs and hands with webbed fingers. These children are often hyperactive, destructive, and self-mutilating, and typically fall within the severe range of mental retardation.

Although the etiology of Cornelia de Lange syndrome is unknown, there is some indication that it may be a genetic trait and may therefore warrant genetic counseling (Franklin, 1971). The syndrome is found in numerous ethnic and racial groups and does not appear to be correlated with parental age, consanguinity, birth order, sex, or abnormalities of pregnancy or delivery. The incidence is basically unknown, although it is estimated to be fewer than 1 per 10,000 births (McArthur & Edwards, 1967; Schuster & Johnson, 1966).

Microcephaly is another type of craniofacial anomaly, also with no known etiology. It is characterized by an abnormally small head, and often exists in conjunction with another syndrome, such as Down syndrome. However microcephaly is only classified within the category of unknown prenatal causes when it exists as an isolated syndrome. Microcephaly may also be primary or secondary. Primary microcephaly is due to genetic causes, and may be hereditary or the result of mutations as in Down syndrome. Secondary microcephaly is not related to genetics but is caused by prenatal irradiation, infection, oxygen deprivation, or unknown factors (Menolascino & Egger, 1978). In theory, only cases in which primary microcephaly is diagnosed, but where the condition does not exist as part of a larger syndrome, are classified within this category. It is often difficult, however, to separate primary microcephaly from other forms (Warkany & Dignan, 1973).

In appearance, the base of the skull of primary microcephalics is typically of normal size. The head gradually gets smaller toward the top, and the forehead is narrow and slants back. The top of the head, or the cranium, is typically very small. In contrast, the only consistent characteristic of nongenetic microcephalics is a small head.

It is often reported that microcephalics who are mentally retarded range from the moderate to severe range of mental retardation (Menolascino & Egger, 1978). Other authors, however, have reported that mental levels vary from mild to profound (Penrose, 1963; Tredgold, 1956), and still others assert that most microcephalics manifest severe mental retardation and often never walk or talk (Lawrence & Weeks, 1971). Prognosis depends on etiology, treatment, and associated handicaps. Many microcephalics survive adulthood, although the childhood mortality rate is fairly high.

There is some disagreement as to the appropriate diagnosis for microcephaly and no single criterion has been accepted. It has been suggested that head circumference of less than 13 inches at six months or less than 18 inches at adulthood indicates microcephaly (Menolascino & Egger, 1978). Böök, Schut, and Reed (1953) recommended that head circumference should be at least three standard deviations below the age mean for appropriate diagnosis, although other authors have reported using two standard deviations as a cutoff point (Warkany & Dignan, 1973).

True microcephaly is a relatively rare condition; only about 15 per 10,000 births (Böök et al., 1953; Kock, 1959). Furthermore, because many microcephalic children die young, the prevalence is estimated to be between 1 in 25,000 and 1 in 50,000. Microcephaly is also relatively rare in comparison with other conditions associated with mental retardation, constituting between .5 and 2 percent of the institutional population (Böök, Schut & Reed, 1953; Penrose, 1956).

No treatment is available for microcephaly. At one time, surgery was performed to expand the skull; however, because microcephaly is primarily a failure of brain growth rather than skull growth, surgery is no longer done (Menolascino & Egger, 1978).

Hydrocephalus is a fourth condition existing at or prior to birth in which there is no known etiology. It is defined as an abnormal accumulation of cereberospinal fluid in the brain cavities due to an overproduction or an underabsorption of fluid. This results in the compression of the brain and the enlargement of the upper part of the head. The overall incidence of hydrocephaly is probably between 1 and 3 per 1,000 births (Menolascino & Egger, 1978; Robinson & Robinson, 1976). In addition to a large head, early signs of hydrocephaly include a failure to progress, irritability, and loss of interest in surroundings (Lawrence & Weeks, 1971). Motor development is often impaired. Mental functioning sometimes remains good, but mental retardation is not unusual and exists in varying degrees.

Lawrence and Coates (1962) estimated that fewer than half the children born with hydrocephaly survive, and of these children 14 percent are physically and mentally within normal limits, 30 percent are within the mild range of mental retardation, and 56 percent are at least moderately retarded. These statistics may be somewhat better today, however, because in some cases it is possible to drain the excess cerebrospinal fluid by means of a shunt (a shunt involves a plastic tube which runs from the brain into another part of the body, such as the abdominal cavity). Although this treatment has reached a fairly high degree of sophistication, complications still occur, such as infections, clogging valves or hardening tubes (Kirman, 1973). Prognosis for children with hydrocephalus depends on the extent of involvement, age of onset, other damage and the mode of management (Menolascino & Egger, 1978).

Altogether, there are over twenty syndromes classified within the category of unknown prenatal causes. Of these, the four mentioned are the most common, though all are extremely rare. Very few anencephalic infants survive, and Cornelia de Lange syndrome and microcephaly occur in fewer than 1.6 per 10,000 live births. Hydrocephalus is the most common condition within this category but it too is rare. Nevertheless, this category is important. For one thing, all these conditions are quite dramatic and involve clear-cut and severe instances of brain damage. For another, the causes of these conditions are all unknown and are present prenatally. Finally, as with most conditions associated with mental retardation, there are no cures once the damage has occurred.

Chromosomal Abnormalities. A sixth category includes syndromes associated with chromosomal or genetic abnormalities. These conditions may involve numerical (e.g., too many or too few chromosomes) or structural (e.g., part of one chromosome attaching to another chromosome) aberrations in the chromosome, or both. Causes of chromosomal abnormalities are many, and include gene mutation, radiation, drugs, viruses, aged gametes, existing aberrations, and a group of conditions involving thermal, temporal, geographic and economic factors (Grossman, 1983).

There are at least nine syndromes included within this category but only six will be discussed. These include Cri-du-chat (cat-cry) syndrome, several types of

Down syndrome, Klinefelter syndrome, and Turner syndrome.

Cri-du-chat syndrome is an extremely rare form of mental retardation caused by a structural aberration in the form of a part of chromosome 5. It was first described by Lejeune and his colleagues in 1963 (Lejeune et al., 1963) and only twenty-four cases had been discovered by 1978 (Menolascino & Egger, 1978). Prevalence estimates vary from 1 in 50,000 to 1 in 100,000; 2/3 of the cases reported are female (Norman, 1971).

Cri-du-chat syndrome is characterized by a high-pitched cat-like cry immediately after birth and during infancy. Other symptoms include microencephaly, epicanthalfold and downward slant of the eyes, a wide-spread nose, abnormal surface markings of the skin, poor growth, and severe mental retardation. Diagnosis is based on chromosomal studies showing that part of chromosome 5 is missing. Furthermore, although it is difficult to determine because so few cases have been noted, the extent of abnormality may be correlated with the extent of deletion of chromosome 5 (Norman, 1971).

Down syndrome was first noted by John Langdon Down, a British physician, in 1866. He advanced a racial hypothesis, in which he suggested that this type of mental retardation was due to a resurgence of Mongolian traits. This hypothesis was based solely on the physical resemblance between persons with Down syndrome and persons of the Mongolian race, and is no longer accepted (Gibson, 1978). In 1959, Lejeune and Turpin discovered that the cells of many individuals with Down syndrome have forty-seven rather than the normal forty-six chromosomes (Menolascino & Egger, 1978).

Down syndrome is characterized by numerous physical symptoms, of which the most commonly cited are: large fissured tongue; short squared hands; epicanthal fold at the inner corner of the eye; single transverse crease across the flabby hands; short and inward curving little fingers, with one lateral crease; nose with flattened bridge and upturned nostrils; fused ear lobes; deep cleft between big toe and second toe; small, flattened skull; smooth simple cluster ear lobe; congenital heart problems (occurring in about 25 percent of the Down population); coarse, dry skin; delayed eruption of teeth; sparse, fine, straight hair; short stature; low-pitched voice; and chronic myelogenic leukemia (a condition that is rare, but more frequent in Down syndrome than in the normal population) (Gibson, 1978; Gibson & Frank, 1961).

In addition to the physical stigmata, there are certain physiological problems associated with Down syndrome involving circulatory, sensory, neurological, and structural limitations. Down babies have twice the premature rate of normal babies, and 50 percent of all Down syndrome pregnancies involve labor and delivery complications. There is a high frequency of hypotonia, hearing loss, and EEG abnormalities associated with Down syndrome. Hypotonia, or poor muscle tone, is very common in Down babies and probably interferes with psychomotor development. It decreases with age, but is generally present until approximately twenty months of age. Although EEG abnormalities are commonly associated with Down syndrome, there are fewer convulsive disorders in this population than among the general mental retardation population.

The Moro reflex tends to be absent in Down infants and other reflexes are often prolonged. With development, there are progressive circulatory, central nervous system, and peripheral nervous system pathologies. Vascular systems' defects occur in approximately one-fourth of the Down population and are often progressive. Persons with Down syndrome also often have certain structural pons and medulla abnormalities (Gibson, 1978). It is important to emphasize that all these problems and pathologies are not present in all Down syndrome individuals, contributing to the enormous amount of variability within the syndrome.

There are three types of Down syndrome, all of which involve a chromosomal aberration in which there is extra chromosomal material present. *Standard trisomy 21* is the most common type of Down syndrome. In this type there are three instead of two chromosomes in position 21 due to a nondisjunction during meiotic division (division of gametes or reproductive cells). Trisomy 21 is not inherited and its occurrence increases with an increase in maternal age, particularly in women over thirty-five. There is also an increased frequency in very young mothers. The risk of having a child with Down syndrome is also increased after the birth of one Down syndrome child, regardless of maternal age.

The second most common type of Down syndrome is *13-15 translocation,* in which a 21st chromosome attaches to pair 13 or 15. With this type there are only 46 chromosomes, but there is extra chromosomal material present. Translocation Down syndrome occurs in mothers of all ages, and 2–3 percent of translocation cases are inherited. Genetic counseling may be appropriate when translocation 13-15 has been identified with prior births.

The least common type of Down syndrome is *mosaicism,* caused by a nondisjunction or failure of a chromosome to divide during mitotic division (normal cell division). This results in an extra chromosome in some cells, but not in others. The proportion of cells affected varies among individuals. That is, one mosaic individual may have 50 percent of his or her cells affected whereas another may have 80 percent affected. This type of Down syndrome is extremely rare, is not related to maternal or paternal age, and is not inheritable (Menolascino & Egger, 1978).

Unfortunately, the specific factors inhibiting cell division are unknown. One hypothesis for trisomy 21 is the eggs of very young women are not fully mature, whereas in older women the eggs are older and are perhaps damaged, increasing the likelihood of a chromosomal aberration. Another hypothesis does not explain errors in cell division but attributes the problem to a failure of the abortive mechanism in older women.

Several studies have looked at the relationship between the three Down syndrome karyotypes (trisomy 21, translocation 13-15, and mosaicism) and various behavior and physical characteristics of Down syndrome. There have been some karyotypic differences found in the overall level of intelligence. Down syndrome individuals with the mosaic karyotype have higher IQs than other syndrome types (Gibson, 1973; Rosecrans, 1968). Overall, there also appears to be a four- to eight-point IQ advantage favoring the translocation karyotype over trisomy 21 (Gibson, 1973). However, this observation may not be directly due to the difference in karyotype because individuals with 13-15 translocation have a higher incidence of heart problems than individuals with trisomy 21 (Gibson, 1978). Hence, these two groups suffer from a differential morality rate which may selectively affect translocation individuals with a lower IQ.

It has been suggested that intelligence varies with the percentage of mosaic (aberrant) cells in individuals with mosaic karyotypes (Zellweger & Abbo, 1963). Research on mosaic individuals is difficult because this karyotype is extremely rare; however Shipe, et al. (1968) combined twenty-one cases of mosaicism reported in the literature and found that individuals with over 50 percent normal cells had a mean IQ of 57, whereas individuals with less than 50 percent had a mean IQ of 35.

Intellectual development and physical growth are both extremely variable within the syndrome. For example, Engler (1949) places the mean age of onset of walking at three years, with a range from ten and a half months to ten years, and the mean age of onset of talking at three and a half years with a range from fifteen months to fourteen years. Similarly, intellectual ability ranges from the severe-profound range to near normal. According to Gibson (1978), variability is due to many factors, including karyotype; secondary organic processes, such as hypotonia; stimulation level; environment; health; sex; structural features of the syndrome; and age. He asserts that the majority of Down syndrome persons fall within the trainable mentally retarded range, a large minority within the custodial range, and a small minority within the EMR range. Furthermore, he states that Down syndrome adults are never within the normal range because they are unable to make abstractions.

There is no cure for Down syndrome, though there is prevention through genetic counseling, amniocentesis, and abortion of positively identified fetuses.

Klinefelter syndrome, like Down syndrome, involves an extra chromosome. In Klinefelter syndrome, however, the abnormality is present only in males and involves an extra female sex chromosome (Baroff, 1974), an XXY constitution, rather than an XY constitution as in normal males. It is not known why the failure in meiotic division occurs, but it may be due to maternal age. It is also correlated to paternal age (Norman, 1971).

The incidence of Klinefelter syndrome is relatively rare, occurring in approximately 1 in 400 live male births (Moore, 1959). Although the majority of persons with Klinefelter syndrome have IQs greater than 50, subnormal IQs have been reported in 25–50 percent of these individuals, and constitute 1–2 percent of the mentally retarded population (Thompson & Thompson, 1966).

Other clinical features include a tall, nonmasculine appearance, decreased secondary sexual characteristics, and high-pitched voice; these become apparent in adolescence. Diagnosis is not usually made until puberty, and requires a chromosome study. Treatment has been done successfully by administering the male hormone, testosterone (Menolascino & Egger, 1978).

Turner syndrome also involves an abnormality in the number of sex chromosomes, but in this case, there is an absence of an X chromosome in girls, making a total 45 chromosomes; this is represented as XO. The syndrome may result from a loss of the second sex chromosome at the first meiotic division in either parent (Robinson & Robinson, 1977). The cause of this loss is unknown and, in this syndrome, does not appear to be related to parental age (Thompson & Thompson, 1966).

The incidence of Turner syndrome is extremely low, occurring in approximately 1 in 2,500 live births (Norman, 1971). Although it is more common at conception, 95–98 percent of the XO fetuses fail to survive to birth (Hetch & MacFarland, 1969).

While mental retardation is not frequently associated with Turner syndrome, it is found more frequently in Turner syndrome than in the normal population, and may result in mild or moderate mental retardation. Other clinical features include a short, stocky build; mature face; webbed neck; low-set ears; low, back-hairline; small jaw; and heart and kidney abnormalities. As in Klinefelter syndrome, this syndrome is usually not identified until puberty, when there is a failure to develop secondary sexual characteristics. Diagnosis requires a chromosomal study, and estrogen replacement therapy is used (Menolascino & Egger, 1978).

Gestational Disorders. Mental retardation may be associated with gestational disorders in which prenatal development was somehow impaired or problematic. Gestational disorders include prematurity, small-for-date or low birth weight babies, and postmaturity. None of these conditions cause mental retardation, though all have been associated with cognitive or learning problems (Parmalee & Schulte, 1970).

There is little consensus concerning the subtle consequences of *prematurity*, defined as delivery before thirty-seven weeks gestational age. Prematurity seems related to the mother's short stature, heavy smoking, presence of certain pathological states, and poor nutrition (Niswander & Gordon, 1972). It may also be related to multiple births and complications at birth, such as toxemia, premature rupture of membranes, early detachment of placenta, and abnormal position of the fetus. Gestational problems are more common in blacks than in whites and in women under 20 years of age, and are twice as likely in low socioeconomic groups than in middle or upper socioeconomic groups (Menolascino & Egger, 1978).

Incidence figures vary considerably in different parts of the world. The percentage of premature live births has been estimated to be 5–7 percent in Sweden, 7–8 percent in the United States, 30 percent in Calcutta, India, and less than 4 percent in Holland (Menolascino & Egger, 1978).

The relationship of gestational problems to mental retardation is extemely complicated. One reason for the complexity is that the definitions of both gestational problems and mental retardation are not clear or consistent from one study to another. Many studies confound socioeconomic status and race with gestational problems, and other controls are often absent or inadequate. Prematurity is also often associated with cerebral palsy. In fact, over 30 percent of patients with cerebral palsy were premature, indicating that prematurity can be associated with both neurological damage and mental retardation. (Menolascino & Egger, 1978). Most studies of other problems, such as intraventricular hemorrhage and respiratory distress syndrome, have shown minimal deficits continuing into middle childhood, evidenced in poor school performance and deficits in performance IQ (Caputo, Goldstein & Taub, 1979; Corrigan et al., 1967; Frances-Williams & Davies, 1974). Thus, although the "catch up" may not be complete, mental retardation is clearly not an inevitable consequence, particularly when prematurity occurs without other complications.

Small-for-date or low birth weight infants are a second group of infants with gestational disorders and at risk for mental retardation. These infants weigh less than 5½ pounds at birth and are delivered at or later than thirty-seven weeks gestational age (Korones, 1976). There are three general etiological factors that can potentially cause fetal growth retardation, resulting in small-for-date infants. First, the mother's general health and health-related problems have been related to fetal growth retardation. Moderate smokers are twice as likely to have such an infant and heavy smokers are three times as likely. Forty percent of the infants born to heroin addicts are small for date. A second source of complications comes from the fetus. Infants born among multiple gestations, such as twins, or triplets, are more likely to be small for date. Similarly, infants born with congenital malformations and chromosomal abnormalities are more likely to be small for date. The third factor causing fetal growth retardation is the placenta, in which, for some medical reason, there is inadequate nutritional and waste exchange between the mother and fetus (Vorherr, 1975).

Low birth weight has also been correlated with impaired school progress and performance measures of mental development, language development, school readiness, and academic achievement from preschool through elementary school. By elementary school, small-for-date babies are more often in special education classes than children who were premature at birth but had appropriate weight for gestational age (Rubin, Rosenblatt, & Balow, 1973). This assertion may be misleading, however, because small-for-date babies also are more likely to have had complications during labor, and are more often born with congenital anomalies. Furthermore, these infants are born to mothers of low socioeconomic status more often than are premature babies, and SES alone is associated with lower mental and performance expectations. Because of all these confounding factors it is unclear whether low birth weight alone is more or less related to developmental problems than prematurity (Menolascino & Egger, 1978).

The third form of gestational disorder often associated with mental retardation is *postmaturity*, defined by Grossman (1983) as a pregnancy lasting seven days past the scheduled birth date. Errors often occur, however, because of the difficulty in exactly specifying length of gestation. Many researchers and obstetricians do not consider an infant postmature until it is at least two weeks overdue (or forty-two weeks gestational age).

While incidence estimates vary from 3.5 to 10.6 percent of all pregnancies, these may be overestimations because of calculation errors. There do not appear to be geographic or ethnic factors related to postmaturity, but the probability of postmaturity is increased in women over thirty-five who are experiencing their first pregnancy.

The literature on mental retardation as a complication of postmaturity is virtually nonexistent. Very few studies have examined the mental development of postmature infants. Many postmaturely born infants appear prematurely aged, looking wrinkled, dry, soft, and puffy. One of the few studies reported that high birth weight and prolonged gestation did not appear to be related to an increased risk of mental retardation (Barker, 1966). Further research is needed to clarify the relationship, if any, between all these gestational disorders, prematurity, small for date, and high birth weight, and mental retardation.

Following Psychiatric Disorder. There is considerable controversy over whether mental retardation can be caused by psychiatric disorders. Furthermore, whenever mental retardation and psychiatric disorders are both diagnosed, it is unclear which one should be categorized as primary. The importance of the primary diagnosis is evident when practical decisions are to be made about a child. The kind of facility to which the child is referred, the type of treatment recommended, and the outcome of the treatment may differ depending on whether the child is characterized as mentally retarded or mentally ill. Despite the importance of these considerations, many feel that accurate differential diagnosis is impossible (Bialer, 1970; Milgram, 1972).

In DSM-III it does not matter whether mental retardation or psychiatric problems are primary; the goal is to detemine the depth and nature of both problems in order to address each as well as the interaction between the two. Furthermore, it must be recognized that mental retardation may be a symptom and not a syndrome. Therefore, if a child is "acting" mentally retarded, i.e., is showing significantly subaverage IQ and adaptive behavior, he or she is classified as mentally retarded.

In cases of psychosis or autism, children are extremely withdrawn and do not interact with the environment or other people. As a result, they do not learn behavioral and cognitive skills necessary to facilitate the development of their intellectual abilities. In these cases, emotional factors may be said to produce decrements in intellectual development, e.g., children with mild mental retardation may be considered of borderline or average ability, except for their behavior due to emotional or psychiatric problems.

This category is an essential one, in that a small percentage of mental retardation is both associated with a psychiatric disorder and has no other etiological features. Nevertheless, it is extremely difficult, if not impossible, to determine which disorder is causing which.

Environmental Influences. When there is no evidence of significant organic disease or pathology, but there is evidence of adverse environmental conditions, an individual's retardation may be attributed to environmental influences. There are thought to be two mechanisms whereby environmental influences may lead to mental retardation. These two mechanisms or types of environmental influences are: pyschosocial disadvantage and sensory deprivation. Sensory deprivation involves handicapping conditions, such as blindness and deafness, which can significantly delay development. Unless these conditions are compounded with other factors, such as brain damage or other forms of environmental deprivations, they are unlikely to result in mental retardation. Psychosocial disadvantage is, by far, the more common environmental cause of mental retardation.

Psychosocial Disadvantage. There is a consistent and reliable relationship between socioeconomic status and intelligence (Jensen, 1973) in every modern industrial society where these two factors have been studied. Obviously, not all poor people are retarded; in fact, very few of them are. Nevertheless, poor people are four times more likely to be retarded, and retarded people are more likely to be among the poor. There are actually several theories as to why there is such a reliable relationship between socioeconomic status (SES) and intelligence. One is implied in the categorization "mental retardation which is attributed to psychosocial disadvantge." This category points to the environment as the cause of the retardation.

Indeed, there is ample reason to believe that environmental factors associated with being poor could significantly influence one's IQ score. Birch and Gussow (1970) present an eloquent description of the hardship suffered by the poor:

> The environments in which disadvantaged children develop from conception are far less supportive to growth and health than are those of children who are not disadvantaged, and this relative environmental impoverishment is exaggerated when the disadvantaged child is non-white. The differences are profound and prolonged. Mothers of such children tend to be

less well fed, less well grown, and less well cared for before they reach childbearing age. When they reach it, they begin to bear children younger, more rapidly, and more often, and they continue to bear them to an older age. When such a mother is pregnant both her nutrition and her health will tend to be poorer than that of a woman who is better off, but she will be far less likely to get prenatal care and far more likely to be delivered under substandard conditions.

Children of such mothers are smaller at birth, die more readily, and are generally in poorer condition in infancy than are children born to the more affluent. If they survive the first month of life, their mortality thereafter is excessively high and their illnesses more frequent, more persistent, and more severe. Their early nutrition is negatively influenced by their mother's health, her age, her income level, her education, her habits and attitudes, so that among such children in the preschool years frank malnutrition, as well as subclinical manifestations of depressed nutritional status (reflected in anemia and poor growth), are markedly more prevalent. During the school years they eat irregularly, their health care continues to be almost totally inadequate, their housing is substandard, their family income is low, subsistence on public assistance is high, and family disorganization is commonplace.

In spite of these conditions, not all poor children end up retarded, a fact that provides meat for the genetic theories of intelligence—especially polygenic models (Jensen, 1970). The polygenic theory claims that many genes contribute to intelligence (thus the name "polygenic"). Furthermore, the particular combinations of genes resulting in low intelligence are simply the low end of the normally distributed, polygenetically determined trait of intelligence. Conversely, the particular combination of genes resulting in extremely high intelligence represents the high end of the normally distributed, polygenetically determined trait of intelligence.

Possible genetic contributions to mental retardation are implicitly included within the psychosocial disadvantage classification (sometimes called familial or garden variety retardation) because of its specification that at least one parent or one or more siblings must show evidence of subnormal intelligence functioning. This category also requires that the retardation is not attributable to disease or defect.

Any classification that is defined by the absence of something, in this case, the absence of "significant organic disease or pathology" may have limited usefulness. Only about 20 percent of the residents of a retardation center have identifiable pathology, but this is dependent on our knowing what to look for. It is probable that the category of psychosocial disadvantage will diminish once we are better at identifying and detecting various organic bases of mental retardation.

Case Illustration: Brian was born into an unusual family. Both his parents were deinstitutionalized just three years before he was born. His mother had an IQ of about 45; his father had an IQ of 72; and Brian's siblings were all retarded. If this were not enough, Brian had heart problems, cerebral palsy, seizures that were controlled by phenobarbital, and a hernia. His family was completely dependent on public assistance and home conditions were chaotic. A social worker witnessed a mealtime in which the parents yelled continuously at the children and each other and food was thrown and spilled all over the house.

Brian, at two years old, was eight months retarded. Though he would probably be classified as psychosocially disadvantaged, it is very difficult to specify an exact cause for his retardation. Clearly his environment was a factor, but his history of medical problems and the genetic implications make almost any single factor diagnosis questionable.

Intervention

In order to get a comprehensive picture of intervention approaches we will trace the efforts to prevent retardation or, at least, to reduce its impact. In the first place, there have been many attempts to reduce the incidence of mental retardation by providing better pre- , peri- , and postnatal care to pregnant mothers and their children. The War on Poverty, which began in the 1960s under Presidents Kennedy and Johnson, contained several programs aimed at improving the general health of poorer people, namely the Family Planning Services and Neighborhood Health Centers. Although their positive impact has not been substantiated, the centers have been used extensively by poor residents.

Once a child is born with a high risk of retardation, a number of steps may be taken. One type of intervention may be focused on the parents. Parents may be counseled to help their adjustment to having a handicapped infant and they may be trained to stimulate their infant. The latter approach, stimulation, is based on the assumption that a potentially handicapped infant needs more stimulation than a normal infant in order to develop at an optimal rate—more physical exercise, more cognitive challenge, and more social contact.

A child-focused intervention works primarily with the child, largely bypassing the parents under the assumption that most parents are not qualified to (or do not have the time or do not have the interest in) giving their infants the extra stimulation that they are believed to need. Such child-focused intervention programs are usually educational day care centers where infants and toddlers receive very structured, intensive attention by a cadre of physical therapists, teachers, speech therapists, occupational therapists, public health nurses and interested aides and volunteers.

Some intervention programs involve both parents and children. While most of the special intervention programs are available mainly in large urban areas, rural consortiums have recently evolved to make them available to parents and children in less populated areas. Again, a government agency, formerly Bureau for the Education of the Handicapped, and now Special Education Programs, is largely responsible for the existence of these infant/toddler intervention programs.

Have these programs been successful in preventing or ameliorating mental retardation? The verdict is not yet in. Some findings are positive ("Efficacy studies in early childhood special education," 1981; Simeonsson, Cooper, & Scheiner, 1982); others are more qualified (Dunst & Rheingrover, 1981). It may be the case that mixed findings are valid. Some children may benefit while others may not. Whether a child benefits from intervention may be due to the nature of the disorder or the type and quality of intervention or both. The diversity of causes and severity of mental retardation makes it almost impossible to do a conclusive study of the efficacy of early intervention. There are seldom enough children in any diagnostic category, except Down syndrome, to have a reasonable group size. The ethics of research make it almost impossible to withhold services from a group of children so that there may be a control group with whom to compare a treatment group. The barriers to conducting a definitive study on the effects of early intervention are, therefore, preventing conclusions on which sound policy can be based.

Institutionalization is an option that is being used less and less by parents as a solution to the problems brought on by the birth of a handicapped baby. This change is being encouraged by a number of interrelated factors: (a) the realization that most institutions are not always very humane places for infants, (b) a movement toward community alternatives, (c) the concepts of "normalizations" and "least restrictive alternative" as determining policy, (d) growing beliefs in the ability of families to be effective in increasing their child's capabilities, (e) a general belief in the power of the environment to overcome or offset the disadvantages of handicapping conditions.

In 1973 and 1975 two legislative acts were enacted which had an enormous impact on what happens to retarded children. The Rehabilitation Act of 1973, Sec. 504, and the Education of All Handicapped Children Act (PL 94-142) provide for free public education and freedom from exclusion for all handicapped children (Turnbull & Turnbull, 1978). As a result, school systems all over the country have accommodated, sometimes reluctantly, to an influx of handicapped children who otherwise would not have had educational services. Section 504 regulations specify further that the schools must place handicapped children in the least restrictive environment. This stipulation has led to a number of organizational maneuvers on the part of schools to mainstream and integrate handicapped children. Thus, handicapped children, depending on their degree of handicap and the propensities of their school system, may find themselves in a special school housing only special children; in separate classrooms in regular schools; in regular classrooms in regular schools with supplementary help in designated areas such as speech therapy and reading; or in regular classrooms in regular schools with no extra help.

The major research question in all this has been the efficacy of mainstreaming retarded children and integrating them into regular classrooms. On this issue the data are mixed. In the first place, there are at least two parts to the question. Do we mean socially or academically? Are there differential effects for different levels of ability? Overall the answer to this complicated question is a qualified "yes"; some children (especially mentally retarded) are better off having more educational contact with nonhandicapped children. This is true on two types of dependent variables, achievement and social/personality (Carlberg & Kavale, 1980).

Most schools are mandated to educate handicapped children until they are eighteen or twenty-one years old. Following graduation, there are several options available to an individual. Depending on the individual's capability and the parents' tolerance and ability, a retarded person may live at home, a large institution, a nursing home, a group home, or semi-independently in an apartment. Some day care–vocational training programs are available for retarded adults, especially in larger urban areas. These vary in quality but are becoming more uniform because of government regulation.

Day care programs typically teach self-help skills and provide social-recreational opportunities. Behavioral research has focused on better ways of training self-help like grooming and toileting [see Chapter 8], and ways of eliminating undesirable behaviors, such as rocking [see Chapter 6] and masturbating in public [see Chapter

12]. Ecologically oriented research has been concerned with the effects of deinstitutionalization, what happens when living environments are changed, the improvement of staff morale and performance in facilities for the retarded, friendship patterns among retarded individuals, and the development of valid, comprehensive, nondiscriminatory adaptive behavior scales.

Because of medical advances and humane concern, more retarded children are surviving for longer periods than ever before. Moreover, the quality of their lives has improved as resources and skills have been directed at helping these children live as independently and satisfying lives as possible.

In this chapter we have considered a number of issues in mental retardation, not the least of which were how it is defined and diagnosed and whether it should be a psychiatric disorder. Although we have presented many esoteric forms of retardation, it should be emphasized that the largest category of retarded children, about 75 percent have no identified organic basis for their subaverage intellectual functioning and that they may be no more psychiatric problems because of their intelligence than are children with above average intellectual functioning.

REFERENCES

Barker, D. J. P. Low intelligence: Its relation to length of gestation and rate of fetal growth. *British Journal of Preventive and Social Medicine.* 1966, *20,* 58–66.

Baroff, G. S. *Mental retardation: Nature, cause, and management.* New York: Wiley, 1964.

Baumeister, A. A. The American residential institution: Its history and character. In A. Baumeister & E. Butterfield (Eds.), *Residential facilities for the mentally retarded.* Chicago: Aldine, 1970.

Baumeister, A. A., & Muma, J. R. On defining mental retardation. *Journal of Special Education,* 1975, 9(3), 293–306.

Bayley, N. *Bayley Scales of Infant Development.* New York: Psychological Corporation, 1969.

Bennett, F. C., Robinson, N. M., & Sells, C. S. Growth and development of infants weighing less than 800 grams at birth. *Pediatrics,* 1983, *71*(3), 319–323.

Berman, J. L., & Ford, R. Intelligence quotients and intelligence loss in patients with phenylketonuria and some variant states. *Journal of Pediatrics,* 1970, *77,* 764–770.

Berry, H. K., Butcher, R. E., Brunner, R. L., Bray, N. W., Hunt, M. M., & Wharton, C. H. New approaches to treatment of phenylketonuria. In P. Mittler (Ed.), *Research to practice in mental retardation, biomedical aspects* (Vol. 3). Baltimore: University Park, 1977.

Bialer, I. Emotional disturbance and mental retardation: Etiologic and conceptual relationships. In F. J. Menolascino (Ed.), *Psychiatric approaches to mental retardation.* New York: Basic, 1970.

Birch, H. G., & Gussow, J. D. *Disadvantaged children: Health, nutrition, and school failure.* New York: Grune and Stratton, 1970.

Blattner, R. J. Congenital damage to the central nervous system as a result of intrauterine infection. *Journal of Pediatrics,* 1958, *52,* 620–626.

Böök, J. A., Schut, J. W., & Reed, S. C. A clincal and genetical study of microcephaly. *American Journal of Mental Deficiency,* 1953, *57,* 637–660.

Broman, S. Perinatal anoxia and cognitive development in early childhood. In T. Field (Ed.), *Infants born at risk.* New York: Spectrum, 1979.

Caputo, D. V., Goldstein, K. M., & Taub, H. B. The development of prematurely born children through middle childhood. In T. Field (Ed.), *Infants born at risk.* New York: Spectrum, 1979.

Carlberg, C., & Kavale, K. The efficacy of special versus regular class placement for exceptional children: A meta-analysis. *Journal of Special Education,* 1980, *14*(3), 295–309.

Cattell, P. *Infant Intelligence Scale.* New York: Psychological Corporation, 1940.

Cooper, G., & Cooper, J. B. Radiation hazards to mother and fetus. *Clinical Obstetrics and Gynecology,* 1966, *9,* 11–21.

Corrigan, F. C., Berger, S. I., Dienstbier, R. A., & Strok, E. S. The influence of prematurity on school performance. *American Journal of Mental Deficiency,* 1967, *71,* 533–535.

Dawson, J. Pulmonary tuberous sclerosis and its relationship to other forms of the disease. *Quarterly Journal of Medicine,* 1954, *23,* 11–145.

Dunst, C. J., & Rheingrover, R. M. An analysis of the efficacy of infant intervention programs with organically handicapped children. *Evaluation and Program Planning,* 1981, *4,* 287–327.

Efficacy studies in early childhood special education. *Journal of the Division for Early Childhood,* December 1981, 4.

Engler, M. *Monogolism.* Bristol: Wright, 1949.

Følling, A. Uber Ausscherdund von phenyl brenztraubensaure in den harn als Stoffeuecksensanomalie. *Verbendung mit Imbezellitat Atschrift fur Physiolische Chemistrie,* 1934, *227,* 169–179.

Frances-Williams, J., & Davies, P. A. Very low birthweight and later intelligence. *Developmental Medicine and Child Neurology,* 1974, *16,* 709–725.

Franklin, A. W. Special syndromes. In A. P. Norman (Ed.), *Congenital abnormalities in infancy.* Oxford: Blackwell Scientific Publications, 1971.

Gibson, D. Karyotype variation and behavior in Down's syndrome: Methodological review. *American Journal of Mental Deficiency,* 1973, *78,* 128-133

Gibson, D. *Down's syndrome: The psychology of mongolism.* Cambridge: Cambridge University Press, 1978.

Gibson, D., & Frank H. F. Dimensions of mongolism. I. Age limits for cardinal mongol stigmata. *American Journal of Mental Deficiency,* 1961, *66,* 30–34.

Golden, M., & Birns, B. Social class and infant intelligence. In M. Lewis (Ed.), *Origins of intelligence: Infancy and early childhood.* New York: Plenum Press, 1976.

Graham, F. K., Ernhard, C. B., Craft, M., & Berman, P. W. Brain injury in the preschool child: Some developmental considerations. *Psychological Monographs,* 1963, *77,* 573–574.

Grossman, H. J. *Classification in mental retardation.* Washington, DC: American Association on Mental Deficiency, 1983.

Guthrie, R., & Susi, A. A simple phenylalanine method for detecting phenylketonuria in large population of newborn infants. *Pediatrics,* 1963, *32,* 330–343.

Haviland, J. Looking smart: The relationship between affect and intelligence. In M. Lewis (Ed.), *Orgins of intelligence: Infancy and early childhood.* New York: Plenum Press, 1976.

Hetch, F., & MacFarlane, J. P. Mosaicism in Turner's syndrome reflects the lethality of XO. *Lancet,* 1969, *2,* 1197.

Honzik, M. P. Value and limitations of infant tests: An overview. In M. Lewis (Ed.), *Orgins of intelligence: Infancy and early childhood.* New York: Plenum Press, 1976.

Ingalls, T. H. Causes and prevention of developmental defects. *Journal of the American Medical Association,* 1956, *161,* 1047–1051.

Jensen, A. R. A theory of primary and secondary familial mental retardation. In N. Ellis (Ed.), *International review of research in mental retardation* (Vol. 4). New York: Academic Press, 1970.

Jensen, A. R. *Educability and group differences,* New York: Harper & Row, 1973.

Jervis, G. A. The genetics of phenylpyruvic oligophrenia: The position of the metabolic error. *Journal of Biologic Chemistry,* 1947, *169,* 651.

Jones, H. W., & Neill, W., Jr. Treatment of carcinoma of the cervix during pregnancy. *American Journal of Obstetrics and Gynecology,* 1944, *48,* 447–463.

Kagan, J., Kearsley, R. B., & Zelazo, P. R. *Infancy: its place in human development.* Cambridge: Harvard University Press, 1978.

Kearsley, R. B., & Zelazo, P. R. *Intellectual assessment during infancy and early childhood.* Paper presented at the meeting of the New England Pediatric Society, Boston, March 1975.

Kirman, B. H. Clinical aspects. In J. Wortis (Ed.), *Mental retardation and developmental disabilities.* New York: Brunner/Mazel, 1973.

Koch, G. Genetics of microcephaly in man. *Acta Genetique Medicale,* 1959, *8,* 75–86.

Korones, S. B. *High risk newborn infant.* St. Louis: Mosby, 1976.

Lawrence, K. M. & Coates, S. Further thoughts on the natural history of hydrocephalus. *Developmental Medicine and Child Neurology,* 1962, *4,* 263–267.

Lawrence, K. M., & Weeks, R. Abnormalities of the central nervous system. In A. P. Norman (Ed.), *Congenital abnormalities in infancy.* Oxford: Blackwell Scientific Publications, 1971.

Lagos, J. C., & Gomez, M. R. Tuberous sclerous: Reappraisal of a clinical entity. *Mayo Clinic Proceedings,* 1967, *42,* 26–49.

Lejeune, J., Laforcade, J., Berger, R., Vialatte, J., Boeswillwald, M., Seringe, P., & Turpin, R. Trois cas de deletion partielle du bras court du chromosome 5. *Comples Rendus Academie des Sciences,* 1963, *257,* 3098.

McArthur, R. G., & Edwards, J. H. DeLange syndrome: Report of 20 cases. *Canadian Medical Association Journal,* 1967, *96,* 1185–1198.

McCall, R. B. The development of intellectual functioning in infancy and the prediction of later IQ. In J. D. Osofsky (Ed.), *Handbook of infant development.* New York: Wiley, 1979.

Menolascino, F. J., & Egger, M. L. *Medical dimensions of mental retardation.* Lincoln, NE: University of Nebraska, 1978.

Mercer, J. R., & Lewis, J. F. *System of multidisciplinary pluralistic assessment.* New York: Psychological Corp., 1978.

Meyers, C. E., Nihira, K., & Zetlin, A. The measurement of adaptive behavior. In N. Ellis (Ed.), *Handbook of mental deficiency, psychological theory and research* (2nd ed.). Hillsdale, NJ: Erlbaum, 1979.

Milgram, N. A. MR and mental illness: A proposal for conceptual unity. *Mental Retardation,* 1972, *10*(6), 29–31.

Miller, R. W. Delayed effects occurring within the first decade of the exposure of young individuals to the Hiroshima atomic bomb. *Pediatrics.* 1956, *18,* 1–18.

Moore, K. L. Sex reversal in newborn babies. *Lancet,* 1959, *1,* 217.

Murphy, D. P. The outcome of 625 pregnancies in women subjected to pelvic radium or roentgen radiation. *American Journal of Obstetrics and Gynecology,* 1929, *18,* 179–187.

Neel, J. V. *Changing perspectives on the genetic effects of radiation. Beaumont lecture, Wayne County Medical Society, Detroit.* Springfield, IL: Thomas, 1962.

Niswander, K. R., & Gordon, M. *The women and their pregnancies* (Vol. 1). Philadelphia: Saunders, 1972.

Norman, A. P. Syndromes due to chromosomal abnormalities. In A. P. Norman (Ed.), *Congenital abnormalities in infancy.* Oxford: Blackwell Scientific, 1971.

Parmalee, A. H., & Schulte, F. Developmental testing of pre-term and small-for-date infants. *Pediatrics,* 1970, *45,* 21–28.

Penrose, L. S. Microcephaly. *Folia Hereditary, et Pathologica,* 1956, *5,* 82–85.

Penrose, L. S. *The biology of mental defect.* New York: Grune & Stratton, 1963.

Robinson, N. M., & Robinson, H. B. *The mentally retarded child.* New York: McGraw-Hill, 1976.

Rosecrans, C. J. The relationship of normal/21 trisomy mosaicism and intellectual development. *American Journal of Mental Deficiency,* 1968, *72,* 562–566.

Rubin, A., Rosenblatt, C., & Balow, B. Psychological and educational sequelae of prematurity. *Pediatrics,* 1973, *52,* 352–363.

Schuster, D. S., & Johnson, S. A. Cutaneous manifestations of the Cornelia de Lange syndrome. *Archives of Dermatology,* 1966, *93,* 702–707.

Sechzer, J. A., Faro, M. D., & Windle, W. F. Studies of monkeys asphyxiated at birth: Implications for minimal cerebral dysfunction. *Seminars in Psychiatry,* 1973, *5,* 19–34.

Shipe, D., Reisman, C. E., Chung, C. Y., Darnell, A., & Kelly S. The relationship between cytogenetic constitution, physical stigmata, and intelligence in Down's syndrome. *American Journal of Mental Deficiency,* 1968, *72,* 789–797.

Simeonsson, R. J., Cooper, D. H., & Scheiner, A. P. A review and analysis of the effectiveness of early intervention programs. *Pediatrics,* 1982, *69,* 635–641.

Terman, L. M., & Merrill, M. A. *Binet intelligence scale.* Boston: Houghton-Mifflin, 1973.

Teuber, H. I. Mental retardation after early trauma to the brain: Some issues in search of facts. In C. R. Angle & E. A. Bering, Jr. (Eds.), *Physical trauma as an etiological spent in mental retardation.* Washington, DC: U.S. Government Printing Office, 1970.

Thompson, J. S., & Thompson, M. W. *Genetics in medicine.* Philadelphia: Saunders, 1966.

Tredgold, A. F. *A textbook of mental deficiency.* Baltimore: Williams & Wilkins, 1956.

Turnbull, H. R., & Turnbull, A. *Free appropriate public education: Law and implementation.* Denver: Love, 1978.

U.S. Dept. of Health and Human Services. *Maternal PKU,* 1982.

Vorherr, H. Placental insufficiency in relation to post-term pregnancy and fetal postmaturity. *American Journal of Obstetrics and Gynecology,* 1975, *123,* 67–103.

Warkany, J., & Dignan, P. S. J. Congenital malformations: Microcephaly. In J. Wortis (Ed.), *Mental retardation and developmental disabilities.* New York: Brunner/Mazel, 1973.

Wechsler, D. *Wechsler intelligence scale for children: Manual.* New York: Psychological Corporation, 1949.

Wechsler, D. *Wechsler adult intelligence scale, manual.* New York: Psychological Corporation, 1955.

Wechsler, D. *Manual for the Wechsler preschool and primary scale of intelligence.* New York: Psychological Corporation, 1967.

Wechsler, D. *Wechsler intelligence scale for children—Revised.* New York: Psychological Corporation, 1974.

Yamazaki, J. N. A review of the literature on the radiation dosage required to cause manifest central nervous system disturbances from in utero and postnatal exposure. *Pediatrics (Supplement),* 1966, *37,* 877–897.

Yamazaki, J. N., Wright, S. W., & Wright, P. M. Outcome of pregnancy in women exposed to the atomic bomb in Nagasaki. *American Journal of Diseases of Children*, 1954, *87*, 448–463.

Yannet, H. Mental deficiency due to prenatally determined factors. *Pediatrics*, 1950, *5*, 328–336.

Zelazo, P. R. Reactivity to perceptual-cognitive events: Application for infant assessment. In R. Kearsley & J. Sigel (Eds.), *Infants at risk*. New York: Wiley, 1979.

Zellweger, H., & Abbo, G. Chromosomal mosaicism and mongolism. *Lancet*, 1963, *1*, 827.

CHAPTER 5

Pervasive Developmental Disorders and Schizophrenia

Gary B. Mesibov and Geraldine Dawson

The term *psychosis* has historically been used to described the most severe forms of mental disturbance, characterized by an extreme lack of contact with the surrounding environment. Kraepelin (1904) noted that dementia praecox, or schizophrenia, often began in adolescence, and that a small percentage of cases could be traced to early childhood. Although Bleuler (1950) did not believe in the adolescent onset of schizophrenia, he did report that 5 percent of his cases could be traced to childhood and occasionally to the first five years of life. Potter (1933) was the first to study systematically and write about childhood psychoses, emphasizing the social, cognitive, language, affective, and motor difficulties of afflicted children.

More recent efforts have focused on defining childhood psychoses (Creak, 1963; Goldfarb, 1970; Rutter, 1978), and that, of course, is what DSM-III does do. Although DSM-III differs somewhat from other nomenclatures, such as the system advocated by the Group for the Advancement of Psychiatry in their definitions and descriptions of these very serious disorders, there is consistency in viewing them as extensively incapacitating, with uncertain etiologies, and involving serious distortions of reality. Moreover, there is also general agreement in regarding the two most common forms of psychosis in childhood as infantile autism and schizophrenia. Therefore, these will represent the main areas of discussion in the chapter.

We shall also discuss childhood onset pervasive developmental disorder, a new category in DSM-III for psychotic children who do not have the symptoms of schizophrenia but become severely withdrawn after 30 months of age, and schizotypal personality disorder (borderline child), another new category, which can apply to children whose behavior is decidedly odd but not quite schizophrenic. Although investigators agree the schizotypal child does not have a psychosis, the behaviors and treatments for these children are similar to those for psychotic children and will be discussed in this chapter.

Technically, DSM-III includes only infantile autism and childhood onset pervasive developmental disorder among the pervasive developmental disorders.

Infantile Autism

The term *early infantile autism* was first used by Leo Kanner (1943) to describe a group of eleven psychotic children who appeared more similar to one another than to other children with psychiatric disorders. The common characteristics of these eleven children included mutism, or delayed speech acquisition and the inability to use communicative speech after it did develop, echolalia, pronoun reversals, severely impaired relationships with other people, repetitive and stereotyped play activities, obsessive insistence on maintaining sameness, a lack of imagination, good rote memory skills, and normal physical appearance. In addition, Kanner noted that this disorder has its onset in early infancy, which was unlike all previously described forms of childhood psychosis which tended to develop much later in life. In fact, the parents reported peculiarities in the child's development virtually from birth.

In 1956, Eisenberg and Kanner had reduced the number of essential symptoms to only two: extreme aloneness and a preoccupation with the preservation of sameness. Although a more clear and concise definition of the autistic syndrome was needed and this consolidation was helpful, it, unfortunately, left out an important defining characteristic, the abnormalities of language and communications.

Since this original description and later clarification, there have been many attempts to clarify the diagnostic criteria of autism (Ornitz & Ritvo, 1968; Rendle-Short, 1969; Schain & Yannet, 1960; Tinbergen & Tinbergen, 1972; Wing & Ricks, 1976). The most influential of these has been the work of Rutter and his colleagues (Rutter, 1966; Rutter & Lockyer, 1967), who made systematic comparisons between autistic children and children of the same sex, age, and general intelligence level with other psychiatric disorders. They found three symptoms present in all autistic children and seen much less frequently in control children: a profound and general failure to develop social relationships; language retardation with impaired comprehension, echolalia, and pronoun reversals; and ritualistic or compulsive behaviors. They also noted four additional symptoms, which though more frequent in the autistic group, did not occur in all autistic children: stereotyped, repetitive movements (particularly hand and finger mannerisms); short attention span; self-injury; and delayed bowel control. The symptoms delineated by Rutter closely resemble those used in DSM-III, which are:

1. Onset before 30 months
2. Pervasive lack of responsiveness to other people
3. Gross deficits in language development
4. If speech is present, peculiar speech patterns such as immediate and delayed echolalia, metaphorical language, and pronoun reversals

5. Bizarre responses to various aspects of the environment, e.g., resistance to change, peculiar interest in or attachment to animate or inanimate objects
6. Absence of delusions, hallucinations, loosening of associations and incoherence as in schizophrenia

This definition is based upon behavioral symptoms in early childhood. Thus, autistic children will most clearly fit the abovementioned diagnostic criteria before the age of five (Wing, 1971). Many investigators have noted that these characteristics tend to change significantly with age (Kanner & Eisenberg, 1956; Schopler & Mesibov, 1983). Although marked social and behavioral handicaps usually persist, older autistic individuals typically exhibit less stereotyped movements, fewer compulsive and perseverative behaviors, and show an increased interest in relating to people (Mesibov, 1983); though disabilities of speech and language remain major handicaps (approximately one half of all autistic people never develop functional language), there also seems to be significant improvement in these skills with age. However, there continue to be significant social problems, even among those exhibiting the highest language skills (Rutter, 1966; Simmons & Baltaxe, 1975).

The prevalence of infantile autism, using the definition based on behavioral symptoms of early childhood, has been estimated as 4–5 cases per 10,000 population (Brask, 1967; Lotter, 1966; Ritvo & Freeman, 1977; Rutter, 1978). Because Kanner's (1943) original sample had a disproportionate number of autistic children from professional families with high IQs and excellent rote memory skills, many have believed that autistic children have the potential for normal intellectual functioning. Unfortunately, current estimates are quite different, with studies reporting that approximately 70 percent of autistic people are functioning intellectually within the mentally retarded range (DeMyer, et al., 1974; Schopler & Dalldorf, 1980). These IQ scores are as stable in autistic children as in their nonhandicapped peers (DeMyer, et al., 1974; Lockyer & Rutter, 1969) and are a relatively accurate predictor of later educational performance (Bartak & Rutter, 1971; Lockyer & Rutter, 1969).

Along with IQ, the other characteristic distinguishing autistic children from the nonhandicapped population is sex ratio; infantile autism occurs more frequently in males than in females, by 3 or 4 to 1 (Gittelmen & Birch, 1967; Kanner, 1957; Kolvin, 1971; Rutter & Lockyer, 1967). This is similar to the sex ratios reported for most other developmental disabilities (Robinson & Robinson, 1976).

Although the distribution of social class was also thought to differ between families of autistic and nonhandicapped children, recent data have shown this to be incorrect. This misconception also grew out of Kanner's original sample, which consisted mainly of professional families, with four out of the eleven having a physician as one of the parents. Recent research has shown that this overrepresentation of upper-class families was a function of their educational and financial positions, which enabled them to find and participate in the highly specialized programs that were available for autistic children in the 1940s and 1950s. Current data, controlling for this self-selection factor (Schopler, Andrews, & Strupp, 1979), show about the same social class distribution for families of autistic children as exists for the population from which they were taken.

Case Illustration: Bob was a ten-year-old boy who was the product of a normal pregnancy, labor, and delivery. He was very fussy in infancy, crying for long periods of time and never appearing content. Holding and cuddling did not help but in fact were reported to have made him more irritable.

Although Bob's parents were frustrated by his unhappiness, they thought he might be okay since his motor skills were developing normally. They first became seriously concerned when he evidenced no language by two years of age. Although he imitated certain sounds and words around the age of one, these dropped out over the next six months. Moreover, Bob did not even try to communicate by gesture.

When tested by a psychologist at the age of ten, Bob was found to be functioning at around a two-year level. His strongest skill was in manipulating objects. He could place pegs in a board, stack blocks, and do simple puzzles. He was most deficient in relating to others socially, with little eye contact, poor imitation, and limited responsiveness to people.

In addition Bob engaged in some unusual behaviors, such as whirling his body, playing with string, and spinning objects for long periods. If interrupted, he would become extremely upset and showed great distress to loud noises, closing his eyes and placing his hands over his ears.

Neurological Correlates

The behaviors characterizing infantile autism strongly suggest this disorder relates to some form of neurological dysfunction. However, the precise nature of the difficulty is not known. Current research is focused on two aspects of this problem: first, the identification of the neurological correlates of autism; and second, attempts at identifying the cause of this handicapping condition. Identified neurological correlates have included soft neurological signs, seizure disorders, abnormal EEGs, unusual sleep patterns, and several conditions known to be related to brain damage.

It has been well documented that autistic children evidence more "soft" neurological signs (e.g., hypotonia, poor coordination) than normal controls. Studies have reported 40–100 percent of autistic children show some evidence of neurological disturbance as indicated by these soft signs (DeMyer et al., 1973; Goldfarb, 1961; Gubbay, Lobaschen, & Ringerlee, 1970; Hinton, 1963; Knoblock & Pasamanick, 1975). Although there is some disagreement as to the relevance of neurological soft signs, many professionals claim that their presence suggests damage, immaturity, and/or poor organization of the brain (Adams & Jenkins, 1981).

A second neurological correlate of autism is the higher incidence of abnormal electroencephalograms (EEGs) in these children as compared with nonhandicapped children. DeMyer (1975) compared a sample of autistic and retarded children and found that 65% of the autistic children had EEG abnormalities as compared to only 39% of the retarded sample. Other studies have reported from 20–30 percent of abnormal EEGs in autistic children (Gubbay, Lobaschen, & Ringerlee, 1970; Kolvin et al. 1971c) to 60–80 percent (Creak & Pampiglione, 1969; White, DeMyer, & DeMyer, 1964). The discrepancy in the figures is probably based on different criteria for autism and also for EEG abnormalities. The abnormal EEGs found in autistic children in these studies were generally characterized by focal slowing, spiking, or paroxysmal spike-wave discharges.

In addition to the higher incidence of abnormal EEGs, autistic children more frequently have seizure disorder (Creak, 1963a). Kolvin, Ounsted, and Roth (1971) found histories of seizures in ten of their sample of forty-six autistic children. Deykin and MacMahon (1979) also report an increased risk of developing seizures for autistic people. However, they make a distinction between totally autistic children (impairments in relatedness, language, the presence of sterotypies) and partially autistic children who show impairments in only two of the three areas. They found that both partially and totally autistic children had an increased risk of seizures starting up to the age of ten, but that only the totally autistic children had an increased risk of seizures starting during adolescence. Bartak & Rutter (1976) have also documented a greater incidence of adolescent onset of seizures in autistic as compared with nonautistic children. In their sample one-fourth to one-third of the autistic children who were seizure-free in childhood developed seizures during adolescence, but this rarely occurred in children with IQs greater than 70. Perhaps the children with lower IQs in this study are similar to the totally autistic children described by Deykin and MacMahon. Rutter argues that the adolescent onset of seizures is related to the physical maturation process occurring during that time.

Finally, autism has frequently been found in association with several central nervous system difficulties. Among those that have been documented are retrolental fibroplasia (Keeler, 1958), tuberous sclerosis (Lotter, 1974), congenital syphilis (Rutter and Lockyer, 1967), phenylketonuria (Knoblock & Pasamanick, 1975), and widespread neurolipidosis (Creak, 1963).

Theories Of Autism

The large number of neurological correlates has led investigators to theorize concerning the neurological mechanisms underlying the autistic syndrome. However, this emphasis on neurological explanations is relatively recent. Historically, autism was thought to be an emotional disorder and many of the earlier causal theories were based on this assumption.

The early psychogenic theories emphasized Kanner's observation that many parents of autistic children were highly intelligent and obsessive individuals lacking in warmth. Kanner's group postulated infantile autism resulted from an interaction between these specific family environments and innate deficits (Eisenberg, 1957; Kanner, 1949).

Following these observations, theorists stressed pathological traits in parents including emotional coldness, obsessiveness, introversion, intellectuality, and schizophrenic features (Ounsted, 1970; van Krevelen, 1963, 1971). Others have attributed autism to a pathological parent-child interaction, lacking in either maternal communication (Goldfarb, Goldfarb, & Scholl, 1966), adequate stimulation (Anthony, 1958; Tinbergen & Tinbergen, 1972; Ward, 1970; Zaslow & Breger, 1969), or caused by earlier parental rejection or separation (Bettelheim, 1969; Despert, 1951).

In general, the research investigating the psychogenic hypothesis has failed to support it. (Ornitz, 1972; Ornitz & Ritvo, 1976). The only consistent finding has been a high prevalence of parents with significantly higher educational and occupational levels than parents of nonhandicapped children (Cox et al., 1975; Kolvin et al., 1971,a, c; Lotter, 1966; Rutter & Lockyer, 1967). However, even this finding has been refuted more recently and attributed to various selection factors (Schopler, Andrews, & Strupp, 1979). At this point, the only conclusive statement concerning the emotional status of parents is that the extreme stress of being a parent of an autistic child can precipitate emotional difficulties (Creak & Ini, 1960;

Schopler, 1971) for these fathers and mothers.

The lack of support for psychogenic theories and the accumulating evidence that infantile autism is a developmental and not an emotional disorder have led to the promotion of several neurological theories. These theories postulate one or more of the following neurological dysfunctions: overarousal of the reticular system, perceptual inconstancy associated with dysfunction in the brain stem, dysfunction of the limbic system, and left hemisphere dysfunction.

Possible problems with the reticular system were first hypothesized by Rimland (1964) and Hutt et al. (1964); the latter speculated that the nonspecific activity of the reticular system might be chronically high in autistic children. Claiming evidence of high levels of low voltage irregularity in the resting EEGs of autistic children, Hutt et al. postulated that this indication of high arousal could be a chronic problem in autistic children and that many of the bizarre behaviors were simply an attempt to maintain some continuity in the environment as a defense against overarousal. However, subsequent experimental investigations comparing autistic children with carefully matched controls did not show any evidence of the postulated relationship between arousal as measured by the EEG and overt behaviors (Churchill, 1971; Hermelin & O'Connor, 1968; Ornitz et al., 1970).

A theory of perceptual inconstancy, advanced by Ornitz and Ritvo (1968), stresses an inability to regulate sensory input as underlying the deficits of these children. This inability to maintain stable percepts precludes the establishment of a coherent, meaningful external reality. Ornitz and Ritvo based their theory upon behavioral observations reflecting fluctuating over- and under-arousal and also on research indicating that vestibularly-induced nystagmus is suppressed in autistic children (Colbert, Koegler, & Markham, 1959; Pollack & Krieger, 1958; Ritvo, Ornitz, & Eviator, 1969). One weakness of the perceptual inconstancy theory is that the precise nature of the proposed "instability in perception" and its effects on development are not clearly delineated. Moreover, the theory does not account for why many autistic children are relatively unimpaired in certain perceptual areas, such as visual-motor skills.

A third neuropsychological explanation for infantile autism was proposed by Boucher and Warrington (1976) and DeLong (1978); they suggested autism may be similar to the amnesic syndrome arising from a lesion in the limbic system. Boucher and Warrington demonstrated that animals with hippocampal lesions show motor stereotypy associated with increased general activity, reduced exploration, and inability to learn from errors. Studies with children, however, have not fully supported this hypothesis (Boucher and Warrington, 1976). While there do seem to be some parallels between autism and amnesia, there also seem to be some significant differences.

Several investigators (Blackstock, 1978; Dawson, 1979; Prior & Bradshaw, 1979; Tanguay, 1976) noted that the specific cognitive and language impairments found in autism are typical of those functions for which the left hemisphere is specialized. In addition, many autistic children show normal or superior abilities in right hemisphere functions (Lockyer & Rutter, 1970). For example, Blackstock (1978) found autistic children attend more readily to a story which is sung rather than read to them. Moreover, they attend predominantly with the left ear, suggesting that they prefer to process information in a "right hemisphere mode."

Using EEG and dichotic listening measures, several investigators have found that many autistic children have an atypical pattern of hemisphere specialization; namely, a preference for right hemisphere dominance for both non-verbal and verbal stimuli (Dawson, Warrenburg, & Fuller, 1982; Prior & Bradshaw, 1979). Rutter (1978), in contrast, has argued that a selective left hemispheric dysfunction in autism is implausible because the plasticity of the infant brain would make right hemisphere compensation for such dysfunction very likely. The apparent lack of right hemisphere compensation for left-sided dysfunction suggests the possibility of bilateral dysfunction, at least in some cases.

Etiological Factors

There has been considerable investigation of potential causal mechanisms of autism. Following refutations of psychogenic theories of causation, recent efforts have focused on biological causes. Three factors have been studied most extensively: difficulties during pregnancy and/or birth; genetic factors; and biochemical and medical studies.

Difficulties during Pregnancy and/or Birth. Several studies of birth histories of autistic children have found an increased incidence of complications as compared with control groups (Knoblock & Pasamanick, 1962; Ornitz & Ritvo, 1976): difficult labors, Rh incompatibility, toxemia, vaginal bleeding, and severe maternal illness. Although research in this area is complex and difficult to interpret, it appears that the findings are most suggestive for prenatal factors, as compared with abnormalities of birth and the neonatal period (Links et al., 1980). For example, although most of the above mentioned prenatal difficulties result in a high incidence of autism, the evidence is not as strong that prematurity or other neonatal factors have the same effect. Gillberg (1980) suggests that, as with Down syndrome, there is an increased risk for infantile autism with increasing maternal and paternal age.

Genetic Factors. In describing his original sample, Kanner suggested that genetic factors may contribute to the etiology of autism. Although the popularity of the psychogenic hypothesis interrupted this area of inquiry, more recent investigators have been examining genetic factors closely.

Bartak, Rutter, and Cox (1975) studied a group of autistic children and found a family history of speech delay in about 25 percent of this sample. They also observed that the rate of autism in the siblings was about fifty times that of the general populations (Rutter, 1967). The most influential and careful study in this area was done by Folstein and Rutter (1977), who studied twenty-one same-sex twins, of whom at least one twin in each pair was diagnosed as autistic. In this study, four of the eleven monozygotic pairs (MZ) but none of the 10 dizygotic pairs (DZ) were concordant for autism. In addition, six nonautistic co-twins (five MZ and one DZ) showed a cognitive abnormality in the form of severe speech delay, learning disability, or mental retardation. Further, in twelve of the seventeen pairs of twins discordant for autism, there was evidence that the autistic member had suffered some form of brain injury whereas in none of the discordant pairs did this occur only in the nonautistic member.

Other investigators are finding similar evidence of the genetic transmission of autism. Ritvo (1981) has found a proportion of monozygotic twins with autism that is similar to Folstein and Rutter (1977) and has also found a high incidence of learning disabilities and other developmental problems in families with autistic children. Tsai, Stewart, and August (1981) have further evidence supporting a genetic hypothesis and their results suggest the transmission of autism is multifactorial.

Biochemical and Medical Studies. Studies of blood levels of indoleamine serotonin have received the most attention. Schain and Freeman (1961) compared twenty-three autistic children to those whose primary diagnosis was mental retardation and found abnormally high levels of blood serotonin in association with autism and severe mental retardation. These authors did not find a relationship between elevated serotonin levels and presenting symptoms in the children.

In a series of studies, Ritvo and his colleagues (Ritvo et al., 1971; Ritvo et al., 1970) have found that while mean serotonin levels and platelet counts were significantly higher in autistic children than in age-matched controls, mean serotonin per platelet levels were not significantly different. The blood serotonin levels appear to be an age-related phenomenon; serotonin levels decrease with age, which suggests a possible maturational basis for elevated serotonin levels in autism. Other studies (Campbell et al., 1976) have indicated that higher serotonin levels are most clearly related to low intellectual functioning. The administration of L-Dopa, which lowers blood serotonin, does not appear to produce behavioral changes in autistic children (Campbell et al., 1976; Ritvo et al., 1971).

Cohen and his colleagues (Cohen et al., 1974; Cohen et al., 1977; Cohen et al., 1978) have postulated that autism is related to dopaminergic overactivity and, furthermore, that there exists a reciprocal relationship between dopaminergic and serotonergic functioning. Another promising lead is Coleman's (1978) report of zinc deficiencies in autistic children.

In addition to the advances in biochemical research, investigators are currently exploring the possibility that autism is caused by a virus. Chess (1971) reported that autism frequently occurs in association with central nervous system viral infection, and more recently, Peterson and Torrey (1976) have postulated a viral cause for autism. Although a study by Stubbs and Magenis (1980) was unable to confirm this, the sample size was too small to make theirs an adequate test of the hypothesis. Future research efforts will, no doubt, be exploring this possibility more carefully.

To date autism has not been definitely related to any biochemical or viral abnormality. This is, no doubt, partly because of poor diagnostic classification, small samples and inadequate control groups. Given the emerging consensus on diagnostic classification with DSM-III and the current emphasis on controlled investigations, these approaches may be more fruitful in the years ahead.

Cognitive Deficit. Although investigators have not been able to identify the basic cause or causes of autism and there is still some disagreement concerning its specific correlates, there is an emerging consensus that autism, above all, represents some form of fundamental cognitive deficit. Parents of autistic children note that the behaviors which normally elicit social responses in others, such as smiling, eye contact, and cuddling, are lacking in their autistic infants. Hermelin and O'Connor (1970) suggest that the social unresponsiveness of autistic children is not due to active avoidance of social contact. Instead, it is supposed that poor communication skills due to underlying perceptual and cognitive deficiencies contribute greatly to the appearance of social indifference in these children. The nature of these perceptual and/or cognitive deficits is under investigation (Prior, 1984). Although the precise nature of this deficit remains to be determined, language and communication processes are certainly involved.

By definition, gross deficits in language development are a central aspect of infantile autism. What we shall do is review and consider the research that has been done to specify the nature of what is wrong with the communication of these children. On a global level, estimates of the prevalence of mutism in infantile autism range from 28 percent (Wolff & Chess, 1965) to 61 percent (Fish, Shapiro, & Campbell, 1966). When speech is present, its onset is usually markedly delayed and its acquisition is very gradual. Even when autistic children do learn to speak, they often fail to use language spontaneously or creatively. Instead, their speech tends to be stereotyped and repetitive and fails to incorporate social nuances. A study by Bartak, Rutter, and Cox (1975) demonstrated that the communication problem in autism extends beyond spoken language to involve a general impairment in the use of symbols. These authors found that, unlike children with developmental receptive aphasia, autistic children do not spontaneously use symbolic gestures to communicate or engage in symbolic play. Ricks and Wing (1975) have argued that the central problem for autistic people is a difficulty in using symbols, which would account for their impairments in language, nonverbal communication, and other cognitive and social skills; while Schwartz and Johnson (1982, p.153) specify an impairment in linking meaning to environmental stimuli caused by deficits in encoding and abstracting.

Prelinguistic Development. The process of learning to communicate normally begins at birth. Prelinguistic vocalizations, social games, and other forms of reciprocal interaction between infants and their caretakers are believed to play important roles in language acquisition (Bruner, 1975, 1977; Snyder, 1978; Uzgiris, 1979). Although research on prelinguistic development in autistic children is relatively sparse, the few studies which have been done, as well as clinical observations, suggest that autistic children are impaired at this early level of development. Ricks (1972) and Ricks and Wing (1975) found that, unlike normal infants and retarded children, autistic children do not use expressive noises to convey meaning and have personal, idiosyncratic ways of expressing emotion. Moreover, the autistic child does not spontaneously participate in social games, such as peek-a-boo or pat-a-cake, in which a child normally learns about his or her role in an interactive process. Most of these social games involve imitating another's movements. Motor imitation and the use of gestures appear to be particularly deficient in autistic children as compared to other developmentally-disabled children (DeMyer et al., 1972; Tubbs, 1966). Lacking these early social experiences in which the basic rules of communication are acquired causes autistic children to have difficulty in learning to use speech in a meaningful and communicative manner.

Deviant Versus Delayed Lanuage. Because the majority of autistic children are also mentally retarded, the speech of autistic children usually reflects both of these conditions. In order to determine which language impairments are unique to autistic individuals, comparisons of autistic children with younger normal, mentally retarded, and aphasic children have been made. Based upon this research, it appears that there are a number of characteristics which, if not unique to autism, are at least found much more frequently in this population than in other kinds of developmental disorders. These include the presence of echolalic speech, pronoun reversals, deficits in some aspects of semantic processing, and an impairment in the social usage of language. Each of these characteristics will be discussed separately.

Echolalia. Research on normal language development indicates that there is no stage in which young children exhibit purely echolalic speech as do many autistic children (Bloom, 1970; McNeill, 1966; 1970). Comparing the elicited verbal imitations of autistic and younger normal children, Shapiro and his colleagues (Shapiro & Lucy, 1978; Shapiro, Roberts, and Fish, 1970) found that the autistic children's imitations were less different from the model and their response latencies were briefer. These findings indicate that echolalic speech depends on a different, more limited decoding of utterances than creative speech. Shapiro and others (Baltaxe & Simmons, 1975; Fay, 1969) have suggested that echolalic speech represents an attempt to communicate on the part of a child who can register speech on a phonetic level but has difficulty understanding certain semantic components of speech. Thus, rather than decoding heard utterances in terms of their basic semantic relationships, the child appears to use the entire utterance as a label for an associated situation or event. Echolalic speech is often the first manner in which language is used by autistic children and its existence, particularly if it occurs before age 5, is associated with a more positive response to language intervention (Howlin, 1981; Rutter & Lockyer, 1967).

Pronoun Reversal. From a psychoanalytic viewpoint, some authors (Bettelheim, 1967; Bosch, 1970) regard the autistic child's tendency not to use "I" as a psychological defense against self-recognition. Bosch has reported that autistic children will even use more developmentally advanced pronouns in order to avoid the use of "I." Careful studies of pronoun usage in autistic children have not supported Bosch's original claim. Silberg (1978) found that autistic children followed a normal progression in developing pronouns. She reported that, while pronoun reversal and echolalia were common in autistic children with shorter mean lengths of utterance, as their sentence complexity increased, the pronoun "I" was used. In fact, the pronoun "I" was the most frequently used pronoun by the children in Silberg's study. Bartak and Rutter (1974) also found no tendency by autistic children to avoid repetition of "I." Their study showed that both normal and autistic children exhibit a recency effect when asked to recall sentences. Since "I" normally occurs at the beginning of a sentence, a failure to repeat "I" could be a function of this memory factor. When the position of "I" in the sentence was controlled, Bartak and Rutter found that autistic children did not fail to echo it.

Fay (1979) argued that the problem of personal pronouns is too complex to be accounted for entirely in terms of "reversal" secondary to echolalia. He pointed out that normal children, as well as retarded children, have difficulty changing the form of a message to take into account another's perspective. Fay further suggested that autistic children may have a deitic (those features of language which require a shift in orientation) disability, particularly with regard to shifting person perspectives. He points out that linguistic deixis probably develops out of earlier gestural deixis (Bates, 1976; Clark, 1978). For example, one early form of gestural deixis is pointing, which assumes joint attention to the object indicated. Given that autistic children are lacking in these early gestures, a deitic disability is likely to prevail. Similarly, Charney (1980) suggests that autistic children may reverse pronouns due to impaired social relationships stemming from an inability to represent self as separate from, or in relation to, others.

In sum, it appears that pronoun reversal can be accounted for in terms of the various linguistic and social handicaps exhibited by autistic children.

Semantics. Although few good studies of semantic development in autistic children exist, those which are reported indicate that these children have difficulty processing semantic information. As stated above, it is likely that autism involves a basic difficulty in handling symbols. Thus, the formation of high-level abstractions and complex linguistic relationships is difficult for autistic persons (Ricks & Wing, 1975). O'Connor and Hermelin (1967a) found that, compared to mentally retarded and normal control subjects, autistic children do not tend to cluster semantically-related words in recall. These authors have also reported that autistic children recall sentences and randomly ordered sequences of words equally well, whereas retarded children are better able to recall meaningful sentences (O'Connor & Hermelin, 1967b). Tager-Flusberg (1981) also found that autistic children have significantly poorer use of semantically-based linguistic strategies than matched mentally retarded children. Simmons and Baltaxe's (1975) analysis of autistic adolescents' language also indicated semantic as well as other linguistic violations. Examples of semantic errors are shown in the following responses:

1. He is getting *rarer and rarer* because *so many of them left.*
2. Q: Do *you* ever get unhappy?
   A: Maybe on the job, maybe *workers* would get unhappy on *their* jobs.
3. —or standing up, just like a—just like *lightening to a fireplace standing up to a fire.*

Bartolucci and Albers (1974) hypothesize that autistic children have particular difficulty with deitic (language involving shifts in orientation) categories. This could include linguistic reference to space (here, there), time (now, then), and person (you, me). For example, they found that autistic children only used the past tense (time orientation) correctly 9 percent of the time whereas matched retarded children showed correct usage 60 percent and normal children 80 percent of the time. Deitic disability has also been suggested as one reason for pronoun difficulties (Fay, 1979), since pronouns are terms which require a shift in perspective from speaker to listener.

Pragmatics. The shift in focus of linguistic research from syntax and semantics to the pragmatics of language has resulted in new insights into the language behavior of autistic persons. Most investigators agree that even when autistic individuals come to possess fairly sophisticated language skills in terms of syntactic complexity, vocabulary, and semantic understanding, the ability to use language in a socially-appropriate and communicative manner remains markedly impaired (Baltaxe & Simmons, 1975). Baltaxe (1977) found that highly verbal autistic adolescents continue to have poor communicative competence. She found the most common difficulty to be an inability to adapt their speaking to the situation or speaker. For example, the subjects were unable to appropriately switch to an informal style of language as shown in these examples:

1. Q: Do you have a girlfriend?
   A: No, I haven't met such a nice lovely young lady as yet.
2. Q: What about the bird?
   A: The pelegrin (*sic*) falcon, it's an endangered species and tragically being wiped out because of insecticide.

As Ricks and Wing (1975) point out, even those children who make good progress continue to be insensitive to the subtleties and complexities of the nonverbal cues which regulate social interaction. These authors cite the common example of the bright autistic child who makes him- or herself conspicuous in public by speaking very loudly or who fails to recognize signs of boredom by the listener in response to topics repeatedly talked about by the child. Ball's (1978) systematic comparisons of the spontaneous speech of autistic, developmental asphasic, and MA-matched normal children (younger normal children with about the same mental ages as the autistic children) have confirmed these clinical observations. Ball found that autistic children were less developed in all spheres of pragmatic competence than either comparison group.

Problems in pragmatic competence are evident in the earliest communicative attempts by autistic children. Seibert and Oller (1981) have offered a model for early communicative assessment of autistic children which focuses on early communicative behaviors such as gaining and sustaining another's attention to oneself, directing another's attention to an object, and regulating another's behavior to achieve an environmental end. These behaviors typically emerge between birth and two years of age in normal children but are rarely observed in the spontaneous behavior of young autistic children (Ball, 1978).

Phonology, Prosody and Syntax. Compared with other aspects of language, autistic children appear to show the least deviance in phonological development. Shervanian (1959) found they progress in the normal developmental sequence of phonemes, although at a retarded rate. However, large individual differences were noted, and certain sounds, such as stops, semivowels, and fricatives, were sometimes deficient. Frith (1969) reported that autistic children were as competent as normals in phonological repetition. Recent comparisons of speech from autistic and matched mentally retarded samples have generally confirmed the notion that phonemic development in autistic children parallels that of retarded and younger normal children (Bartolucci & Pierce, 1977; Bartolucci et al., 1976; Boucher & Warrington, 1976).

Researchers do not agree on whether the syntactic and prosodic features of language pose particular problems for autistic children beyond general developmental delays in these areas. The findings with regard to syntactic development in autism are similarly unclear. What appear to be specific syntactic deficiencies may actually reflect the difficulties autistic children have in using language in a complex and changing social context.

Treatment

Treatment approaches for autistic children can be classified in three ways: psychodynamic, medical, and behavioral. The psychodynamically-oriented therapies view infantile autism as an emotional disorder and emphasize intensive psychotherapy. Medical interventions utilize a range of drug and vitamin treatments, while behavioral therapies utilize principles of learning to teach a variety of appropriate behaviors. Although most educational interventions focus on behavioral techniques, they are discussed separately because of their emphasis on academic and school-related skills.

Psychodynamically-Oriented Therapies. Bruno Bettelheim (1974) has been the main proponent of the psychodynamic approach to therapy for autistic children. Arguing that cold and rejecting parents are the main cause of autism in their children, he advocates the removal of the children from their parents' home and their placement in a residential setting. This relocation allows the autistic child to let down his/her psychotic defenses and facilitates the establishment of trust relationships. The combination of a therapeutic, residential milieu, removed from parental control, plus individual psychodynamically-oriented therapy has also been advocated by Ruttenberg (1971) and Goldfarb, Mintz, and Strook (1969).

The residential setting, according to Bettelheim, should be a planned environment which meets the child's needs, alleviates anxieties, provides consistency, and allows the child to exert some control over his/her life. Bettelheim (1974) views this as essential because of the need to remove the child from unconscious parental hostility. He sees the role of twenty-four hours-a-day concerned caretakers as absolutely necessary to undo the psychotic process and establish more appropriate relationships. This allows for psychotic defenses to be relinquished, for trust to be established, for needs to be met, and for the feeling of powerlessness to be undone.

Although DesLauriers (1978) views early infantile autism as a sensory impairment instead of the outgrowth of inadequate parenting, he is described under the psychodynamic approaches because of treatment similarities. DesLauriers argues for *pheraplay*, a form of play therapy, as the best way to provide sensory stimulating experiences, which are intense enough to overcome the child's basic sensory deficit. Pheraplay is somewhat different from traditional play therapy in that the child is not taught anything specifically. Instead, the child learns to enjoy interpersonal interactions because they are of a highly stimulating nature e.g., tickling.

In general, the psychodynamically-oriented therapies are not used by most clinicians working with autistic children today. One reason for this is that the cumulative evidence refutes the assumptions upon which these theories are based. Autism is not seen as the result of inadequate parenting but rather of some nonspecific brain abnormalities (DeMyer, 1979; Ross, 1980; Rutter & Schopler, 1978). Because there is little evidence that autism is an emotional problem, there is little reason to believe that treatments based on this assumption will be effective. Moreover, the few studies done on the effectivness of psychodynamically-oriented psychotherapy with psychotic youngsters have shown no differences in children treated this way as compared with a group of untreated controls (Brown, 1960, 1963).

Biological Interventions. Drugs that have been used most frequently have been anticonvulsants, amphetamines, phenothiazines, and more recently, megavitamins. Anticonvulsant drugs are used to control seizures in autistic people (DeyKin & MacMahon, 1979) in much the same ways that they are used with the general population, and will therefore not be discussed further in this context.

Amphetamines are sometimes helpful in reducing the hyperactivity which often accompanies autism. These drugs do not produce recovery from autism, but can improve the attention spans and activity levels of these children and make them more susceptible to other forms of learning. Although there are many clinical reports of the effectiveness of the amphetamines, the main published studies with autistic children show worsening of behavior when treated with these drugs (Campbell et al., 1972).

Phenothiazines and haloperidol (haldol) have been useful, though unpredictable, in reducing severe aggressive and self-injurious behaviors (Dalldorf & Schopler, 1980). They can also increase learning deficits in autistic children and must be carefully monitored for side-effects, including excessive weight gain, reduced seizure threshold, and tardive dyskinesia (Schiele et al., 1973).

Lithium, generally used with manic-depressive patients, has more recently been used with some autistic children, especially those exhibiting aggressive or self-injurious behaviors, who have not been responsive to other forms of drug treatment. Campbell et al. (1972) found that, in general, lithium produced very small and relatively insignificant improvement in a sample of preschoolers, with the exception of one child whose self-mutilation behaviors were reduced "dramatically." Lithium is probably most appropriate for autistic children who show a cyclical behavior pattern and/or family history of cyclical affective illness. Lithium is especially difficult to monitor and there is a very narrow range between therapeutic and toxic levels.

The administration of megavitamins has been a recent biological intervention strategy. Although rigorous research studies have not demonstrated the effectiveness of megavitamin therapy for autistic children (Greenbaum, 1970), it is being widely used and reports of improvement for individual children are common (Rimland, 1973). In a recent study (Lelord et al., 1981), a double-blind, crossover procedure was used to assess the effects of large doses of vitamin B_6 and magnesium. Of the sample of forty-four children, clinical improvement with the vitamins and the worsening of symptoms after termination of doses was observed in fifteen.

The above findings are representative of the findings on megavitamins. Basically, it appears that some autistic children, though clearly not all and probably not even the majority, benefit. This may be no different from the evidence on most psychoactive drugs, which makes megavitamins preferable because they have many fewer side effects. In any case, more research is needed before conclusive statements can be made.

In summary, biological interventions are apparently less effective with autistic children than with other populations because of these children's unpredictable and idiosyncratic responses. However, when reasonably administered and carefully monitored, they can, at times, represent an important adjunct to other treatment efforts.

Behavioral Interventions. The great advances over the past fifteen years in treating autistic children have resulted from the use of behavioral interventions (Ross, 1980; Rutter & Schopler, 1978). Schopler and Dalldorf (1980) have subdivided these into two major categories; behavior management and special education. Behavior management is primarily concerned with social and interpersonal behaviors, while special education involves more conventional school-related skills, such as language and reading.

The early investigations of autistic social behavior assumed the main problem to be nonresponsiveness to social rewards. Lovaas, Freitag et al. (1966) gave food to autistic children contingent upon their attending and responding to social stimuli. This operant technique has also been used to shape social behaviors such as showing affection and giving friendly greetings (Lovaas, Schreibman, & Koegel, 1974).

Metz (1965) used a similar operant approach to teach imitation skills to autistic children. Using a combination of primary reinforcers, such as food, and secondary reinforcers, such as the word "good," Metz taught such imitative responses as kicking a bean bag, putting a blanket on a doll, and blowing a whistle. He was also able to demonstrate generalization of these behaviors to new tasks.

A more recent study used operant training techniques to teach interactive social behaviors directly (Romanczyk et al., 1975). Using food as a reward, they demonstrated that the cooperative toy play of autistic children could be increased in a group setting and would persist if the reinforcement was gradually faded out instead of abruptly withdrawn.

Severe behavioral difficulties, including aggression and self-injurious behaviors, have led to much effort being put into decreasing these behaviors. Risley and Wolf (1967) demonstrated the effectiveness of behavioral control techniques in regulating mildly disruptive behaviors by looking away from a child until he sat quietly in his chair. When more severe behaviors occurred, the investigators responded by leaving the room. Lovaas and Simmons (1969) effectively used a similar procedure in withdrawing attention for self-injurious behaviors.

The withdrawal of reinforcement or other positive events, contingent upon a child's inappropriate behaviors, is generally referred to as *time-out*. Although this procedure can often be quite effective, there are several drawbacks. Solnick, Rincover, and Peterson (1977) demonstrated that one must be sure the time-out procedure is more negative than the task the child is being asked to complete if it is to be an effective intervention technique. In their study, they found that temper tantrums increased whenever a teacher left the room during a work period. They concluded that the time-out procedure allowed the child to engage in self-stimulatory behaviors, which were more satisfying for the child than the required task and the teacher's presence. Once the investigators became aware of this, they used physical restraint, which was a more effective deterrent than time-out.

Time-out is also an ineffective intervention when the behaviors in question are extremely severe and potentially dangerous. In these instances, several investigators have used aversive techniques like electric shock to suppress these potentially life-threatening behaviors (Lovaas, Schaeffer, & Simmons, 1965; Risley, 1968; Tate & Baroof, 1966). These investigators emphasize that shock should only be used for extremely dangerous behaviors requiring immediate suppression when less intrusive techniques have proven ineffective. In addition to the serious ethical issues involved with the use of shock, there is also the problem that shock only eliminates certain behaviors and must be used in conjunction with more positive techniques, which are designed to build positive behaviors (Lovaas & Newsom, 1976).

Overcorrection is another aversive technique which has more recently been used to suppress aggressive and self-injurious behaviors (Foxx & Azrin, 1973). *Overcorrection* involves following an undesirable behavior with a specified set of activities designed to correct the damage that the inappropriate behavior has caused.

Foxx and Azrin have described two types of overcorrection: restitution and positive practice. Restitution requires the individual to correct the consequences of an inappropriate behavior by making the situation significantly better than it was before the outbreak. For example, a child who knocks a classmate over in a fight might be required to help him up, clean off his clothes, comb his hair, and otherwise tend to the victim's physical needs.

The other type of overcorrection, positive practice, consists of repeated direct or appropriate behaviors following an error. For example, a child who inappropriately hits a peer might be required to smile and shake that person's hand as well as everyone else's in the classroom. The child repeatedly practices the appropriate response and is, therefore, thought to be more likely to perform that behavior in similar situations.

Overcorrection has not been widely used with autistic children. It is very time consuming, often aversive to the staff involved, and frequently inconsistently applied (Koegel, Rincover, & Engel, 1982). Moreover, its effectiveness depends on a child's cognitive ability to see the relationship between his/her behavior and its implications. This understanding is often beyond the capabilities of many autistic children.

More recent efforts to manage aggressive and self-injurious behaviors have emphasized a more positive approach. This new emphasis is certainly more humane and also easier to implement (Mesibov, 1983).

Favell (1983) argues for more comprehensive treatment approaches, emphasizing environmental enrichment as opposed to behavioral suppression. Rincover's (1978) *sensory extinction approach*, based on the notion that self-stimulatory behavior is maintained by its sensory consequences, is another less aversive and potentially useful technique. For example, a boy who punches himself might be fitted with heavy boxing gloves to muffle the blows. In this study, Rincover identified the stimulation that two children were receiving through their self-stimulatory behaviors and eliminated it. As a result, the self-injurious behaviors of these children decreased significantly. Rincover argues this is a most effective way of decreasing inappropriate behaviors and a good way of generating potent reinforcers for more appropriate behaviors. Finally, a recent study suggests that physical exercise might also be an effective way of decreasing self-stimulatory behaviors (Watters & Watters, 1980). Implementing an eight to ten minute daily jogging session significantly decreased the self-stimulatory behaviors in a group of autistic boys.

Special education programs designed specifically for autistic children have also emphasized behavioral intervention techniques. It has always been difficult to assess the effectiveness of any specialized services for autistic children because of their great diversity and the low incidence of the disorder (Bartak, 1978). Most of the early evaluative studies suffered from major methodological shortcomings, making them extremely difficult to evaluate (Yule & Berger, 1972). Bartak and Rutter (1973) assessed their behaviorally-oriented special education interventions as part of their Maudsley study. Their data suggest that autistic children make progress in intensive, behaviorally-oriented, individualized educational programs. There also appears to be a positive correlation between the degree of organization and structure and the amount of progress.

Lansing & Schopler (1978) also advocate a behaviorally-oriented special education program adapted for individual use. In addition, they argue for the involvement of parents in the learning process to promote the transfer of learning from the classroom to the home. In the North Carolina statewide program (TEACCH), they developed organizational structures designed to maximize individualization and generalization. Individualization is facilitated by the direct evaluation of children using the Psychoeducational Profile (1979), which was developed by the program to assess the needs and skills of autistic children. The strength of this measure is the ease with which assessment data can be translated into individualized teaching objectives. Generalization of acquired skills to the home environment is facilitated through the involvement of parents as cotherapists for their autistic children (Schopler & Reichler, 1971). The TEACCH program features five treatment centers around the state of North Carolina where parents are trained to work with their autistic children.

Autistic children seem to need a high degree of structure. Schopler et al. (1971), using a variety of measures, demonstrated more favorable responses in structured as compared to unstructured settings. The educational evaluation program (Bartak, 1978) in the Maudsley study found the most successful curriculum to be the one that had the most structure. More recently, Ferrara and Hill (1980) compared the social responsiveness of autistic children in predictable as compared with unpredictable environments. They found that these children could develop expectancies from environmental events if these events were also found to be more responsive to environmental events. Clark and Rutter (1981) also found positive effects with increasing structure. They exposed ten autistic children to different teaching styles, varying in the extent to which structure was provided. When adequate structure was not provided, autistic behavior patterns and inappropriate interpersonal behaviors appeared to increase.

In addition to identifying conditions that facilitate learning in autistic children, behavioral techniques have also been utilized to teach specific skills more effectively. Operant conditioning has been one of the most common methods used by clinicians to increase language in autistic children (Lovaas, Berberich, et al., 1966; Schell, Stark, & Giddan, 1967; Sloane & MacAulay, 1968). By using techniques such as prompting, modeling, and contingent reinforcement, clinicians have attempted not only to increase a child's vocabulary and the frequency of utterances (Jellis & Grainger, 1975), but also to increase the syntactical complexity of children's speech (Wheeler & Sulzer, 1970; Long & Rasmussen, 1974; Howlin, 1980).

Howlin (1981) reviewed 150 studies of the effectiveness of operant conditioning as a language intervention for autistic children. She noted that children showed highly variable responses to treatment, and that length and intensity of the treatment program were not necessarily predictive of outcome measures. Two factors which do appear to relate to outcome are the age at which therapy commences, and the initial language level of the child. Howlin (1979) found that age at which treatment begins is most critical for children with echolalic speech. Based on findings from 70 studies involving 125 children, she reported that all echolalic children below age five years developed useful phrase speech. Eighty-three percent of the echolalic children who began treatment between five and ten years of age developed phrase speech, and only 66 percent of those children who began treatment after ten years of age did so. The effect of age for children with lower language ability was not as evident.

According to Howlin's review of past outcome research, language level prior to treatment is the most powerful predictor of effectiveness of behavioral treatment. In her own research, Howlin (1980) found that children at the single-word level benefited most from treatment, whereas noncommunicative children made very slow progress. Echolalic children eventually developed phrase speech regardless of whether they received treatment. Howlin concluded that operant conditioning methods were most effective for helping children to use prerequisite skills more frequently and effectively. Using these techniques to increase the syntactical complexity of autistic children's language was a much slower process. The rarity with which behavioral programs result in the use of spontaneous, creative, rule-governed speech which can be generalized to new settings has been a major criticism of this approach (Bonvillian, Nelson, & Rhyne, 1981).

Recently, many clinicians have been using sign language as an alternative to, or in conjunction with, traditional oral training methods (De Villiers & Naughton, 1974; Bonvillian & Nelson, 1976; Offir, 1976; Salvin et al., 1977). Sign language may be particularly appropriate for autistic children who have little or no expressive speech since these children appear to be least responsive to behavioral approaches. Barrera, Lobato-Barrera, and Sulzer-Azaroff (1980) compared the relative effectiveness of three different training methods: signing, signing combined with oral input (total communication), and oral training alone, for teaching expressive speech to a four-and-one-half year-old mute autistic child. The total communication method proved to be most effective. Based on their review of twenty studies on sign language involving about 100 autistic children, Bonvillian, Nelson, and Rhyne (1981) also concluded that sign language can be an effective way of teaching communication skills for even low-functioning autistic children. They noted that almost every child acquired the ability to comprehend trained signs, and the large majority were able to produce five or more signs. Moreover, for many of these children, operant speech training had proven unsuccessful.

While it seems clear that sign language can be helpful to many autistic children, it is likely that its effectiveness is as limited by the cognitive and social impairments of autistic children as are the other therapeutic approaches. For example, compared to deaf children, the rate of acquisition of signs is much slower. In fact, early learning may be very slow until the autistic child acquires the cognitive understanding that objects and actions have labels (Carr et al., 1978). While many autistic children are able to eventually acquire sign labels and even early sign combinations, most children do not progress to long and complex signed utterances (Bonvillian, Nelson, & Rhyne, 1981.)

As language theorists have begun to recognize the importance of preverbal development to the acquisition of language (Bruner, 1975; Bates, 1976), so have they begun to incorporate prelinguistic skills into their intervention strategies. As mentioned earlier, Seibert and Oller (1981) suggested assessing early communicative competencies, such as the ability to gain and sustain another's attention, as a beginning point for therapy. Moreover, they stressed the need for evaluating each child's individual interactive style in natural situations in which spontaneous communicative behaviors are likely to be observed. Several authors (Bonvillian, Nelson, & Rhyne, 1981; Schaeffer, 1978) suggest that communication may be more readily facilitated if teaching occurs in natural environments and is made relevant to the interests or desires of the child. In this context, communication, in itself, should be reinforcing (Yoder & Calculator, 1981).

Finally, behavioral approaches to teaching educational skills have also focused on methods for presenting academic materials to autistic children (Dunlap & Koegel, 1980). Investigators have reduced stimulus overselectivity in autistic children, manipulated the rate of instructional delivery and learning, and varied tasks to improve discrimination and motivation.

The issue of stimulus overselectivity has received considerable attention (Lovaas & Schreibman, 1971; Reynolds, Newsom, & Lovaas, 1974; Schreibman & Lovaas, 1973). *Stimulus overselectivity* refers to the fact that autistic children often respond to one component out of a complex stimulus array and perhaps not the most relevant one. Dunlap and Koegel (1980) minimized the effects of this difficulty by modifying the task requirements. In presenting a complex stimulus they required the children to verbally label the cues that were presented. This seemed to sensitize the youngsters to more aspects of the stimulus situation and to decrease the possibility of overselectivity producing an incorrect response.

A second way of improving learning is by varying the rate of instructional delivery. Speed of presentation is manipulated by varying the *intertrial interval* (ITI) or the duration between trials. In general, with autistic children the shorter the ITI, the more effective the learning (Koegel, Dunlap, & Dyer, 1980); more rapid and frequent presentations of learning tasks result in more effective learning.

A third aspect of instructional presentation that has received considerable attention has been the varying of task instructions to improve discrimination ability. Although the great difficulty that autistic children have in dealing with change leads many investigators to make learning situations as standardized as possible, recent evidence suggests that this can lead to boredom and reduced motivation (Dunlap & Koegel, 1980). In one study learning was facilitated by simply substituting coins for blocks as a part of the stimulus array. Similar strategies might not only increase motivation but also facilitate the generalization of learned responses which is so difficult with autistic children.

Schizophrenia in Childhood and Adolescence

Case Illustration: When about nine years old, this young girl's parents noticed that she was becoming increasingly isolated. She would often exhibit extreme rage reactions and self-destructive behavior, such as scratching her own hand. During one of her tantrums, she bit her mother's hand to the point of bleeding. During the next few years, she became more withdrawn, had many fears, and frequently had nightmares.

By the time she was admitted for psychiatric evaluation, her speech had become disconnected, unrelated to ongoing conversation, and distinctly bizarre. She often seemed to be talking to imaginary characters and made frequent references to crocodiles biting her. Some of her spontaneous remarks were: "I have to hide from the crocodiles," "I'm missing my eyebrows because the crocodile bit them," "People do bad things like kicking, yelling, opening curtains, sobbing, bobbing, and hitting. That's what God likes us to do; start fresh learn new things." At times, she would giggle or laugh uncontrollably, even when unhappy events were being discussed. Conversely, she would often express pronounced hostility when discussing pleasant or innocuous events. Her self-injurious behavior had become more severe. She often scratched her hand to the point of producing abrasions, and bent her fingers back quite vigorously. She also had episodes of pronounced destructive behavior. For example, while playing quietly with a toy dollhouse, she suddenly began ripping pictures off the wall of the psychologist's office. At times like this, she was unresponsive to verbal input and had to be physically restrained.

Her parents complained that she was so anxious and fearful of new situations that she no longer could accompany them to the grocery store. She had many compulsive rituals, such as wearing a certain necklace when she took a bath, and would become extremely anxious if these were disturbed. Her bizarre behavior and self-preoccupation interfered greatly with her teachers' attempts to instruct her. The diagnosis was schizophrenia.

Case Illustration: This young boy's mother had not noticed any unusual behavior until preschool when his teachers remarked that he had poor fine motor control and articulation difficulties, and he tended to prefer being alone. By first grade, he had become excessively nervous and irritable, and increasingly solitary at home and school.

At eight years of age, he was admitted to a psychiatric hospital for evaluation. His mother's main concern was that he had developed "nervous tics" during the past year. These included grimacing, grunting, and making high-pitched squeaky noises. He was socially ostracized at school because of his odd mannerisms and inflexibility in play situations. His mother claimed that he was content to play by himself and that his play behavior tended to be repetitive and stereotyped, such as lining up cars in a row. His speech also tended to be repetitive. He would often express one idea such as, "I want to go swimming," repeatedly for days. Further, his speech had an atonal quality. When he was even mildly frustrated, such as having to wait for a late dinner, he often became extremely agitated. At these times, he would start yelling and his speech became disorganized and unintelligible. In general, he initiated little social contact with peers or adults.

Psychological testing indicated that this boy was of normal intellectual ability but that he had a number of difficulties related to speech. He showed no evidence of hallucinations or delusions. In fact, he tended to be overly concrete and unimaginative when making perceptual judgments. The diagnosis was childhood onset pervasive developmental disorder.

Background

According to DSM-III when the onset of symptoms similar to those of infantile autism occurs after the child is thirty months old and before twelve years of age, the diagnosis of childhood onset pervasive developmental disorder should be made. However, if a child within this age range exhibits hallucinations or delusions, or if an older child meets the appropriate diagnostic criteria, a form of schizophrenia should be diagnosed. Among the symptoms which overlap among all these very serious disorders are: verbal incoherence; seriously impaired interpersonal relations; disturbances in thought processes; cognitive deficits; and inappropriate or blunted affect. The symptoms that DSM-III identifies as peculiar to schizophrenia, at least in this context since it is possible to have drug-induced disorders of this kind, are: delusions, usually patently absurd or bizarre; hallucinations, usually auditory; and catatonic or extremely disorganized behavior. Evidence of some of these symptoms must be present for at least six months and they must constitute a definite deterioration in functioning from a previous level in order for schizophrenia to be diagnosed.

Although poor interpersonal relationships are an important aspect of schizophrenia, they do not represent the central defining characteristic as in autism. In his sample, Kolvin (1971b) found that only half of the children diagnosed as schizophrenic mixed poorly or avoided contact with adults or other children. Although all schizophrenic children do not have profoundly withdrawn interpersonal difficulties, many do stare blankly and unexpressively, and show sudden uncontrolled bursts of anger and assaultiveness both toward themselves and others (Knopf, 1979). It is the presence of hallucinations or delusions that DSM-III makes crucial for the diagnosis of schizophrenia in childhood.

Motor difficulties frequently include bizarre body movements such as whirling, rocking, head banging, rigid posturing, twitching, hand movements, and facial grimacing. Movement abnormalities were present in 18 percent of Kolvin's sample. Bender (1955) proposed that certain physiological differences predispose schizophrenic children toward "whirling": have a child close the eyes and extend the arms; turn the child's head to the side; a schizophrenic child frequently turns the body in line with the moving head, while a nonschizophrenic child generally maintains the body in the same position.

Disturbances in thought processes and affect are similar to those in adult schizophrenia. While auditory hallucinations have been observed in both children and adults (Kolvin, 1971b), the incidence of visual hallucinations is generally higher in children (Eggers, 1978; Kolvin, 1971a). Kolvin (1971b) has also documented the following mood abnormalities in children with schizophrenia: inappropriate giggling, incongruity, blunting of affect, perplexity, rages, self-directed aggression, and ambivalence.

Kolvin, Humphrey, and McNay (1971) have also found clear evidence that IQ scores of schizophrenic children are lower than average, averaging about one standard deviation below the mean. Only half their sample had IQ scores in the normal range. Other investigators have replicated this finding. In reviewing the literature between 1937 and 1965, Pollack (1967) found that at least one-third of the children had IQ scores below 80. A more recent study cites this figure as one-half

(Walker & Birch, 1974). As with most conditions, those schizophrenic children with above-average IQs were more likely to have favorable outcomes; the reverse was true for children of below-average intellectual ability (Eggers, 1978).

Although not as severe as in autism, language disturbances are still a prominent aspect of schizophrenia in childhood. Although some schizophrenic children are mute, most possess adequate language, even though many do not use it to communicate. Schizophrenic children are frequently echolalic, use words in bizarre combinations, and establish highly idiosyncratic meanings for words and sentences. In addition, their communication frequently fails to convey their feelings or thoughts.

Physiological disturbances are also more frequent in children with schizophrenia than in other populations. Bender (1955) found these children to show an upset in normal rhythms which disturbed eating and sleeping patterns. Similar disturbances have been found in bladder and/or bowel control and activity level (Knopf, 1979).

The prevalence of schizophrenia in childhood is unknown with DSM-III, but it is probably more common than infantile autism. Kolvin (1971a) found a predominance of boys with this disorder; the sex ratio in his sample was 2.6:1, which is lower than is typically found with autism. This ratio is similar to that reported by Loew (1966) and Kallman and Roth (1956). Age of onset is prescribed as at least after thirty months and certainly after twelve years. Most children in Kolvin's (1971a) sample were not recognized as clearly schizophrenic until seven years of age or older. Eggers (1978) found that children who were identified before the age of ten were more likely to have a chronic rather than an acute course and were less likely to have an eventual remission. Kolvin (1971a) and Eggers (1978) both reported that at early ages the onset is usually insidious rather than acute.

Differential Diagnosis

There are several features distinguishing schizophrenia in childhood from infantile autism. First is the different age of onset of autism as compared with schizophrenia and the presence of delusions and hallucinations in the latter, but not the former. Second are family history and intellectual differences, with autism less commonly occurring in families and generally accompanied by lower IQs (Kolvin et al., 1971c). Third, remissions and relapses are much more characteristic of schizophrenia than autism (Rutter, 1968), and autistic individuals rarely develop delusions and hallucinations during adulthood (Rutter, 1970). Fourth, there is greater evidence of cerebral dysfunction in autistic as compared with schizophrenic clients, including seizures and the association of autism with known neurological conditions such as tuberous sclerosis and phenyleketonuria (Dalldorf & Schopler, 1981). Finally, whereas schizophrenia frequently represents a withdrawal from social relationships, autistic children seem unable to form these relationships in the first place.

Etiology

The specific cause of schizophrenia has not been determined. Nevertheless progress has been made in determining some important contributing factors, with most of the research focusing on organic, genetic, and environmental determinants.

Organic Factors. Although many investigators argue that schizophrenia is organically based, no consistent organic deficit has yet been found (Davison & Neale, 1974). This is true with children as well as with adults.

There is evidence that pregnancy and birth complications are more common in children with schizophrenia than normal controls. Kolvin (1971a) found these complications in 12 percent of his sample. Mednick (1970) also found a high incidence of pregnancy and delivery complications in his longitudinal sample. He suggests that these complications interfere with the control of the body's stress-response mechanism, which increases avoidance responses, and results in schizophrenic behaviors if other predispositional factors are present. Goldfarb (1970), based on an extensive review of the literature, agrees that there is considerable evidence of some central nervous system impairment.

Biochemical studies, which have been suggestive with schizophrenic adults (Himwich et al., 1972; Narasimachri & Himwich, 1975), have unfortunately been less consistent with children. The few existing studies of schizophrenic children have found no differences in the uptake rates of serotonin by platelets of normal, autistic, or schizophrenic children (Lucas, Rause, & Domino, 1971; Siva-Sankar, 1970). More research on biochemical factors in schizophrenic children is obviously needed.

Genetic and Environmental Factors. To date, most of the research on genetic factors in schizophrenia has focused on adults. The one major study with pre-adolescents found concordance rates of 71 percent for monozygotic twins and 17 percent for dizygotic twins (Kallman & Roth, 1956). These data are consistent with the results obtained for adults and strongly suggest that the genetic data is applicable to both populations.

The increased incidence of schizophrenia in families of schizophrenic patients, estimated to occur in about 11 percent of parents and siblings of schizophrenic individuals (Essen-Moller, 1955), has led investigators to search for a genetic cause for the disorder. The concordance rate for monozygotic twins in which at least one twin was affected is significantly higher than that for dizygotic twins, ranging from 50–80 percent concordance (Gottesman & Shields, 1966; Kallman, 1946; Kringlen, 1967; Rosenthal, 1959; Slater, 1953). The most compelling evidence for a genetic basis comes from a series of Scandinavian studies in which children who were adopted at an early age and who were born of schizophrenic mothers continued to show an increased rate of schizophrenia or other personality disorders (Rosenthal & Kety, 1968).

It is now generally agreed that a genetic predisposition is a necessary but not sufficient condition for schizophrenia. The fact that only one-half of the monozygotic twins are concordant for the disorder indicates that other factors, such as prenatal or perinatal complications and/or environmental stresses during childhood, contribute to the development of schizophrenia. In support of environmental influences, Kringlen (1967) found that concordant twins tended to be raised in more similar environments characterized by less social contact with other children, closer relationships between the twins, and more overprotection by the parents than the environments of discordant twins.

MacSweeney (1970), Pollin and Stabenau (1968) and Medick et al. (1971) found that, in discordant pairs, the schizophrenic twin tended to weigh less at birth, and was more likely to have feeding, sleeping, and other physiological problems during early infancy. However, these findings have not been substantiated in other studies (Kringlen, 1967; Shields, 1968). Several studies of disconcordant twins have reported that personality differences between the twins were apparent from early childhood (Kringlen, 1967; Pollin & Stabenau, 1968; Tienari, 1968). Typically the affected twin was found to be more submissive, fearful, and dependent than the non-affected co-twin.

The question of to what degree, if any, the family environment is a factor in the development of schizophrenia is a difficult one to resolve. The incidence of psychiatric illness is higher in parents of schizophrenic children, which could influence the genetics and the quality of childrearing the child receives. Kolvin, Garside, and Kidd (1971) found that mothers of schizophrenic children tend to be more introverted, sensitive and suspicious than the average. A "disturbed family atmosphere" was reported in thirty-three of the fifty-seven schizophrenic children studied by Eggers (1978). However, family environment did not prove to be of prognostic value and in twenty-four cases, the environment was assessed as normal.

While certain investigators (Singer & Wynne, 1965; Waxler & Mishler, 1970; Wynne, 1968) have documented disturbed communication patterns in families of schizophrenic children, attempts to replicate these findings have failed (Hirsch & Leff, 1971). Also, it is possible that these faulty communication patterns could have developed *in response* to the disturbed child, which is supported by the tendency for the poor communication style to be directed only toward the affected child and not his/her siblings.

It is likely that schizophrenia is the result of a complex interaction between genetic, intrauterine and possibly family factors. There is good evidence that when a constitutional predisposition for schizophrenia exists, environmental factors can play a significant role in the precipitation of schizophrenia. The onset of the disorder and subsequent relapses are often related to significant emotional stresses a person has experienced (Birley & Brown, 1970; Eggers, 1978; Kolvin, 1971a).

Treatment

The prognosis for complete recovery from schizophrenia in childhood is thought to be poor (e.g. Fish, 1971; Rutter, 1967). In a long-term follow-up study of fifty-seven cases, Eggers (1978) found that 20 percent had complete remissions, 30 percent reached a relatively good social adjustment, and 50 percent had a moderate to poor outcome. Early age of onset (below ten years), personality disturbances such as shyness and introversion, and below average intelligence were predictive of poor outcome. Interestingly, family environment and family incidence of schizophrenia were not related to prognosis.

Treatment has generally consisted of a combined approach involving behavioral management, special education, social skills training, individual and family psychotherapy, and drug therapy. Kolvin (1972) and others (Campbell, Shapiro, & Floyd, 1970; Englehardt et al., 1973) have found phenothiazines to be helpful in some cases. However, carefully controlled drug outcome studies are lacking.

Fish (1976) advocates a preventative approach. Her approach to prevention would include:

1. Early identification of high risk or vulnerable infants

2. Stimulation or compensation for development in the areas in which the infant is lacking
3. Remedial help for language and perceptual motor problems
4. Supervision and support to families

Fish and her co-workers (Fish & Shapiro, 1965; Fish et al., 1966, 1968) have found response to treatment and long-term outcome depend upon the severity of the initial developmental impairments. Yet, they reported even the most severely disturbed children could be helped to develop without overt psychosis when treatment was comprehensive and began at an early age.

Individual therapy generally focuses on establishing some form of positive relationship with the child. Because most psychodynamic theories of schizophrenia in childhood view parents as primary causal agents, the establishment of this relationship is generally done by someone outside the family, either the therapist or a housemanager in a residential program. Play and interview techniques are utilized and interpretation of symbolic meanings is stressed. In addition to attempts at establishing positive relationships, attempts are made to reactivate the delayed psychosexual stages.

Goldfarb, Mintz, and Strook (1969) see a residential environment as necessary for corrective socialization. The role of adults in these settings is to clarify confusion, point out reality, and model coping and adaptation skills. If successful, this environment develops self-awareness, identity, and individuality in the schizophrenic children.

Ruttenberg (1971) has described a day treatment program. The goal was to establish a relationship between the psychotic children and a warm and sensitive adult. According to Ruttenberg, this relationship establishes the basis for a child's sense of trust, individuation, and eventual entrance into the adult world. The relationship is fostered by encouraging one-to-one interaction in a small cubicle where the child and caretaker can be alone. This cubicle is consistent and provides a safe retreat from the confusion of the everyday world.

Childhood Onset Pervasive Developmental Disorder

Based on findings from a comprehensive epidemiological study in which 163 children with "difficulties in communication, poor social interaction, or repetitive, stereotyped behavior" were evaluated, Wing (1981) concluded that the syndrome of early infantile autism orginally described by Kanner (1943) was somewhat arbitrary. The abnormalities which most consistently occurred together were impairments in social interaction, communication, and imaginative activities, without regard to an onset from birth. Children falling into this broader framework showed varying degrees of social and intellectual impairment.

The existence of "autistic-like" children led to a new diagnostic category, namely, childhood onset pervasive developmental disorder. This disorder differs from infantile autism in several ways: age of onset is after thirty months; an impairment in social relationships is present, but does not necessarily take the form of a lack of responsiveness; the language deficit may be less severe or different in nature; and motor abnormalities and other behavioral oddities are more common. This diagnostic category was created by the DSM-III Task Force to account for a very heterogeneous group of children who are neither clearly autistic nor schizophrenic, but fall into the overall group of pervasive developmental disorder (Dennis Cantell, personal communication). This heterogeneous group of children with multiple psychological impairments has yet to be clearly described and understood. Moreover, an informal survey of clinicians in child in-patient settings suggests that the diagnostic category childhood onset pervasive developmental disorder is not being used very frequently. Whether this will prove to be just another logical but not very useful diagnostic category is not yet known.

Schizotypal Personality Disorder

The concepts of borderline and schizotypal personality disorders have been marked by confusion, imprecision, and lack of clarity. As Spitzer, Endicott, and Gibbon have written, "Some believed that the borderline concept represents everything that is wrong with American psychiatry because of the confused way in which the term has been used, the heavy reliance in the borderline literature on metapsychological concepts, and the relative paucity of hard data regarding the usefulness (validity) of the concept" (1979, p. 17). The situation becomes even more complex when considering preadolescent children because the question of how applicable the schizotypal syndrome is to this population is still unresolved. Therefore, the focus of this section will be on presenting the concept as it is currently used and speculating as to its appropriateness for explaining certain conditions of childhood.

The term *borderline* was introduced by Knight (1953) to describe those patients who could not be classified as either psychotic or neurotic. Although the term had been used earlier (Stern, 1938), Knight's was the first reasonable approximation of the modern-day usage. Others had referred to this condition as ambulatory schizophrenia (Zilboorg, 1941) latent schizophrenia (Federn, 1952), and pseudoneurotic schizophrenia (Dunaif & Hoch, 1955).

Although the term *borderline* is now generally accepted, there still exists considerable disagreement over its definition. The two most common uses are: to categorize a constellation of neurotic and psychotic personality features, though the individual is not regarded as psychotic; or to describe a constellation of characteristics that seem related to chronic schizophrenia. Because the former concept, relating to personality disorder, appears more relevant to those interested in the childhood psychoses, that meaning is involved in the DSM-III diagnostic category of schizotypal, which is to be used instead of borderline for children and adolescents meeting four of these criteria for the disorder: magical thinking; ideas of reference; socially withdrawn; odd speech; recurrent illusions, such as sensing the presence of a person; depersonalization, or derealization; inadequate rapport due to constricted or inappropriate affect; suspiciousness; and undue social anxiety or hypersensitivity to criticism.

Since this is a new diagnostic category there has been little research on schizotypal personality and the discussion must draw from the clinical impressions of borderline children.

Case Illustration: At the age of twelve Ron was found to be functioning in the low normal range on the WISC–R. He was not particularly cooperative during the testing, lashing out at the examiner in anger at one point and later being extremely pleasant and ingratiating. On the Rorschach his performance deteriorated considerably. Ron was totally unable and unwilling to complete this test, giggling inappropriately at times and running around the room.

Ron's motor behavior during testing was excessive and unusual. At times he seemed quite immature or inappropriate, such as when he kissed the examiner's hand and put his arm around her shoulder. He also ran to the window, looked in the mirror, and lay on the floor.

Ron's mother was depressed and isolated. She was overly enmeshed with Ron and had great difficulty letting him grow up, or be independent and autonomous. Ron alternated between accepting this seeming infantilization and exploding in anger. He appeared to be extremely anxious and generally unhappy. He also appeared quite immature and had no friends to play with. The diagnostic impression was of a schizotypal personality disorder.

Differential Diagnosis

In general, the major diagnostic issues are to differentiate schizotypal children from those who are schizophrenic and severely anxious. There are several characteristics that tend to differentiate these disorders. First, most schizotypal children are thought to function adequately on more objective assessment instruments such as the WISC–R. Their performance only deteriorates in the absence of external structure as is generally seen on the Rorschach. This discrepancy between their functioning on these two assessment instruments is one characteristic that has been identified.

A second distinguishing characteristic is that manipulation and intense dependence more frequently characterize the interpersonal relationships of schizotypal children. This is in contrast to the more socially isolated and withdrawn behavior of children with schizophrenia. Finally, psychotic episodes, when they occur in schizotypal children, seem brief and related to stress. These are not pervasive as in schizophrenic children.

Etiology

In adults, there seems to be general agreement that the borderline personality disorder results from an incomplete development of internalized representations of self. These are generally attributed to an arrest in psychological development (Masterson, 1976). According to Kernberg (1972), inaccurate personal representations (self-image) would occur in schizotypal children because they, biologically, have an excess of aggressive impulses which make positive integration difficult to achieve. Mahler, Pine, and Bergman (1975) also recognized the existence of aggressive impulses but view a pathological mother-child relationship during the period of separation-individuation as even more significant. Specifically, the mother, who they find is often borderline herself, does not perceive the developing child as being separate from herself. For this reason, she consistently fosters an unhealthy degree of dependency in the child and hinders the normal separation-individuation process.

Although other investigators differ in how they think this developmental arrest occurs, most agree that the outcome of this arrest is an individual who is cognitively aware of differences between self and nonself but affectively unable to make a complete separation from others or to integrate representations of good and bad. Although most of the theorizing relates to adults, similar processes are postulated in children.

More recently, a rival hypothesis concerning etiology in children has been proposed. Examining the referrals for a full diagnostic evaluation at a major teaching hospital in-patient setting over an eighteen month period, Gualtieri, Koriath, and Van Bourgondien (1981) reviewed the records of the sixteen children who had been referred with the diagnosis of borderline. In this sample, the children were found to be multiply handicapped with combinations of intellectual, cognitive, linguistic, attentional, perceptual, and motor difficulties. These often occurred in the context of a severely disorganized home situation. Moreover, these cognitive and behavioral peculiarities were understandable in terms of the developmental handicaps and difficult life situations the children presented. The conclusion of this study is that in many cases the borderline or schizotypal syndrome results more from developmental handicaps than from psychosocial factors. This hypothesis is certainly worthy of further investigation, especially when one considers the importance of a similar theory for the current understanding of infantile autism.

Treatment

Treatment is similar to that described under childhood schizophrenia. However, there are several modifications to accommodate the differences between this disorder and schizophrenia. Medication is not frequently used with young children, but when drugs are prescribed, the neuroleptics (e.g. Mellaril), or even lithium, might be considered. Lithium would be more likely for those children evidencing wide mood swings or severe aggressive and/or self-destructive behaviors.

In working with these children, it would be important to avoid either underestimating or overestimating their potential. One characteristic of schizotypal children is the wide variation between their abilities and the performance of various skills. For example, although they often appear to have good intellectual ability, they rarely perform at that level in school.

A final implication of this diagnosis would be that social learning programs might be needed in conjunction with more insight-oriented therapeutic approaches. Since most of the difficulties of borderline personalities involve their interactions with others, these would probably need more direct interventions.

If one accepts the hypothesis of Gualtieri et al. (1981) and views most borderline personalities as resulting from developmental handicaps, the treatment implications are quite different. Viewing the schizotypal personality as a developmental handicap would make most of the biological and insight-oriented treatment approaches to childhood schizophrenia much less relevant. In these instances, the psychoeducational approaches discussed under the topic of autism would be much more productive.

REFERENCES

Adams, R. L., & Jenkins, R. L. Basic principles of the neuropsychological examination. In C. E. Walker (Ed.), *Clinical practice of psychology.* New York: Pergamon, 1981.

Anthony, J. An experimental approach to the psychopathology of childhood: Autism. *British Journal of Medical Psychology,* 1958, *31,* 211–215.

Ball, J. *A pragmatic analysis of autistic children's lan-*

guage with respect to aphasic and normal language development. Unpublished doctoral dissertation, Melbourne University, 1978.

Baltaxe, C. A. Pragmatic deficits in the language of autistic adolescents. *Journal of Pediatric Psychology,* 1977, *2,* 176–180.

Baltaxe, C. A., & Simmons, J. Q. Language in childhood psychosis: A review. *Journal of Speech and Hearing Disorders,* 1975, *30,* 439–458.

Barrera, R. D., Lobato-Barrera, D., & Sulzer-Azaroff, B. A simultaneous treatment comparison of three expressive language training programs with a mute autistic child. *Journal of Autism and Developmental Disorders,* 1980, *10,* 21–37.

Bartak, L. Educational approaches. In M. Rutter and E. Schopler (Eds.), *Autism: A reappraisal of concepts and treatment.* New York: Plenum, 1978.

Bartak, L., & Pickering, C. Aims and methods of teaching. In M. P. Everard (Ed.), *Some approaches to teaching autistic children.* Oxford: Pergamon, 1976.

Bartak, L., & Rutter, M. Educational treatment of autistic children. In M. Rutter (Ed.), *Infantile autism: Concepts, characteristics, and treatment.* London: Churchill, 1971.

Bartak, L., & Rutter, M. Special educational treatment of autistic children: A comparative study. I. Design of study and characteristics of units. *Journal of Child Psychology and Psychiatry,* 1973, *14,* 161–179.

Bartak, L., & Rutter M. Differences between mentally retarded and normally intelligent autistic children. *Journal of Autism and Childhood Schizophrenia,* 1976, *6,* 109-120.

Bartak, L., & Rutter, M. The use of personal pronouns by autistic children. *Journal of Autism and Childhood Schizophrenia,* 1974, *4,* 217–222.

Bartak, L., Rutter, M., & Cox A. A comparative study of infantile autism and specific developmental receptive language disorder. I. The children. *British Journal of Psychiatry,* 1975, *126,* 127-145.

Bartolucci, G., & Albers, R. J. Deitic categories in the language of autistic children. *Journal of Autism and Childhood Schizophrenia,* 1974, *4,* 131-141.

Bartolucci, G., & Pierce, S. J. A preliminary comparison of phonological development in autistic, normal, and mentally retarded subjects. *British Journal of Disorders of Communication,* 1977, *12,* 137–147.

Bartolucci, G., Pierce, S. J., Streiner, D., & Eppel, P. T. Phonological investigation of verbal autistic and mentally retarded subjects. *Journal of Autism and Childhood Schizophrenia,* 1976, *6,* 303–316.

Bates, E. Pragmatics and sociolinguistics in child language. In D. Morehead & A. Morehead (Eds.), *Normal and deficient child language.* Baltimore: University Park, 1976.

Bender, L. Twenty years of research on schizophrenic children with special reference to those under twenty years of age. In G. Kaplan (Ed.), *Emotional problems of early childhood.* New York: Basic Books, 1955.

Bettelheim, B. *The empty fortress: Infantile autism and the birth of the self.* New York: The Free Press, 1967.

Bettelheim, B. *A home for the heart.* New York: Knopf, 1974.

Birley, J. L. T., & Brown, G. W. Crisis and life changes preceding the onset or relapse of acute schizophrenia: Clinical aspects. *British Journal of Psychiatry,* 1970, *116,* 327–333.

Blackstock, E. G. Cerebral asymmetry and the development of infantile autism. *Journal of Autism and Childhood Schizophrenia,* 1978, *8,* 339–353.

Bleuler, E. *Dementia Praecox or the group of schizophrenias* (1911). New York: International Universities Press, 1950.

Bloom, L. *Language development: Form and function in emerging grammars.* Cambridge, MA: MIT Press, 1970.

Bonvillian, J. D., & Nelson, K. E. Sign language acquisition in a mute autistic boy. *Journal of Speech and Hearing Disorders, 1976,* **41,** *339–347.*

Bonvillian, J. D., Nelson, K. E., & Rhyne, J. M. Sign language and autism. *Journal of Autism and Developmental Disorders,* 1981, *11,* 125–138.

Boucher, J., & Warrington, E. K. Memory deficits in early infantile autism: Some similarities to the amnesic syndrome. *British Journal of Psychology,* 1976, *67,* 73–87.

Brask, B. H. The need for hospital beds for psychotic children. *Ugerkr Laeg,* 1967, *129,* 1559–1570.

Brown, J. L. Prognosis from presenting symptoms of preschool children with atypical development. *American Journal of Orthopsychiatry,* 1960, *30,* 382–390.

Brown, J. L. Follow-up of children with atypical development. *American Journal of Orthopsychiatry,* 1963, *33,* 855–861.

Bruner, J. S. From communication to language—A psychological perspective. *Cognition,* 1975, *3,* 255–287.

Campbell, M., Fish, B., David, R., Shapiro, T., Collins, P., & Koh, C. Response to triiodothyronine and dextroamphetamine: A study of preschool schizophrenic children. *Journal of Autism and Childhood Schizophrenia,* 1972, *2,* 343–358.

Campbell, M., Fish, B., Shapiro, T., & Floyd, A. Thiotnixene in young disturbed children. *Archives of General Psychiatry,* 1970, *23,* 70–72.

Campbell, M., Small, A., Collins, P., Friedman, E., David, R., & Genieser, N. Levodopa and levoamphetamine: A crossover study in young schizophrenic children. *Current Therapeutic Research,* 1976, *19,* 70–86.

Carr, E. G., Binkoff, J. A., Kologinsky, E., & Eddy, M. Acquisition of sign language by autistic children. I. Expressive labelling. *Journal of Applied Behavior Analysis,* 1978, *11,* 489-501.

Charney, R. Pronoun errors in autistic children: Support for a social explanation. *British Journal of Disorders in Communication,* 1980, 15, 39–43.

Chess, S. Autism in children with congenital rubella. *Journal of Autism and Childhood Schizophrenia,* 1971, *1,* 33–47.

Churchill, D. W. Effects of success and failure in psychotic children. *Archives of General Psychiatry,* 1971, *25,* 208–214.

Clark, E. From gesture to word: On the natural history of deixis in language acquisition. In J. S. Bruner & A. Garton (Eds.), *Human growth and development: Wolfson College lectures 1976.* Oxford: Clarendon Press, 1978.

Clark, P., & Rutter, M. Autistic children's responses to structure and to interpersonal demands. *Journal of Autism and Developmental Disorders,* 1981, *11,* 201–217.

Cohen, D. J., Caparulo, B. K., & Shaywitz, B. A. Neurochemical and developmental models of childhood autism. In G. Serban (Ed.), *Cognitive defects in the development of mental illness.* New York: Brunner/Mazel, 1978.

Cohen, D. J., Caparulo, B. K., Shaywitz, B. A., & Bowers, M. B., Jr. Dopamine and serotonin in neuropsychiatrically disturbed children: Cerebrospinal fluid homovanillic acid and 5-hydroxyindoleacetic acid. *Archives of General Psychiatry,* 1977, *34,* 561–567.

Cohen, D. J., Johnson, W. T., & Browers, M. B., Jr. Biogenic amines in autistic and atypical children: Cerebrospinal fluid measures of homovanillic acid and 5-hydroxyindoleacetic acid. *Archives of General Psychiatry,* 1974, *31,* 845–

Colbert, E. G., Koegler, R. R., & Markham, C. H. Vestibular dysfunction in childhood schizophrenia. *Archives of General Psychiatry,* 1959, *1,* 600–617.

Coleman, M. A report on the autistic syndromes. In M. Rutter & E. Schopler (Eds.), *Autism: A reappraisal of concepts and treatment.* New York: Plenum Press, 1978.

Cox, A., Rutter, M., Newman, S., & Bartak, L. A comparative study of infantile autism and specific developmental receptive language disorder: II. Parental characteristics. *British Journal of Psychiatry,* 1975, *126,* 146–159.

Creak, M. Childhood psychosis: A review of 100 cases. *British Journal of Psychiatry,* 1963, *109,* 84–89.

Creak, M., & Pampiglione, G. Clinical and EEG studies on a group of 35 psychotic children. *Developmental Medicine and Child Neurology,* 1969, *11,* 218–227.

Dalldorf, J. S., & Schopler, E. Diagnosis and management of autism. *Comprehensive Therapy,* 1981, *7,* 67–73.

Davison, G. C., & Neale, J. M. *Abnormal psychology: An experimental clinical approach.* New York: Wiley, 1974.

Dawson, G. D. *Early Infantile Autism and Hemispheric Specialization.* Unpublished doctoral dissertation. University of Washington, 1979.

Dawson. G., Warrenburg, S., & Fuller, P. Cerebral lateralization in individuals diagnosed as autistic in early childhood. *Brain and Language,* 1982, *15,* 353–368.

DeLong, G. R. A neuropsychological interpretation of infantile autism. In M. Rutter & E. Schopler (Eds.), *Autism: A reappraisal of concepts and treatment.* New York: Plenum Press, 1978.

DeMyer, M. K. Research in infantile autism: A strategy and its results. *Biological Psychiatry,* 1975, *10,* 433–450.

DeMyer, M. K., Alpern, G. D., Barton, S., DeMyer, W. E., Churchill, D. W., Hingtgen, J. N., Bryson, C. Q., Pontius, W., & Kimberlin, C. Imitation in autistic, early schizophrenic and non-psychotic subnormal children. *Journal of Autism and Childhood Schizophrenia,* 1972, *2,* 264–287.

DeMyer, M. K., Barton, S., Alpern, G. D., Kimberlin, C., Allen, J., Yang, E., & Steele, R. The measured intelligence of autistic children: A follow-up study. *Journal of Autism and Childhood Schizophrenia,* 1974, *4,* 42–60.

DeMyer, M. K., Barton, S., DeMyer, W. E., Norton, J. A., Allen, J., & Steele, R. Prognosis in autism: A follow-up study. *Journal of Autism and Childhood Schizophrenia,* 1973, *3,* 199–246.

DesLauriers, A. M. Play, symbols, and the development of language. In M. Rutter and E. Schopler (Eds.), *Autism: A reappraisal of concepts and treatment.* New York: Plenum, 1978.

Despert, J. L. Some considerations relating to the genesis of autistic behavior in children. *American Journal of Orthopsychiatry,* 1951, *21,* 335–350.

De Villiers, J. G., & Naughton, J. M. Teaching a symbol language to autistic children. *Journal of Con-*

sulting and Clinical Psychology, 1974, *42*, 111-117.

Deykin, E. Y., & MacMahon, B. The incidence of seizures among children with autistic symptoms. *American Journal of Psychiatry*, 1979, *136*, 1310–1312.

Dunaif, S., & Hoch, P. H. Pseudopsychopathic schizophrenia. In P. H. Hoch & J. Zubin (Eds.), *Psychiatry and the Law*. New York: Grune & Stratton, 1955.

Dunlap, G., & Koegel, R. L. Motivating autistic children through stimulus variation. *Journal of Applied Behavior Analysis*, 1980, *13*, 619–627.

Eggers, C. Course and prognosis of childhood schizophrenia. *Journal of Autism and Childhood Schizophrenia*, 1978, *8*, 21–36.

Eisenberg, L. The course of childhood schizophrenia. *Archives of Neurological Psychiatry*, 1957, *78*, 69–83.

Eisenberg, L., & Kanner, L. Early infantile autism. *American Journal of Orthopsychiatry*, 1956, *26*, 556-566.

Engelhardt, D. M., Polizos, P., Waizer, J., & Hoffman, S. P. A double-blind comparison of fluphenazine and haloperidol in out-patient schizophrenic children. *Journal of Autism and Childhood Schizophrenia*, 1973, *3*, 128–137.

Essen-Moller, E. The calculation of morbid risk in parents of index cases, as applied to a family sample of schizophrenics. *Acta Genetica et Statistica Medica (Basel)*, 1955, *5*, 334–342.

Favell, J. E. The management of aggressive behavior. In E. Schopler & G. B. Mesibov (Eds.), *Autism in adolescents and adults*. New York: Plenum, 1983.

Fay, W. On the basis of autistic echolalia. *Journal of Communication Disorders*, 1969, *2*, 38–47.

Fay, W. Personal pronouns and the autistic child. *Journal of Autism and Developmental Disorders*, 1979, *9*, 247–260.

Federn, P. *Ego psychology and the psychoses*. New York: Basic Books, 1952.

Ferrara, C., & Hill, S. D. The responsiveness of autistic children to the predictability of social and nonsocial toys. *Journal of Autism and Developmental Disorders*, 1980, *10*, 51–57.

Fish, B. Contributions of developmental research to a theory of schizophrenia. In J. Wellmath (Ed.), *Exceptional infant*, Vol. 2. New York: Brunner/Mazel, 1971.

Fish, B. An approach to prevention in infants at risk for schizophrenia. *Journal of Child Psychiatry*, 1976, *15*, 62–82.

Fish, B., & Shapiro, T. A typology of children's psychiatric disorders. *Journal of Child Psychiatry*, 1965, *4*, 32–52.

Fish, B., Shapiro, T., Campbell. M., & Wile, R. A classification of schizophrenic children under five years. *American Journal of Psychiatry*, 1968, *124*, 1415-1423.

Fish, B., Shapiro, T., & Campbell, M. Long-term prognosis and the response of schizophrenic children to drug therapy: A controlled study of trifluoperazine. *American Journal of Psychiatry*, 1966, *123*, 32–39.

Folstein, S., & Rutter, M. Genetic influences and infantile autism. *Nature*, 1977, *265*, 726–728.

Foxx, R., & Azrin, N. The elimination of autistic self-stimulatory behavior by overcorrection. *Journal of Applied Behavior Analysis*, 1973, *6*, 1–14.

Frith, U. Emphasis and meaning in recall in normal and autistic children. *Language and Speech*, 1969, *12*, 29–38.

Gillberg, C. Maternal age and infantile autism. *Journal of Autism and Developmental Disorders*, 1980, *10*, 293–297.

Gittelman, M., & Birch, H. G. Childhood schizophrenia: Intellect, neurological status, perinatal risk, prognosis and family pathology. *Archives of General Psychiatry*, 1967, *17*, 16–25.

Goldfarb, W. *Childhood schizophrenia*. Cambridge, MA: Harvard University Press, 1961.

Goldfarb, W. Childhood psychoses. In P. M. Mussen (Ed.) *Carmichael's manual of child psychology* (Vol. 2). New York: Wiley, 1970.

Goldfarb, W., Goldfarb, N., & Scholl, H. The speech of mothers of schizophrenic children. *American Journal of Psychiatry*, 1966, *122*, 1220-1227.

Goldfarb, W., Mintz, I., & Strook, K. *A time to heal*. New York: International Universities, 1969.

Gottesman, I. I., & Shields, J. Contributions of twin studies to perspectives on schizophrenia. In B. A. Maher (Ed.), *Progress in experimental personality* (Vol. 3). New York: Academic Press, 1966.

Greenbaum, G. H. An evaluation of niacinamide in the treatment of childhood schizophrenia. *American Journal of Psychiatry*, 1970, *127*, 129–132.

Gualtieri, C. T., Koriath, U., & Van Bourgondien, M. E. *"Borderline" children*. Paper presented at the meeting of the American Association of Psychiatric Services for Children, San Francisco, November 1981.

Gubbay, S. S., Lobaschen, M., & Kingerlee, P. A neurological appraisal of autistic children: Results of a Western Australian survey. *Developmental Medicine and Child Neurology*, 1970, *12*, 422–429.

Hermelin, B., & O'Connor, N. Measures of the occipital alpha rhythm in normal, subnormal and autistic children. *British Journal of Psychiatry*, 1968, *114*, 603–610.

Hermelin, B., & O'Connor, N. *Psychological experiments with autistic children.* Oxford: Pergamon, 1970.

Himwich, H., Jenkins, R., Fujimori, M., & Narasimachari, N. A biochemical study of early infantile autisms. *Journal of Autism and Childhood Schizophrenia,* 1972, *2,* 114–126.

Hinton, G. G. Childhood psychosis or mental retardation: A diagnostic dilemma. II. Pediatric and neurological aspects. *Canadian Medical Association Journal,* 1963, *87,* 1020–1024.

Hirsch, S. R., & Leff, J. P. Parental abnormalities of verbal communication in the transmission of schizophrenia. *Psychological Medicine,* 1971, *1,* 118–127.

Howlin, P. Training parents to modify the language of their autistic children: A home based approach. Unpublished doctoral dissertation, London University, 1979.

Howlin, P. Language training with the severely retarded. In W. Yule & J. Carr (Eds.), *Behavior modification with the severely retarded.* London: Croom Helm, 1980.

Howlin, P. A. The effectiveness of operant language training with autistic children. *Journal of Autism and Developmental Disorders,* 1981, *11,* 89–106.

Hutt, S. J., Hutt, C., Lee, D., & Ounsted, C. Arousal and childhood autism. *Nature,* 1964, *204,* 908–909.

Jellis, T., & Grainger, S. The back projection of kaleidoscopic patterns as a technique for electing verbalization in an autistic child. *British Journal of Disorders of Communication,* 1972, *7,* 157-162.

Kallmann, F. J. The genetic theory of schizophrenia: An analysis of 691 schizophrenic twin index families. *American Journal of Psychiatry,* 1946, *103,* 309–322.

Kallmann, F. J., & Roth, B. Genetic aspects of preadolescent schizophrenia. *American Journal of Psychiatry,* 1956, *112,* 599–606.

Kanner, L. Autistic disturbances of affective contact. *Nervous Child,* 1943, *2,* 217–250.

Kanner, L. Problems of nosology and psychodynamics of early infantile autism. *American Journal of Orthopsychiatry,* 1949, *19,* 416–426.

Kanner, L. *Child psychiatry,* (3d ed.). Springfield, IL: Thomas, 1957.

Kanner, L., & Eisenberg, L. Early infantile autism, 1943–1955. *American Journal of Orthopsychiatry,* 1956, *26,* 55–65.

Keeler, W. R. Autistic patterns and defective communication in blind children with retrolental fibroplasia. In P. H. Hoch & J. Zubin (Eds.), *Psychopathology of communication.* New York: Grune & Stratton, 1958.

Kernberg, O. F. Early ego integration and object relations. *Annals of the New York Academy of Sciences,* 1972, *193,* 233–247.

Knight, R. Borderline states. *Bulletin of the Menninger Clinic,* 1953, *17,* 1–12.

Knoblock, H., & Pasamanick, B. *Etiologic factors in "early infantile autism" and "childhood schizophrenia."* Presented at the 10th International Congress of Pediatrics. Lisbon, September 1962.

Knoblock, H., & Pasamanick, B. Some etiological and prognostic factors in early infantile autism and psychosis. *Pediatrics,* 1975, *55,* 182–191.

Knopf, I. J. *Childhood psychopathology: A developmental approach.* Englewood Cliffs, NJ: Prentice-Hall, 1979.

Koegel, R. L., Dunlap, G., & Dyer, K. Intertrial interval duration and learning in autistic children. *Journal of Applied Behavior Analysis,* 1980, *13,* 91–99.

Koegel, R. L., Rincover, A., & Engel, A. L. *Educating and understanding autistic children.* San Diego: College-Hill Press, 1982.

Kolvin, I. Psychoses in childhood - a comparative study. In M. Rutter (Ed.), *Infantile autism: Concepts, characteristics and treatment.* Edinburgh: Churchill Livingstone, 1971. (a)

Kolvin, I. Studies in childhood psychoses. I. Diagnostic criteria and classification. *British Journal of Psychiatry,* 1971, *118,* 381–384.(b)

Kolvin, I. Late onset psychoses. *British Medical Journal,* 1972, *3,* 816–817.

Kolvin, I., Garside, R. F., & Kidd, J. S. Studies in childhood psychoses. IV. Parental personality and attitude and childhood psychoses. *British Journal of Psychiatry,* 1971, *118,* 403–406.(a)

Kolvin, I., Humphrey, M., & McNay, A. Studies in childhood psychoses. VI. Cognitive factors in childhood psychoses. *British Journal of Psychiatry,* 1971, *118,* 415-419.(b)

Kolvin, I., Ounsted, C., & Roth, A. Studies in childhood psychoses. V. Cerebral dysfunction and childhood psychoses. *British Journal of Psychiatry,* 1971, *118,* 407–414.(c)

Kraepelin, E. *Lectures on clinical psychiatry.* New York: Hafner, 1904.

Kringlen, E. *Heredity and environment in the functional psychoses.* London: Heinemann, 1967.

Lansing, M. D., & Schopler, E. Individualized education: A public school model. In M. Rutter & E. Schopler (Eds.), *Autism: A reappraisal of concepts and treatment.* New York: Plenum Press, 1978.

Links, P. S., Stockwell, M., Abichandani, F., & Simeon, J. Minor physical anomalies in childhood autism. Part I. Their relationship to pre- and perinatal complications. *Journal of Autism and Developmental Disorders*, 1980, *10*, 273–285.

Lockyer, L., & Rutter, M. A five to fifteen year follow-up study of infantile psychosis. III. Psychological aspects. *British Journal of Psychiatry*, 1969, *115*, 865–882.

Lockyer, L., & Rutter, M. A five to fifteen year follow-up study of infantile psychosis: IV. Patterns of cognitive ability. *British Journal of Social and Clinical Psychology*, 1970, *9*, 152–163.

Loew, L. H. Families of children with early childhood schizophrenia. *Archives of General Psychiatry*, 1966, *14*, 26–30.

Long, J. S., & Rasmussen, M. The acquisition of simple and compound sentence structure in an autistic child. *Journal of Applied Behavior Analysis*, 1974, *7*, 473–479.

Lotter, V. Epidemiology of autistic conditions in young children. I. Prevalence. *Social Psychiatry*, 1966, *1*, 124–137.

Lotter, V. Factors related to outcome in autistic children. *Journal of Autism and Childhood Schizophrenia*, 1974, *4*, 263–277.

Lovaas, O. I., Berberich, J. P., Perloff, B. F., & Schaeffer, B. Acquistion of imitative speech by schizophrenic children. *Science*, 1966, *151*, 705-707.

Lovaas, O. I., Freitag, G., Kinder, M. I., Rubenstein, B. D., Schaeffer, B., & Simmons, J. O. Establishment of social reinforcers in two schizophrenic children on the basis of food. *Journal of Experimental Child Psychology*, 1966, *4*, 109-125.

Lovaas, O. I., & Newsom, C. D. Behavior modification with psychotic children. In H. Leitenberg (Ed.), *Handbook of behavior modification and behavior therapy*. Englewood Cliffs, NJ: Prentice-Hall, 1976.

Lovaas, O. I., Schaeffer, B., & Simmons, J. Q. Experimental studies in childhood schizophrenia: Building social behavior in autistic children by use of electric shock. *Journal of Experimental Research in Personality*, 1965, *1*, 99-109.

Lovaas, O. I., & Schreibman, L. Stimulus overselectivity of autistic children in a two-stimulus situation. *Behavior Research and Therapy*, 1971, *9*, 305–310.

Lovaas, O. I., Schreibman, L., & Koegel, R. L. A behavior modification approach to the treatment of autistic children. *Journal of Autism and Childhood Schizophrenia*, 1974, *4*, 111–129.

Lovaas, O. I., & Simmons, J. Q. Manipulation of self-destruction in three retarded children. *Journal of Applied Behavior Analysis*, 1969, *2*, 143–157.

Lucas, A., Krause, R., & Domino, E. Biological studies in childhood schizophrenia: Plasma and RBC cholinesterase activity. *Journal of Autism and Childhood Schizophrenia*, 1971, *1*, 172–181.

MacSweeney, D. A. A report on a pair of male MZ twins discordant for schizophrenia. *British Journal of Psychiatry*, 1970, *116*, 315–322.

Mahler, M. S., Pine, F., & Bergman, A. *The psychological birth of the human infant*. New York: Basic Books, 1975.

Masterson, J. F., *Psychotherapy of the borderline adult*. New York: Brunner/Mazel, 1976.

McNeill, D. Developmental psycholinguistics. In F. Smith & G. A. Miller (Eds.). *The genesis of language*. Cambridge, MA: MIT Press, 1966.

McNeill, D. *The acquisition of language*. New York: Harper & Row, 1970.

Mednick, S. A. Breakdown in individuals at high risk for schizophrenia: Possible predispositional perinatal factors. *Mental Hygiene*, 1970, *54*, 50–63.

Mednick, S. A., Mura, M., Schulzinger, F., & Mednick, B. Perinatal conditions and infant development in children with schizophrenic parents. *Social Biology*, 1971, *18*, 5103–5113.

Mesibov, G. B. Current perspectives and issues in autism and adolescence. In E. Schopler & G. B. Mesibov (Eds.), *Autism in adolescents and adults*. New York: Plenum, 1983.

Metz, J. R. Conditioning generalized imitation in autistic children. *Journal of Experimental Child Psychology*, 1965, *2*, 389–399.

Narasimachari, N., & Himwich, H. Biochemical study in early infantile autism. *Biological Psychiatry*, 1975, *10*, 425–432.

O'Connor, N., & Hermelin, B. Auditory and visual memory in autistic and normal children. *Journal of Mental Deficiency Research*, 1967, *11*, 126-131.(a)

O'Connor, N., & Hermelin, B. The selective visual attention of psychotic children. *Journal of Child Psychology and Psychiatry*, 1967, *8*, 167–179.(b)

Offir, C. W. Visual speech: Their fingers do the talking. *Psychology Today*, June 1976, 72-78.

Ornitz, E. M. Development of sleep patterns in autistic children. In C. D. Clemente, E. Purpura, F. Mayer (Eds.), *Sleep and the maturing nervous system*. New York: Academic Press, 1972.

Ornitz, E. M., Brown, M. B., Sorosky, A. D., Ritvo, E. R., & Dietrich, L. Environmental modification of autistic behavior. *Archives of General Psychiatry*, 1970, *22*, 560–565.

Ornitz, E. M., & Ritvo, E. R. Perceptual inconstancy in early infantile autism. *Archives of General Psychiatry*, 1968, *18*, 76–98.

Ornitz, E. M., & Ritvo, E. R. The syndrome of autism: A critical review. *American Journal of Psychiatry*, 1976, *133*, 609–621.

Ounsted, C. A biological approach to autistic and hyperkinetic syndromes. In J. Apley (Ed.), *Modern trends in pediatrics*. London: Butterworths, 1970.

Peterson, M. R., & Torrey, E. F. Viruses and other infectious agents as behavioral teratogens. In M. Coleman (Ed.), *The autistic syndromes*. New York: American Elsevier, 1976.

Pollack, M. Mental subnormality and "childhood schizophrenia." In J. Zubin & G. A. Jervis (Eds.), *Psychopathology of mental development*. New York: Grune and Stratton, 1967.

Pollack, M., & Krieger, H. P. Oculomotor and postural patterns in schizophrenic children. *Archives of Neurology and Psychiatry*, 1958, *79*, 720–726.

Pollin, W., & Stabenau, J. R. Biological, psychological, and historical differences in a series of MZ twins discordant for schizophrenia. In D. Rosenthal and S. S. Kety (Eds.), *The transmission of schizophrenia*. New York: Pergamon, 1968.

Potter, H. Schizophrenia in children. *American Journal of Psychiatry*, 1933, *12*, 1253–1268.

Prior, M. Developing concepts 6f childhood autism: the influence of experimental cognitive research. *Journal of Consulting and Clinical Psychology*, 1984, 52, 4-16.

Prior, M. R., & Bradshaw, J. L. Hemisphere functioning in autistic children. *Cortex*, 1979, 15, 73–81.

Rendle-Short, J. Infantile autism in Australia. *Medical Journal of Australia*, 1969, 2, 245–249.

Reynolds, B. S., Newsom, C. D., & Lovaas, O. I. Auditory overselectivity in autistic children. *Journal of Child Psychology*, 1974, 2, 253–263.

Ricks, D. M., & Wing, L. Language, communication, and the use of symbols in normal and autistic children. *Journal of Autism and Childhood Schizophrenia*, 1975, 5, 191–221.

Rimland, B. *Infantile autism*. New York: Appleton-Century-Crofts, 1964.

Rimland, B. High dosage levels of certain vitamins in the treatment of children with severe mental disorders. In D. Hawkins and L. Pauling (Eds.), *Orthomolecular psychiatry*. San Francisco: Freeman, 1973.

Rincover, A. Sensory extinction: A procedure for eliminating self-stimulatory behavior in developmentally disabled children. *Journal of Abnormal Child Psychology*, 1978, *6*, 299–310.

Risley, T. R. The effects and side effects of punishing autistic behaviors of a deviant child. *Journal of Applied Behavior Analysis*, 1968, *1*, 20–34.

Risley, T. R., & Wolf, M. Establishing functional speech in echolalic children. *Behaviour Research and Therapy*, 1967, *5*, 73–88.

Ritvo, E. R. *Genetic and immuno-hematologic studies on the syndrome of autism*. Paper presented at the International Conference on Autism, Boston, July 1981.

Ritvo, E. R., & Freeman, B. J. National Society for Autistic Children definition of the syndrome of autism. *Journal of Pediatric Psychology*, 1977, *2*, 146–148.

Ritvo, E. R., Yuwiler, A., Geller, E., Kales, A., Rashkis, S., Schicor, A., Plotkin, A., Axelrod, R., & Howard, C. Effects of L-dopa on autism. *Journal of Autism and Childhood Schizophrenia*, 1971, *1*, 190–205.

Robinson, N. M., & Robinson, H. B. *The mentally retarded child: A psychological approach* (2d ed.). New York: McGraw-Hill, 1976.

Romanczyk, R. G., Diament, C., Coren, E. R., Trunell, G., & Harris, S. L. Increasing isolate and social play in severely disturbed children: Intervention and post-intervention effectiveness. *Journal of Autism and Childhood Schizophrenia*, 1975, *5*, 57–70.

Rosenthal, D. Some factors associated with concordance and discordance with respect to schizophrenia in MZ twins. *Journal of Nervous and Mental Disease*, 1959, *129*, 1–10.

Rosenthal, D., & Kety, S. S. (Eds.). *The transmission of schizophrenia*. New York: Pergamon, 1968.

Ross A. O. *Psychological disorders of children*. New York: McGraw-Hill, 1980.

Ruttenberg, B. A psychoanalytic understanding of infantile autism and its treatment. In D. Churchill, G. Alpern, & M. DeMyer (Eds.), *Infantile autism: Proceedings, Indiana University Colloquium*. Springfield, IL: Charles C. Thomas, 1971.

Rutter, M. Behavioural and cognitive characteristics of a series of psychotic children. In J. Wing (Ed.), *Early childhood autism*. Oxford: Pergamon, 1966.

Rutter, M. Psychotic disorders in early childhood. In A. Coppen & A. Walk (Eds.), *Recent developments in schizophrenia*. British Journal of Psychiatry Special Publication. Ashford, Kent: Headley Bros., 1967.

Rutter, M. Concepts of autism: A review of research. *Journal of Child Psychology and Psychiatry*, 1968, *9*, 1–25.

Rutter, M. Autistic children: Infancy to adulthood. *Seminars in Psychiatry*, 1970, *2*, 435–450.

Rutter, M. Diagnosis and definition. In M. Rutter & E. Schopler (Eds.), *Autism: A reappraisal of concepts and treatment.* New York: Plenum Press, 1978.

Rutter, M., & Lockyer, L. A five to fifteen year follow-up study of infantile psychosis. I. Description of sample. *British Journal of Psychiatry,* 1967, *113,* 1169–1182.

Rutter, M., & Schopler, E. (Eds.). *Autism: A reappraisal of concepts and treatment.* New York: Plenum Press, 1978.

Salvin, A., Routh, D. K., Foster, R. E., & Lovejoy, K. M. Acquisition of modified American Sign Language by a mute autistic child. *Journal of Autism and Childhood Schizophrenia,* 1977, *7,* 359–371.

Schaeffer, B. Teaching spontaneous sign language to nonverbal children: Theory and method. *Sign Language Studies,* 1978, *21,* 317–352.

Schain, R. J., & Freedman, D. Studies on 5-hydroxyindole metabolism in autistic and other mentally retarded children. *Journal of Pediatrics,* 1961, *58,* 315–320.

Schain, R. J., & Yannet, H. Infantile autism: An analysis of 50 cases and a consideration of certain relevant neurophysiologic concepts. *Journal of Pediatrics,* 1960, *57,* 560–567.

Schell, R. E., Stark, J., & Giddan, J. J. Development of language behavior in an autistic child. *Journal of Speech and Hearing Disorders,* 1967, *32,* 51–64.

Schiele, B. C., Gallant, D., Simpson, G., Gardner, E. A., & Cole, J. O. Tardive dyskinesia. *American Journal of Orthopsychiatry,* 1973, *43,* 506, 888.

Schopler, E. Parents of psychotic children as scapegoats. *Journal of Contemporary Psychotherapy,* 1971, *4,* 17-22.

Schopler, E., Andrews, C. E., & Strupp, K. Do autistic children come from upper middle-class parents? *Journal of Autism and Developmental Disorders,* 1979, *9,* 139–152.

Schopler, E., Brehm, S. S., Kinsbourne, M., & Reichler, R. J. Effect of treatment structure on development in autistic children. *Archives of General Psychiatry,* 1971, *24,* 415–421.

Schopler, E., & Dalldorf, J. Autism: Definition, diagnosis, and management. *Hospital Practice,* June 1980, 64–73.

Schopler, E., & Reichler, R. J. Parents as cotherapists in the treatment of psychotic children. *Journal of Autism and Childhood Schizophrenia,* 1971, *1,* 87–102.

Schreibman, L., & Lovaas, O. I. Overselective response to social stimuli by autistic children. *Journal of Abnormal Child Psychology,* 1973, *1,* 152–168.

Schwartz, S., & Johnson, J. H. *Psychopathology of childhood.* New York: Pergamon, 1982.

Seibert, J. M., & Oller, D. K. Linguistic pragmatics and language intervention strategies. *Journal of Autism and Developmental Disorders,* 1981, *11,* 75–88.

Shapiro, T., & Lucy, P. Echoing in autistic children: A chronometric study of semantic processing. *Journal of Child Psychology and Psychiatry,* 1978, *19,* 373–378.

Shapiro, T., Roberts, A., & Fish, B. Imitation and echoing in young schizophrenic children. *Journal of American Child Psychiatry,* 1970, *9,* 548–567.

Shervanian, C. *The speech development of pre-communicative psychotic children.* Unpublished Doctoral Dissertation. University of Pittsburgh, 1959.

Shields, J. Summary of the genetic evidence. In D. Rosenthal & S. S. Kety (Eds.), *The transmission of schizophrenia.* New York: Pergamon, 1968.

Silberg, J. The development of pronoun usage in the psychotic child. *Journal of Autism and Childhood Schizophrenia,* 1978, *8,* 413–425.

Simmons, J. Q., & Baltaxe, C. Language patterns of adolescent autistics. *Journal of Autism and Childhood Schizophrenia,* 1975, *5,* 333–351.

Singer, M., & Wynne, L. Thought disorders and family relations of schizophrenics. *Archives of General Psychiatry,* 1965, *12,* 201–212.

Siva-Sankar, D. Biogenic amine uptake by blood platelets and RBC in childhood schizophrenia. *Acta Paedopsychiatra,* 1970, *37,* 174–182.

Slater, E. *Psychotic and Neurotic Illnesses in Twins.* London: Her Majesty's Stationery Office, 1953.

Sloane, H. N., & MacAulay, B. D. *Operant procedures in remedial speech and language training.* Boston: Houghton Mifflin, 1968.

Snyder, L. Communicative and cognitive abilities and disabilities in the sensorimotor period. *Merrill-Palmer Quarterly,* 1978, *24,* 161–180.

Solnick, J. V., Rincover, A., & Peterson, C. R. Some determinants of the reinforcing and punishing effects of timeout. *Journal of Applied Behavior Analysis,* 1977, *10,* 415–424.

Spitzer, R. L., Endicott, J., & Gibbon, M. Crossing the border into borderline personality and borderline schizophrenia. The development of criteria. *Archives of General Psychiatry,* 1979, *36,* 17–24.

Stern, A. Psychoanalytic investigation of and therapy in the borderline group of neuroses. *Psychoanalytic Quarterly,* 1938, *7,* 467–489.

Stubbs, E. G., & Magenis, R. E. HLA and autism. *Journal of Autism and Developmental Disorders,* 1980, *10,* 15–19.

Tager-Flusberg, H. On the nature of linguistic functioning in early infantile autism. *Journal of Autism and Developmental Disorders,* 1981, *11*,45-56.

Tanguay, P. E. Clinical and electro-physiological research. In E. R. Ritvo (Ed.), *Autism: Diagnosis, current research and management.* New York: Spectrum, 1976.

Tate, B. G., & Baroff, G. S. Aversive control of self-injurious behavior in a psychotic boy. *Behavioral Research and Therapy,* 1966, *4,* 281–287.

Tienari, P. Schizophrenia in monozygotic male twins. In D. Rosenthal & S. S. Kety (Eds.), *The tranmission of schizophrenia.* New York: Pergamon, 1968.

Tinbergen, E. A., & Tinbergen, N. Early childhood autism: An etiological approach. In Advances in Ethology, 10, Supplement to *Journal of Comparative Ethology.* Berlin and Hamburg: Verlag Paul Pany, 1972.

Tsai, L., Stewart, M. A., & August, G. Implication of sex differences in the familial transmission of infantile autism. *Journal of Autism and Developmental Disorders,* 1981, *11,* 165–173.

Tubbs, V. K. Types of linguistic disability in psychotic children. *Journal of Mental Deficiency research,* 1966, *10,* 230–240.

Uzgiris, I. C. (Ed.). *Social interaction and communication during infancy.* San Francisco: Jossey-Bass, 1979.

van Krevelen, D. A. On the relationship between early infantile autism and autistic psychopathy. *Acta Paedopsychiatric,* 1963, *30,* 303–323.

van Krevelen, D. A. Early infantile autism and autistic psychopathy. *Journal of Autism and Childhood Schizophrenia,* 1971, *1,* 82–86.

Walker, H. A., & Birch, H. G. Neurointegrative deficiency in schizophrenic children. *Journal of Nervous and Mental Disease,* 1970, *151,* 104–113.

Walker, H., & Birch, H. G. Intellectual patterning in schizophrenic children. *Journal of Autism and Childhood Schizophrenia,* 1974, *4,* 143–161.

Ward, A. J. Early infantile autism: Diagnosis, etiology and treatment. *Psychological Bulletin,* 1970, *73,* 350–362.

Watters, R. G., & Watters, W. E. Decreasing self-stimulatory behavior with physical exercise in a group of autistic boys. *Journal of Autism and Developmental Disorders,* 1980, *10,* 379–387.

Waxler, N. E., & Mishler, E. G. Experimental studies of families. In L. Berkowitz (Ed.), *Advances in experimental social psychology.* Vol. 5. New York: Academic, 1970.

Wheeler, A. J., & Sulzer, B. Operant training and generalization of a verbal response form in a speech deficient child. *Journal of Applied Behavior Analysis,* 1970, *3,* 139–147.

White, P. T., DeMyer, W., & DeMyer, M. EEG abnormalities in early childhood schizophrenia: A double-blind study of psychiatrically-disturbed and normal children during promazine sedation. *American Journal of Psychiatry,* 1964, *120,* 950–958.

Wing, L. Language, social, and cognitive impairments in autism and severe mental retardation. *Journal of Autism and Developmental Disorders,* 1981, *11,* 31-44.

Wing, L., & Ricks, D. M. The aetiology of childhood autism: A criticism of the Tinbergens' ethological theory. *Psychological Medicine,* 1976, *6,* 533–544.

Wolff, S., & Chess, S. An analysis of the language of fourteen schizophrenic children. *Journal of Child Psychology and Psychiatry,* 1965, *6,* 29–41.

Wynne, L. C. Methodologic and conceptual issues in the study of schizophrenics and their families. In D. Rosenthal & S. Kety (Eds.), *The transmission of schizophrenia.* New York: Pergamon, 1968.

Yoder, D. E., & Calculator, S. Some perspectives on intervention strategies for persons with developmental disorders. *Journal of Autism and Developmental Disorders,* 1981, *11,* 107–124.

Yule, W., & Berger, M. Behavior modification principles and speed delay. In M. Rutter & J. A. M. Martin (Eds.), *The child with delayed speed.* London: Simp/Heinemann, 1972.

Zaslow, R. W., & Berger, L. A theory and treatment of autism. In L. Berger (Ed.), *Clinical-cognitive psychology.* Englewood Cliffs, NJ: Prentice-Hall, 1969.

Zilboorg, G. Ambulatory schizophrenia. *Psychiatry,* 1941, *4,* 149–155.

CHAPTER 6

Disorders of Attention and Movement

Donald K. Routh and James E. Patton

The problems discussed in this chapter, namely hyperactivity, tics, and stereotyped movements, are behaviorally quite distinct from each other and have hardly ever been discussed together. (An exception to this neglect is a far-ranging article by Levy, 1944, "On the Problem of Movement Restraint: Tics, Stereotyped Movements, Hyperactivity.") These disorders have in common the fact that they usually originate in childhood, involve excessive movement of some kind, and have been successfully treated either by drugs or by behavioral management techniques. As the following case histories suggest, the relation of these three types of disorder to certain drug treatments indicates that some common physiological mechanisms may be involved in them.

Two "Pharmacological" Case Histories

Golden (1974) presented the case of a hyperactive child treated with a stimulant drug, methylphenidate (Ritalin), who as a result developed Gilles de la Tourette syndrome, a condition involving multiple bodily and vocal tics:

This nine-year-old white boy was first seen two years previously because of "learning difficulty" and behavior problems at school. The latter were characterized by hyperactive, disruptive behavior and constant intrusions into other children's activities. Examination showed a hyperactive child with an extremely short attention span, who was distracted by almost any extraneous stimulus. Motor abnormalities included mild incoordination, clumsiness, difficulty with skilled large muscle movements, and pinch synkinesis. There were no adventitious movements at rest. Psychological testing showed a full-scale IQ (WISC) of 92 with marked scatter in performance sub-test scores. There was also impaired graphomotor incoordination, constructional apraxia and right-left disorientation. With these test data and the "soft" neurological signs, a diagnosis of "minimal brain dysfunction" was made. Medication was not initiated at that time, but because of an increase in his hyperactivity and disruptiveness in school, the boy was later begun on methylphenidate ('Ritalin'), 10 mg twice a day. There was marked improvement in his behavior at home and in the classroom. Approximately eight weeks later, the child suddenly began to produce loud explosive noises, somewhat resembling a cough, and to make multiple "tic" movements involving the face, arms, and body. All movements occurred with the patient fully alert and conscious. He was greatly disturbed by these tics, especially by the vocalization. His symptoms could be partially controlled voluntarily, but they then returned with a transient increase in intensity and frequency. His mother discontinued the methylphenidate for several days and there was some decrease in the symptoms, but they did not disappear entirely. The drug was reinstituted and the severity of the symptoms again increased. Neurological examination at this time revealed almost continuous, random, large and small amplitude movements of the extremities. Grimacing movements of the face were also almost constant. The most striking feature, however, was a noise produced by involuntary forced expiration of air through the nose and mouth. This produced a loud sound that sounded like a combination of a grunt, a cough, and a bark. The results of the remainder of the neurological examination were unchanged. Methylphenidate was discontinued. As the boy was extremely upset by his symptoms and because the previous withdrawal of medication had not produced a complete remission, he was immediately begun on haloperidol (Haldol) 0.5 mg twice a day. The following day, the motor manifestations had disappeared entirely and the vocalizations greatly decreased in frequency and intensity. Haloperidol was increased to 0.5 mg three times daily and on this dose he remains free of tics. The respiratory component still breaks through several times a day, especially when the child is under stress. Attempts to discontinue haloperidol are still unsuccessful and lead to an exacerbation of his symptoms (Golden, 1974, pp. 76–77).

Stereotyped movements, such as body rocking or repetitive hand motions, are most commonly seen in institutionalized individuals with moderate, severe, or profound retardation. Such behaviors can respond rather specifically to antipsychotic drugs such as chlorpromazine.

Hollis (1968), for example, set up a situation in which a severely retarded female was conditioned to pull a ball on a reinforcement schedule with a fixed ratio of rewarded to nonrewarded responses. Intervals of extinction (no rewards for ball pulling) with this individual were associated with high rate stereotyped body rocking movements. When she was given 150 mg of chlorpromazine two hours before the start of a session, there was complete blockage of the rocking movements during extinction but no effect on the ball pulling response rate during rewarded periods.

One possible side effect of drugs like chlorpromazine, however, especially when given in high dosages over long periods of time, is an organic condition known as tardive dyskinesia, which involves lip smacking and facial grimacing. Another possible side effect is one resembling Gilles de la Tourette syndrome, with bodily tics (e.g., eye blinks) and vocal tics, including cursing or so-called coprolalia ("dirty words").

Let us now turn to a more systematic discussion of each of the disorders of attention and movement covered by this chapter. In the terminology of DSM-III (American Psychiatric Association, 1980), they are as follows: attention deficit disorder with and without hyperactivity; and stereotyped movement disorders, including transient tic disorder, chronic motor tic disorder, Tourette's disorder, and atypical stereotyped movement disorder.

Attention Deficit Disorder with Hyperactivity

DEFINITION

Attention deficit disorder with hyperactivity is the DSM-III designation for the problem previously known as hyperactivity or hyperkinetic behavior. Hyperactivity is most apparent in a traditional classroom setting where the child, instead of remaining seated and attending quietly to school work, is often out of seat, running around, and otherwise bothering children. Although the high level of inappropriate activity is the most dramatic manifestation of the disorder, many clinicians have felt that the inability to pay attention or concentrate was basic, hence the change in terminology. Let us begin with the DSM-III definition of attention deficit disorder with hyperactivity:

> The child displays signs of developmentally inappropriate inattention, impulsivity, and hyperactivity. . . . Symptoms typically worsen in situations that require self-application, as in the classroom. Signs of the disorder may be absent when the child is in a new or a one-to-one situation.
>
> The number of symptoms specified in order to make the diagnosis is for children between the ages of eight and ten, the peak age range for referral. In younger children, more severe forms of the symptoms or a greater number of symptoms need to be present. The opposite is true of older children.
>
> A. Inattention. At least three of the following:
>   1. Fails to finish things
>   2. Doesn't seem to listen
>   3. Is easily distracted
>   4. Has difficulty concentrating
>   5. Has difficulty sticking to a play activity
>
> B. Impulsivity. At least three of the following:
>   1. Often acts before thinking
>   2. Shifts about excessively
>   3. Has difficulty organizing work (not due to a cognitive impairment)
>   4. Needs much supervision
>   5. Frequently calls out in class
>   6. Doesn't wait turn in games or group situations
>
> C. Hyperactivity. At least two of the following:
>   1. Runs about or climbs on things excessively
>   2. Can't sit still or fidgets
>   3. Can't remain seated
>   4. Very restless sleep
>   5. Is always "on the go" or acts as if "driven by a motor"
>
> D. Onset before the age of seven.
>
> E. Duration of at least six months.
>
> F. Not due to schizophrenia, affective disorder, or severe or profound mental retardation (American Psychiatric Association, 1980, pp. 43–44)

An illustrative case history was given above. However, it should be remarked in connection with that illustration that the development of tics as a side effect of stimulant drugs, though it is perhaps of considerable theoretical interest and has been reported by others, is actually not a common occurrence.

PREVALENCE

At present in the United States, though attention deficit disorder with hyperactivity is one of the most frequent psychiatric diagnoses applied to school-age children, good data on prevalence are not easy to find.

A parent and teacher survey in Grand Rapids, Michigan (Bosco & Robin, 1980) indicated that teachers considered 3.38 percent of elementary and junior high school students to be hyperactive, parents considered 3.16 percent of them to be so, and the parents indicated that 2.92 percent had been so diagnosed by a physician. So a rule of thumb estimate of 3 percent of the school age population would not be far wrong. Another community prevalence survey was carried out in the San Francisco Bay area. (Lambert, Sandoval, & Sassone, 1978, 1979). Of children surveyed in kindergarten through fifth grade, 4.92 percent were considered hyperactive by one or more definers. Of these, 3.30 percent were considered hyperactive by the school only, and only 1.19 percent were agreed to be hyperactive by teachers, parents, and physicians. It should be noted that neither of these studies used the DSM-III definition, and we do not yet have information on the prevalence of attention deficit disorder with hyperactivity so defined.

The disorder is agreed to be considerably more common in boys than in girls, by ratios of 3 or 4 to 1 (Achenbach, 1982, pp. 368–369).

Diagnostic Considerations

DSM-III describes the various symptoms of inattention, impulsivity, and hyperactivity but does not specify them in complete operational detail. How much activity is hyperactivity? Another conceptual definition of hyperactivity (also not providing operational details) was given by Routh (1978); "a child's consistent failure to comply in age appropriate fashion with situational demands for restrained activity, sustained attention, and inhibition of impulsive response" (p. 3).

A commonly used procedure for operationalizing the diagnosis of hyperactivity has been a score of 15 or above on the abbreviated version of the Conners (1969) Teacher Rating Scale. The use of this scale has helped produce some comparability in populations of children selected for research studies but it does have its limitations. One limitation of the Conners Scale is that its ratings are based on recollections rather than upon direct behavioral observations of the child. Some procedures do exist for directly observing inattentive, hyperactive, and impulsive behaviors, either in a standardized playroom situation (Barkley, 1981; Roberts, 1979; Routh, 1980; Routh & Schroeder, 1976) or in the classroom (Abikoff, Gittelman, & Klein, 1980), but these are probably too expensive for routine clinical use and must be reserved for research purposes.

A second major difficulty with both the above definitions and the use of the Conners Scale is a lack of discriminant validity, i.e., the fact that there is not an adequate distinction between hyperactivity and unsocialized aggressive behavior in children. Although hyperactivity and aggression are related difficulties (i.e., two-thirds of hyperactive children are also aggressive, while three-fourths of unsocialized aggressive children are also hyperactive according to Stewart, DeBlois, and Cummings, 1980), the distinction between them is an important one. It seems the aggressive children rather than the hyperactive ones have a worse long-term prognosis (Milich & Loney, 1979). Also, if children are divided into four groups (hyperactive only, aggressive only, those who are both hyperactive and aggressive, and controls), and observed in a standard academic task situation (Roberts, 1979), the hyperactives and hyperactive-aggressives have great difficulty staying on task, while the children who are aggressive only are indistinguishable from controls.

Loney and Milich (1982) have developed a new version of the Conners Scale, called the IOWA Conners (*I*nattention *O*veractivity *W*ith *A*ggression) which promises to provide a solution to this problem of discriminant validity, yielding separate indices for hyperactivity and aggression and deleting items that confuse the two.

Distractibility. DSM-III lists sixteen separate symptoms of attention deficit disorder with hyperactivity. A more detailed discussion singling out one of these, distractibility, will suggest some of the complexities involved in understanding this disorder.

"Distractibility" implies that the child's performance of a task (for example, doing arithmetic computations in school) is interfered with by some extraneous stimulus. However, the classroom teacher usually observes only that the child is "off task" a lot and *attributes* this to distraction. This reasonable but unverified assumption has had far-reaching effects on educational practices with hyperactive children, such as seating them away from windows and play equipment (Clements, 1966), the use of isolation cubicles (Cruickshank et al., 1961), reducing the number of problems on math worksheets or using color to highlight critical written information (Hallahan & Kaufman, 1976), and even on the design of school buildings (Evans & Lovell, 1979.) But evidence is lacking that the child's inattention is actually due to distraction, or that a hyperactive child is any more subject to particular distracting influences than other children in the same situation.

An experiment (Patton, Routh, & Offenbach, 1981), for example, exposed reading-disabled children (no doubt including some hyperactive ones) and non-reading-disabled controls to videotaped classroom sights and sounds; and both groups were equally impaired by these stimuli in their academic performance. The only difference was that when given the opportunity to avoid this distraction, the reading disabled children were significantly more likely not to do so or to make the distraction worse by turning up the sound. Actually, well-behaved, normally achieving school children often prefer to study with the radio on, or if they are doing math, even with the TV on (Patton, Stinard, & Routh, 1981).

It is true that some laboratory work with hyperactive children has demonstrated differential distractibility in some situations. Denton and McIntyre (1978), for example, presented a span of apprehension task, such as seeing how many letters can be recognized in a given exposure, to normal and hyperactive boys and found that in the absence of visual "noise," the span of both groups was the same. When the amount of "noise" in the form of irrelevant letters in the display was increased, the hyperactive boys' performance was significantly more impaired. Future research on the distractibility of hyperactive children needs to be extended to more representative academic and home situations.

Etiologies

It was once widely assumed that what is now called attention deficit disorder with hyperactivity was part of an organically based syndrome of minimal brain dysfunction (MBD) (e.g., Clements, 1966). This view was undermined: on the one hand because the different behaviors presumed to be part of the syndrome did not correlate with each other (Nichols & Chen, 1981; Routh & Roberts, 1972); and on the other hand, by the fact that attention deficits and hyperactivity were found to have only a nonspecific relationship with known neurological disorder (e.g., Rutter, 1977), that is, neurologically impaired children are at increased risk for all kinds of behavior disorders, not just hyperactivity.

Another argument for the organic basis of attention deficit disorder with hyperactivity was the fact that its symptoms were "paradoxically" responsive to stimulant medications, such as amphetamine and methylphenidate. However, it has been shown that normal, healthy children respond the same way to such drugs as do hyperactive children (Rapoport et al., 1978). For these reasons, the hypothesis that MBD is generally responsible for attention deficit disorder with hyperactivity has been disputed

In the recent past, evidence was presented to show hyperactivity runs in families and that disorders in the so-called *St. Louis triad* of alcoholism, antisocial personality, and hysteria are more common among the biological relatives of hyperactive children than among the relatives of control subjects. However, many of these family studies (e.g., Cantwell, 1972; Morrison & Stewart, 1971, 1973) did not make the important distinction between hyperactivity and unsocialized aggressive behavior. Stewart and his colleagues (e.g., Stewart, DeBlois, and Cummings, 1980) are beginning to find evidence that it is unsocialized aggression and *not* hyperactivity that is truly associated with such disorders in biological relatives. So it may be that attention deficit disorder with hyperactivity is neither part of an MBD syndrome nor part of a familial disorder, once the presence of aggressive behavior is taken into account.

What does this leave? It must be admitted that we do not know the etiology in most specific cases of attention deficit disorder with hyperactivity, though of course there are psychodynamic, behavioral, and medical explanations (See Chapter 1). Presently the strongest evidence points to various chemical and toxic substances in the environment. Among the suspected, but still unproven, possible influences are subclinical lead intoxication (e.g., Needleman, 1982) and food dyes or other food additives (Weiss, 1982). Another factor being studied more intensively is maternal cigarette smoking.

One study (Denson, Nanson, & McWatters, 1975) implicated maternal smoking—mothers of hyperactive children reported two to three times as many cigarettes a day as mothers of control children, and reported significantly higher prenatal smoking rates as well. There were no differences in the fathers' rates of smoking. Nichols and Chen (1981) reported analysis of prospective data from the Collaborative Perinatal Project on a group of nearly 30,000 seven-year-old children. Mothers of hyperactive children smoked significantly more cigarettes during pregnancy than mothers in the comparison group. In fact, in a discriminant function analysis, the length of maternal smoking history was the best single predictor of hyperactive behavior in the child at age seven.

Outcome

It was once thought that hyperactivity was a problem seen only in the preadolescent age group, that it resolved when the child became a teen-ager. As follow-up data began to be more extensively reported, however, it became apparent that many hyperactive children continue to have difficulties well into their adolescent and adult years. They often get failing grades in school, continue to have trouble making friends, and have a difficult time staying on task at school and perhaps later at work as well. Even their hyperactive behaviors may not entirely abate.

One longitudinal study (Loney, Kramer, & Milich, 1979) reported that the predictive values of childhood hyperactivity and aggression as judged by chart raters were quite different. The hyperactivity factor was a significant predictor only of adolescent academic achievement. Childhood aggression, on the other hand, predicted adolescent hyperactive symptoms (even better than did childhood hyperactivity), adolescent aggressive symptoms, and delinquent behavior. So, once more there is evidence for the importance of evaluating both of these factors in children with attention deficit disorder with hyperactivity.

Treatment

Drugs. The favorable effect of stimulant drugs on children's attention was discovered somewhat serendipitously by Bradley (1937) with an inpatient population of delinquent boys, who referred to the benzedrine Bradley used as "smart pills." However, the first double blind, placebo controlled studies evaluating the efficacy of stimulant drugs such as dextroamphetamine (Dexedrine) and methylphenidate (Ritalin) did not begin to appear until the late 1950s and 1960s. Another drug, pemoline (Cylert) was developed which does not have to be administered so frequently during the day.

Barkley's (1977) definitive review of these medications indicates that about three out of four hyperactive children show a favorable response to stimulant drugs in terms of, for example, teacher ratings on the Conners (1969) Scale or on various laboratory tasks sampling attentional processes. Of course, as already noted, the effects of stimulant drugs on normal children are similar, i.e., the efficacy of the medication is not specific to the hyperactive child (Rapoport et al., 1978).

One hope for stimulant drugs was that they would facilitate the child's attention in the classroom and produce a long-term favorable effect on learning. Unfortunately, this hope is not yet fulfilled (e.g., Rie & Rie, 1977). The effect of the drugs on academic performance, for example, on handwriting (Lerer, Lerer, & Artner, 1977), seems only transient.

In fact, the major clinical justification for the use of stimulants with these children is social rather than academic. There is good evidence that while the child is on medication, his or her behavior becomes more acceptable both to the parents (Barkley & Cunningham, 1980) and to the teacher (Whalen, Henker, & Dotemoto, 1980, 1981). Though research continues (Barkley et al., 1983; Chatoor et al., 1982), it needs to address drug effects on these children's peer relations; but it is probable that the social effects of stimulant drugs, like the academic ones, are transient rather than lasting.

A study by Varley (1983) examined the effects of methylphenidate on adolescents with attention deficit disorder. The effects were favorable in terms of both teacher and parent ratings, belying the traditional assumption that stimulant drug treatment was indicated only for prepubescent children.

Diet. The question of the effects of diet on hyperactivity continues to be a controversial one. Feingold (1975) claimed that a large proportion of the problem of hyperactivity was due to dietary factors, including artificial colors and flavors, but the research evidence on this issue so far is equivocal. Diet may benefit some hyperactive children, though certainly not the large majority. In January 1982 a Consensus Development Conference was held at the National Institutes of Health on this topic, and the interested reader may consult the resulting report (NIH, 1982). There has also been interest in whether the ingestion of refined sugar might not be a factor in producing hyperactivity, at least for some children. A correlation has been found (Prinz, Roberts, & Hantman, 1980) between the amount of sugar products consumed by hyperactive children and the destructive-aggressive or restless behavior observed during their free play. However, the consensus of other investigators, including animal researchers and some who have done double-blind experimental studies with children, is that sugar and other carbohydrates are more likely to induce slowed activity or sleepiness than activation (Kolata, 1982).

Behavior Therapy. Considerable research has been done on behavioral approaches to attention and conduct problems of the type presented by children with attention deficit disorder with hyperactivity. These were reviewed in some detail by Routh and Mesibov (1980). This research may be briefly summarized by stating that: Using the principles of reward, punishment, modeling, and so on, it is clearly possible to decelerate a child's overactivity, lengthen time on task, and reduce disruptive behaviors. If a therapist is specifically interested in increasing the quality or amount of academic work produced, it is better to focus the rewards on those goals instead of trying to influence academic performance indirectly through activity and attentional changes.

The drawbacks to behavioral approaches consist of their expense (certainly higher than that of pharmacological approaches) and their situational specificity. Like other treatment approaches, behavioral ones have yet to be established as having any significant effect on the long term outcomes of these children.

If one accepts the premise that at present pharmacological treatment is more cost-effective than a behavioral approach (and both are palliative rather than curative), then the focus of behavioral treatment research might shift toward the study of factors influencing adherence to a prescribed medical regimen such as stimulant medication. Firestone (1982) found that 20 percent of a sample of hyperactive children and their families had discontinued medication by the fourth month of treatment, and 44 percent had done so by the tenth month. Varley and Trupin (1983) proposed the use of double-blind assessment of stimulant medication, not as a research tool but as a clinical procedure for dealing with individual families' concerns about whether the drug was benefiting their child. This is a refreshingly rational approach to the problem of adherence given that the drug is indeed helpful for only about three out of four hyperactive children.

Conclusions

The DSM-III definition of attention deficit disorder is a relatively new one. It needs to be translated into clearer operational criteria; its reliability needs to be established; and above all its validity needs to be better studied. It is already clear from what has been said that the definition pays too little heed to the important distinction between attention deficit/hyperactivity and unsocialized aggressive behavior. In this respect the new teacher rating scale developed by Loney and Milich (1982) seems to be a step in the right direction.

Once there is consensus about the definition and operational assessment of this disorder, it should be possible to collect more meaningful data on incidence and prevalence, and of course to study etiology, outcome, and treatment efficacy. However, such consensus cannot be established by the fiat of any committee; it can only emerge from a wider base of knowledge than we presently have concerning attention deficit disorder with hyperactivity.

Attention Deficit Disorder without Hyperactivity

According to DSM-III the criteria for this disorder are the same as those for attention deficit disorder with hyperactivity except that the child never met the criteria for hyperactivity (part C). This category seems an invention of the DSM-III committee and has not been the subject of much research. It therefore seems best to reserve judgment as to whether it will prove to be a useful or valid diagnostic classification.

The Tic Disorders

The tic disorders include transient tic disorder, chronic motor tic disorder, and Tourette disorder. The authors of DSM-III admit that it is unknown whether the three as ordered represent distinct conditions or a continuum of severity.

Transient Tic Disorder

DSM-III criteria for transient tic disorder are as follows:

A. Onset during childhood or early adolescence
B. Presence of recurrent, involuntary, repetitive, rapid, purposeless motor movements (tics)
C. Ability to suppress the movements voluntarily for minutes to hours
D. Variation in the intensity of the symptoms over weeks or months
E. Duration of at least one month but not more than one year (American Psychiatric Association, 1980, p. 75)

Prevalence. Lapouse and Monk (1958, 1964) found that 12 percent of a sample of children between the ages of six and twelve had a history of some kind of tic, with about equal frequency in males and females. It is not known how many of these tics would meet the criteria for transient tic disorder.

Diagnostic Considerations. Ordinarily when a person engages in movement, it appears purposeful, as when someone blinks an eye in response to bright light or a bit of dust on the cornea. The same movement may be regarded as a tic if it is made repeatedly in the absence of any apparent stimulus or voluntary intention of the individual. Even though it is not strictly speaking a voluntary movement, a tic may usually be suppressed by the individual through effort. However, continued suppression requires vigilant attention and cannot be maintained indefinitely. Tics do not occur during sleep.

The most common type of tic is an eye blink or other facial movement. However, the whole head, torso, or limbs may be involved. An individual may have a single tic or a number of them, and they may be performed together or separately. The onset may be as young as two years of age.

Etiologies. The etiologies of transient tics are unknown.

Outcome. By definition, transient tic disorder has a duration of less than one year. The presence of variation in intensity may be a good prognostic sign, since this is not characteristic of chronic motor tic disorder (see below).

Treatment. The present authors have been unable to discover published reports of attempts to treat transient tic disorder. In practice, the usual way of dealing with the problem is to reassure the child and parents that the tics will likely disappear with time.

Conclusions. If a problem behavior is known to be transient, the best counsel may indeed be to wait for it to go away. However, as will be seen, it is possible for the more severe tic disorders to begin with one or a few simple tics, which become progressive and chronic. What is needed are prospective longitudinal studies of simple tics in children to identify criteria which will predict these different outcomes.

Chronic Motor Tic Disorder

DSM-III diagnostic criteria for this disorder are:

A. Presence of recurrent, involuntary movements (tics) involving no more than three muscle groups
B. Ability to suppress the movements voluntarily for minutes to hours
C. Duration of at least one year (American Psychiatric Association, 1980, p. 75)

Prevalence. The prevalence of chronic motor tic disorder is not known.

Diagnostic Considerations. By definition, chronic motor tic disorder lasts longer than the transient variety. It may be delayed in its onset until adulthood, e.g., after age forty (in which case usually only a single muscle group tends to be involved), and also chronic tics are less variable in intensity. In contrast to Tourette disorder, vocal tics are either not present or are less prominent in chronic motor tic disorder.

Etiologies. It is not known what causes chronic motor tic disorder, though there are psychodynamic, behavioral, and medical explanations (See Chapter 1).

Outcome. The course of this disorder is, by definition, chronic.

Treatment. Although well controlled treatment studies of chronic motor tic disorder have not appeared, there are a number of case reports using behavioral treatment methods and reporting favorable outcomes. The oldest and best known behavioral approach is Dunlap's (1932) method of "negative practice," in which the person is asked to perform the tic voluntarily and repeatedly, in massed sessions.

A successful example of this type of treatment, provided by Nicassio et al. (1972), is of a twenty-two-year-old male college student who since age seven had a neck-jerk tic. He was asked to record the frequency of his neck tic in a small notebook for two days of baseline recording and also throughout treatment. Without the patient's knowledge, a psychiatric technician also recorded the frequency of his tics during social evenings at the mental health center, providing a check on the accuracy of his records. The treatment involved voluntary practice of the neck tic for ten-minute sessions, six times per day. The rate of practice was thirty-five to fifty tics per minute. By the eighth day of treatment, the spontaneous frequency of the tic was reduced from about 200 to 50 per day. By the conclusion of treatment (slightly over a month in all), the frequency of the tics was almost nil, and their amplitude when they did occur was attenuated to the point that strangers would not identify them as such. At eighteen month follow-up the neck tic had not returned, nor had others developed.

As encouraging as the above report may seem, it is an uncontrolled study. The tic might have disappeared spontaneously without treatment at that point, or other concurrent events may have been responsible for the change. Even in the published literature, negative practice is hardly always successful as a treatment for tics. In fact, Nicassio et al. (1972) also reported a treatment failure.

Barrett (1962), in a single subject operant design, was able to demonstrate experimental control over her adult male subject's rates of tic behaviors. This man's tics seem to meet the criteria for chronic motor tic disorder. She found that noncontingent presentation of loud noise increased the tic rate over baseline, but noise contingent upon tics (i.e., punishment) reduced the rates. It was found that the subject could lower his rate of tics or suppress them in order to be able to listen to continuous music on earphones.

Conclusions. Some of the behavioral treatment studies of patients with chronic motor tic disorder are suggestive, but they typically lack proper control procedures and adequate follow-up data. More rigorous behavioral treatment studies are needed.

In view of the success of haloperidol with Tourette's Disorder (see below), pharmacological approaches to chronic motor tic disorder may also be useful.

TOURETTE'S DISORDER

DSM-III diagnostic criteria for Tourette's disorder are:

A. Onset between two and fifteen years

B. Recurrent, involuntary movements affecting multiple muscle groups

C. Involuntary utterances

D. Ability to suppress movements voluntarily for minutes to hours

E. Variations in the intensity of the symptoms over weeks or months

F. Duration of more than one year (American Psychiatric Association, 1980, p. 77).

Illustrative Case The best known case of this disorder was that of the Marquise de Dampierre in France, first published in 1825 by J. M. G. Itard, the famous physician who had worked with Victor, the "Wild Boy of Aveyron." This woman was subsequently seen by Charcot, and the case was discussed by Georges Gilles de la Tourette, for whom the syndrome was named (Shapiro et al., 1978). Her symptoms began at age seven and persisted until her death at eighty-five. Her coprolalia, which forced her to become a recluse, was described as follows:

> It occurs suddenly in the middle of an interesting conversation. Her words are in extraordinary contrast to her refined manners. For the

most part they are vulgar swear words, obscene epithets, and no less embarrassing for those who hear them, expressions that lack judgment or that are unfavorable for someone who is present. The patient herself gives the explanation that is the most plausible: the more she herself thinks that her vulgarities would be revolting, the more she is tortured by the fear that she would utter them, and it precisely this preoccupation that when she can no longer control it puts these words at the tip of her tongue (Itard, 1825, cited by Stevens, 1964, p. 227).

Prevalence. The prevalence of Tourette's disorder is estimated at from 1 in 2000 to 1 in 1000. Despite the fact that this disorder was first identified over 150 years ago, until recent years it was considered a somewhat rare or exotic syndrome, and cases often went unrecognized by clinicians. Therefore, it may actually be more prevalent than the above estimates suggest.

Tourette's disorder is about three times as common in boys as in girls (Shapiro et al., 1978).

Diagnostic Considerations. Tourette's disorder has a childhood onset, most commonly about age seven (Shapiro et al., 1978) and almost always before age thirteen (American Psychiatric Association, 1980, p. 76). It is distinguished from chronic motor tic disorder by this fact and also in that its symptoms fluctuate over time, but most of all by the presence of vocal tics such as grunts, throat clearing noises, shrieks, barks, etc. Coprolalia, the irresistable urge to utter obscenities, such as (to mention the most common ones) "fuck," "shit," "cunt," etc., is present as a vocal tic in only about 60 percent of the cases but when it occurs is considered to confirm the diagnosis. Coprolalia may not be present at first, and it is not uncommon for it to develop only in adolescence. Other symptoms which may occur include copropraxia (e.g., giving "the finger" or pointing to the genitals) and echolalia (repeating the phrases of others).

The early stages of Tourette's disorder may be impossible to distinguish from transient tic disorder in that in about half the cases Tourette's begins with a single tic, such as an eye blink, head movement tic, or facial grimace (Shapiro et al., 1978); it may be some time before the vocal tics which are more diagnostic appear. On the other hand, vocal tics including coprolalia may be present right from the first, as in the case of the four-year-old boy whose first tic symptom was the word "fuck."

Persons with Tourette's disorder are commonly distressed by their symptoms and usually try to suppress them in public, in a physician's office, or in other places where they might prove embarrassing. The individual may be able to vocalize some inarticulate noise instead of an obscenity in such circumstances. Thus, the tics are most likely to occur when the person is alone and thinks himself or herself to be unobserved. It is not unusual for a Tourette patient to go into the bathroom and there release a burst of foul language.

Etiologies. The causes of Tourette's disorder are not known.

The prominence of the symptom of coprolalia in Tourette's disorder, involving as it does the violation of ordinary social norms prohibiting obscene language, has long suggested the importance of psychological and social factors in the etiology of the condition. On the other hand, it can be argued that some disorders of undisputed organic etiology, such as aphasia, can be manifested in a similar way—for example, during recovery from a stroke, an aphasic's first linguistic accomplishments may well be swear words.

Any plausible account of the etiology of Tourette's disorder will have to explain the 3:1 male to female sex ratio.

Although cases of Tourette's disorder have been reported in all parts of the world, Shapiro et al. (1978) reported that about 43 percent of their sample of 145 Tourette patients were of eastern European Jewish (Ashkenazi) background. The reasons for this disproportionate frequency are not yet clear and could be partly explained by sampling bias. Systematic epidemiological surveys will be necessary to investigate this matter further.

A particularly interesting finding in terms of the focus of the present chapter is Shapiro et al.'s report that about 58 percent of their sample of Tourette patients had signs and symptoms of minimal brain dysfunction using Clements' (1966) criteria. Although most hyperactive, learning disabled, or clumsy children do not have tics, children with Tourette's disorder often appear to exhibit the symptoms of MBD.

As the case histories presented at the outset of this chapter suggest, pharmacology has given us some of the most interesting leads as to the possible physiological mechanisms underlying Tourette's disorder. Haloperidol (Haldol) seems to have specific value in decreasing all of the types of tics which are seen in Tourette's disorder. Since haloperidol is known to block dopamine receptors in the nervous system, some mechanism involving dopamine might be inferred to be responsible for the disorder. This idea is supported by the fact that stimulant drugs such as methylphenidate and the amphetamines, which can cause Tourette's symptoms as a side effect, are known to potentiate dopamine action.

Finally, Tourette's symptoms may be seen alongside tardive dyskinesia as a sequel to long-term high dosages of neuroleptic drugs. The mechanism causing tardive dyskinesia has been suggested to be hypersensitivity of neural dopamine receptors caused by their long blockade. One puzzle in all of this pharmacological reasoning is why haloperidol and not other drugs, such as chlorpromazine, can be used to treat Tourette's disorder. After all, these other drugs block dopamine action, too. If dopamine is the only key, these drugs should be equally therapeutic, and they are not.

Outcome. Tourette's disorder usually has a lifelong course. Individual tic symptoms wax and wane with time; some disappear, while new ones develop. The intensity of the condition fluctuates, and total remission may occur, with or without later reappearance of the disorder. So far no factors have been identified which permit prediction of differential outcome.

Treatment. Comparative treatment results with Tourette's disorder, summarized in a review of the literature by Abuzzahab and Anderson (1973), based on 430 patients and 586 treatment trials, indicated an improvement rate of 89 percent for haloperidol, 48 percent for other antipsychotic or neuroleptic drugs, and 35 percent for psychological treatments. Although these are not controlled studies, the differential results seem to be quite compelling.

For treatment of Tourette's disorder, haloperidol is generally given in daily dosages averaging 5 mg (significantly lower dosages than the 25 to 200 mg or more used in treating schizophrenia with the same drug). This dosage seems to be low enough so that tardive dyskinesia is not a significant risk (Shapiro et al., 1978, p. 318), but significant cognitive impairment or obtunding is reported to be a common complication. Shapiro et al. consider this to be serious enough to render an "A" student into a "D" student while on the drug, and a "B" student might begin to fail courses. In children who already have significant learning difficulties, as many with Tourette's disorder do, this is a very worrisome side effect indeed.

A number of behavior therapy studies have been carried out with Tourette's disorder patients, and the above figure of 35 percent success rate for psychological treatments may be an underestimate of what is possible with behavioral methods. Shapiro et al. are, however, quite critical of some commonly used behavioral research strategies in relation to this disorder. Studies with a simple design involving baseline, then treatment, may suggest treatment "success" due only to the well-known variability of the disorder over time. If the behavior of the patient only during treatment sessions is observed, temporary suppression of the tics may be mistaken for true generalized changes in symptom rates. The therapist must assess tic rates in other locales and times of the day. Finally, Shapiro et al. suggest that even a multiple baseline design (in which the frequency of some tics might be used as a "control" while other tics are treated) is inappropriate because it does not consider possible placebo artifacts. In general, one has to agree with the view that considerably better treatment research is needed (and that goes for pharmacological as well as behavioral studies).

Conclusion. In a classic article on the application of learning theory to the treatment of tics, Yates (1958) apparently did not even recognize that his subject had Tourette's disorder. Thanks to the work of such people as Abuzzahab and Anderson (1973) and Shapiro et al. (1978), Tourette's disorder has been brought from obscurity to the point of recognition, even by members of the public. One factor which no doubt gave an impetus to the clinical recognition of this problem was the discovery of haloperidol treatment for it in the early 1960s. It seems that anything that can be treated will begin to be diagnosed more frequently!

Atypical Stereotyped Movement Disorder

DSM-III does not give an explicit set of diagnostic criteria for stereotyped movement disorder but states that this category is for head banging, rocking, repetitive hand or voluntary movements of usually the fingers or arms. These disorders are distinguished from tics in that they are voluntary and not spasmodic. Further, the children seem to be unconcerned about the symptom and may even appear to enjoy it. This disorder is often found among children who are retarded or severely withdrawn, though it may occur in isolation. (American Psychiatric Association, 1980, p. 77).

Prevalence

No definitive information is available on the prevalence of stereotyped movement disorder. Rhythmical behavior or rhythmical habit patterns similar to those described above seem to be nearly universal in infants and are certainly not abnormal in them. For example, Kravits and Boehm (1971) noted body rocking in 182 of a sample of 200 normal infants (91 percent) who were observed from one month to one year of age. The median age of onset of body rocking was 6.1 months, and in fact what characterized abnormal infants in this study was a delay in the onset of such common rhythmic habit patterns as body rocking, head banging, head rolling, thumb and finger sucking, lip biting, toe sucking, and teeth grinding.

Thelen's (1981) longitudinal observational study of twenty normal infants in their homes from ages four weeks to one year confirmed that the peak frequency of rhythmical stereotypies was seen at six to seven months of age, with a small but real decline thereafter. These stereotypies were regarded as transitional behaviors between uncoordinated activity and complex, coordinated, voluntary motor control. For example, rocking on the hands and knees appeared just before crawling, and rhythmical hand and arm movements appeared before complex manual skills developed.

After infancy these stereotyped behaviors disappear, except in certain special populations of children, such as the retarded and psychotic, and thus become statistically infrequent enough to be considered a disorder when they do occur. Exactly how infrequent is unclear. One of the present authors (Routh) wanted to carry out a study of stereotyped movement disorder and canvassed teachers and principals throughout a whole school system. No instances of children with such movements could be located in the system, except in a special school for severely and profoundly retarded individuals, and there several cases were readily found.

Berkson and Davenport (1962) found that stereotyped movements and postures were present in two-thirds of a population of seventy-one institutionalized, severely retarded people. Baumeister (1978) surveyed about 500 admission records taken at random from a mental retardation institution's files and found that approximately 15 percent made reference to stereotyped or self-injurious activities. Klaber and Butterfield (1968) carried out observations in wards serving preponderantly ambulatory patients who were severely retarded in four large state institutions and found that at any given time somewhere between 5.3 to 15.7 percent of the residents were engaged in stereotyped body rocking.

Diagnostic Considerations

It does not seem to be difficult to identify stereotyped movements. As noted above, they appear to be voluntary and are extremely repetitive, although they are often of an idiosyncratic character. To dramatize the uniqueness of some of these activities, Berkson (1964) describes a retarded individual who always kept a shoe lace and a sort of disc with him:

> He played with no other objects and became disturbed if the lace and disc were taken from him. He ordinarily threaded the lace through the disc and engaged in complex play which consisted mainly in twirling the disc around the axis of the string. If the toy was taken from him, he would immediately pull a button from his overalls and shred a leg of the overalls to obtain a string. He would thread the string through the button and immediately resume his play. All this would occur within about sixty seconds (p. 260).

Such behaviors may not always be a cause for concern in themselves. An important additional feature of stereotyped movements, however, is that they often seem to be part of a state of unresponsiveness to the environment (Berkson & Mason, 1964).

Etiologies

In a sense, what needs to be explained is not why stereotypes develop (since these behaviors seem to be a part of normal infancy), but why they persist and become such a pervasive feature of the behavior of some older individuals. One obvious correlate is a deprivation of opportunities for social interaction, whether imposed externally or by the individual's own social withdrawal.

The importance of social deprivation is suggested by Berkson's (1973) research with infant monkeys. Noting that stereotyped behaviors are often seen in the blind and attributed to visual defect, Berkson did an experiment in which infant monkeys were either blinded soon after birth or not blinded, and then either raised in social isolation or not socially isolated. As expected, the blinded, socially isolated monkeys routinely developed pervasive stereotyped behaviors, but it was the social isolation and not the blindness that was responsible. Monkeys which were blinded but had normal social experiences did not have any more stereotypies than nonblind control animals. The applicability of this animal work to humans is supported by Fraiberg's (1977) studies with blind human infants. Because the blind infant does not return its mother's smile, it may seem bland and unresponsive. It is therefore at greater risk for being left alone than a nonblind infant; and it is apparently this relative social isolation rather than the sensory deficit per se which is responsible for the stereotypies sometimes called "blindisms."

Similarly, in the severely retarded, the day-to-day frequency of stereotyped rocking is to some extent related to the opportunities the setting offers for alternative behaviors. In an institution the lowest rates of stereotyped behaviors are consistently at snack or meal time, or in other words, when there is most clearly something else to do (Baumeister et al., 1980). In fact, the amount of body rocking observed could be regarded as a measure of institutional and ward attentiveness: the more attentive the care, the less stereotypic rocking (Klaber & Butterfield, 1968).

As noted in the paragraph quoted from DSM-III, stereotyped behaviors often seem to be rewarding to the individuals. It is not really mysterious that socially isolated or bored children, especially in an institution, would soon discover this fact. Studies of infants (e.g., Ter Vrugt & Pederson, 1973) have demonstrated a positive relationship between the frequency with which a baby is rocked and the effectiveness of the rocking in ending crying and facilitating sleep. As Baumeister (1978) says, "The invention of the rocking chair was certainly no accident!" (p. 378). Rincover, Newsome, and Carr (1979) showed experimentally that for one developmentally disabled child a light-switching ritual was maintained by the contingent visual feedback provided (the light going on and off) and for another child by the auditory stimulation (clicking sound) the switch provided.

Also, part of the cause of stereotyped movement disorder surely lies in the limited repertoire of other behaviors possessed by the individual, thus the association between these behaviors and severe mental retardation. Even in institutionalized persons, Berkson and Davenport (1962) found a correlation of −.33 between IQ and stereotyped movements. A severely retarded child may be nonambulatory and nonverbal and have only limited skills at play or social interaction. An autistic child's alternative behaviors are also limited by the pervasive impairment of social relationships seen among such children.

Other factors which have been found to increase rates of stereotyped behaviors in the retarded include intensive noise (Hollis, 1971), frustration (Forehand & Baumeister, 1971), movement restraint (Forehand & Baumeister, 1970) and various aspects of ward routines (Klaber & Butterfield, 1968).

Outcome

Stereotyped movement disorder seems to be a rather chronic condition. In his survey of the admission records of 500 retarded individuals, Baumeister (1978) reports that in no instance did he locate an individual who at admission exhibited stereotyped activities and subsequently ceased to do so. In other words, if the stereotyped behavior was sufficiently salient to be noted in admission records, it continued unless some specific treatment was instituted to try to change it.

Treatment

The Hollis (1968) study on the specific responsiveness of the stereotypies of one retarded child to the drug chlorpromazine was already mentioned at the beginning of the chapter. Davis, Sprague, and Werry (1969) confirmed that a similar neuroleptic drug, thioridazine, significantly decreased stereotyped behavior in profoundly retarded individuals without affecting nonstereotyped behaviors. The use of such drugs has become widespread. In fact, surveys by Lipman (1970) and Sprague and Baxley (1978) indicated that about half of the retarded people in U.S. institutions are receiving psychotropic medications, with one of these two drugs (chlorpromazine or thioridazine) being used with about six out of ten individuals who are so medicated.

An extensive and increasingly sophisticated literature also exists on the behavioral management of stereotyped movements. One well-established way to decrease stereotyped responding is simply to provide the individual with novel objects, toys, or opportunities to interact with another person (Berkson & Mason, 1964; Davenport & Berkson, 1963). A second, perhaps more cumbersome method might involve rewarding the person for sitting still, i.e., for not engaging in stereotyped behaviors. Mulhern and Baumeister (1969), for example, successfully did this using M&M candies as the rewards.

Or one might use the response-contingent withdrawal of some rewarding event to suppress stereotyped behaviors. Murphy, Nunes, and Hutchings-Ruprecht (1977) successfully used access to a vibrator as the item to be withdrawn in this kind of situation. Finally, quite a number of studies have demonstrated that stereotyped behaviors in retarded individuals may be suppressed by response-contingent punishment of one kind or another, for example, physical restraint (Reid, Tombaugh, & Van den Heuvel, 1981), requiring the person to engage in "overcorrection" behaviors (Foxx & Azrin, 1977), slapping the child's hand (Romanczyk, 1977), or even electric shock (Baumeister & Forehand, 1972).

In considering any of the more coercive of these treatments (e.g., powerful drugs or punitive behavioral methods), one has to weigh carefully the decision as to whether treatment is justified at all. If the individual appears to enjoy engaging in stereotyped behaviors, and if more satisfying alternative experiences are not being made available as a replacement, a depriving and punitive attitude on the part of the therapist may be ethically questionable.

Conclusion

Stereotyped movement disorder is frequently encountered in severely and profoundly mentally retarded individuals, whether inside or outside of institutions. The management of this problem is therefore best viewed not narrowly, but as an aspect of the rehabilitation of the retarded and of their quality of life. If stereotyped behaviors are not directly interfering with the rehabilitation process, it may be better to tolerate them than to engage in overly intrusive treatment activities. We should ponder questions such as the following: Do we really have something better for Berkson's (1964) patient to do than to play with his disc and shoelace? If we do not, should our efforts be directed at the symptom or at devising that better something?

REFERENCES

Abikoff, H., Gittelman, R., & Klein, D. F. Classroom observation code for hyperactive children: A replication of validity. *Journal of Consulting and Clinical Psychology*, 1980, *48*, 555–565.

Abuzzahab, F. S., & Anderson, F. O. Gilles de la Tourette's syndrome: International registry. *Minnesota Medicine*, 1973, *56*, 492–496.

Achenbach, T. M. *Developmental psychopathology.* New York: Wiley, 1982.

American Psychiatric Association. *DSM-III*: *Diagnostic and statistical manual of mental disorders* (3d ed.). Washington, DC: A.P.A., 1980.

Barkley, R. A. A review of stimulant drug research with hyperactive children. *Journal of Child Psychology and Psychiatry*, 1977, *18*, 137–165.

Barkley, R. A. *Hyperactive children.* New York: Guilford, 1981.

Barkley, R. A., & Cunningham, C. E. The parent-child interactions of hyperactive children and their modification by stimulant drugs. In R. M. Knights & D. J. Bakker (Eds.), *Treatment of hyperactive and learning disordered children.* Baltimore: University Park, 1980.

Barkley, R. A., Cunningham, C. E., & Karlsson, J. The speech of hyperactive children and their mothers: Comparison with normal children and stimulant drug effects. *Journal of Learning Disabilities*, 1983 *16*, 105–110.

Barrett, B. H. Reduction in rate of multiple tics by free operant conditioning. *Journal of Nervous and Mental Disease*, 1962, *135*, 187–195.

Baumeister, A. A. Origins and control of stereotyped movements. In C. E. Meyers (Ed.), *Quality of life in severely and profoundly retarded people: Research foundations for improvement.* Washington, DC: American Association on Mental Deficiency, 1978.

Baumeister, A. A., & Forehand, R. Effects of contingent shock and verbal command on body rocking of retardates. *Journal of Clinical Psychology*, 1972, *28*, 586–590.

Baumeister, A. A., MacLean, W. E., Jr., Kelly, J., & Kasari, C. Observational studies of retarded children with multiple stereotyped movements. *Journal of Abnormal Child Psychology*, 1980, *8*, 501–521.

Berkson, G. Stereotyped movements of mental defectives: V. Ward behavior and its relation to an experimental task. *American Journal of Mental Deficiency*, 1964, *69*, 253–264.

Berkson, G. Visual defect does not produce stereotyped movements. *American Journal of Mental Deficiency*, 1973, *78*, 89–94.

Berkson, G., & Davenport, R. K., Jr. Stereotyped movements of mental defectives: I. Initial survey. *American Journal of Mental Deficiency*, 1962, *66*, 849–852.

Berkson, G., & Mason, W. A. Stereotyped movements of mental defectives: IV. The effects of toys and the character of the acts. *American Journal of Mental Deficiency*, 1964, *68*, 511–524.

Bosco, J. J., & Robin, S. S. Hyperkinesis: Prevalence and treatment. In C. K. Whalen & B. Henker (Eds.), *Hyperactive children: The social ecology of identification and treatment.* New York: Academic Press, 1980.

Bradley, C. The behavior of children receiving benzedrine. *American Journal of Psychiatry*, 1937, *94*, 577–585.

Cantwell, D. P. Psychiatric illness in the families of hyperactive children. *Archives of General Psychiatry*, 1972, *27*, 414–417.

Chatoor, I., Wells, K. C., Connors, C. K., Seidel, W. T., & Shaw, D. The effects of nocturnally administered stimulant medication on EEG sleep and behavior in hyperactive children. *Journal of the American Academy of Child Psychiatry,* 1982, *22,* 337–342.

Clements, S. D. *Minimal brain dysfunction in children: Terminology and identification.* Washington, DC: U.S. Department of Health, Education, and Welfare, 1966.

Conners, C. K. A teacher rating scale for use in drug studies with children. *American Journal of Psychiatry,* 1969, *126,* 884–888.

Cruickshank, W. M., Bentzen, F. A., Ratzburg, F. H., & Tannhauser, M. T. *A teaching method for brain-injured and hyperactive children.* Syracuse, NY: Syracuse University Press, 1961.

Davenport, R. K., & Berkson, G. Stereotyped movements of mental defectives: II. Effects of novel objects. *American Journal of Mental Deficiency,* 1963, *67,* 879–882.

Davis, K. V., Sprague, R. C., & Werry, J. S. Stereotyped behavior and activity level in severe retardates: The effect of drugs. *American Journal of Mental Deficiency,* 1969, *73,* 721–727.

Denson, R., Nanson, J. L., & McWatters, M. A. Hyperkinesis and maternal smoking. *Canadian Psychiatric Association Journal,* 1975, *20,* 183–187.

Denton, C. L., & McIntyre, C. W. Span of apprehension in hyperactive boys. *Journal of Abnormal Child Psychology,* 1978, *6,* 19–24.

Dunlap, K. *Habits: Their making and unmaking.* New York: Liveright, 1932.

Evans, G. W., & Lovell, B. Design modification in an open plan school. *Journal of Educational Psychology,* 1979, *71,* 41–49.

Feingold, B. F. *Why your child is hyperactive.* New York: Random House, 1975.

Firestone, P. Factors associated with children's adherence to stimulant medication. *American Journal of Orthopsychiatry,* 1982, *52,* 447–456.

Forehand, R., & Baumeister, A. A. Body rocking and activity level as a function of prior movement restraint. *American Journal of Mental Deficiency,* 1970, *74,* 608–610.

Forehand, R., & Baumeister, A. A. Rate of stereotyped body rocking of severe retardates as a function of frustration of goal-directed behavior. *Journal of Abnormal Psychology,* 1971, *78,* 35–42.

Foxx, R. M., & Azrin, N. H. The elimination of autistic self-stimulatory behavior by overcorrection. *Journal of Applied Behavior Analysis,* 1973, *6,* 1–14.

Fraiberg, S. *Insights from the blind.* New York: Basic, 1977.

Golden, G. S. Gilles de la Tourette's syndrome following methylphenidate administration. *Developmental Medicine and Child Neurology,* 1974, *16,* 76–78.

Hallahan, D. P., & Kaufman, J. M. *Introduction to learning disabilities.* Englewood Cliffs, NJ: Prentice-Hall, 1976.

Hollis, J. H. Chlorpromazine: Direct measurement of differential behavioral effect. *Science,* 1968, *159,* 1487–1489.

Hollis, J. H. Body-rocking: Effects of sound and reinforcement. *American Journal of Mental Deficiency,* 1971, *75,* 642–644.

Klaber, M. M., & Butterfield, E. C. Stereotyped rocking: A measure of institution and ward effectiveness. *American Journal of Mental Deficiency,* 1968, *73,* 13–20.

Kolata, G. Food affects human behavior. *Science,* 1982, *218,* 1209–1210.

Kravitz, H., & Boehm, J. J. Rhythmic habit patterns in infancy: Their sequence, age of onset, and frequency. *Child Development,* 1971, *42,* 399–413.

Lambert, N. M., Sandoval, J., & Sassone, D. Prevalence of hyperactivity in elementary school children as a function of social system definers. *American Journal of Orthopsychiatry,* 1978, *48,* 446–463.

Lambert, N. M., Sandoval, J., & Sassone, D. Prevalence of treatment regimens for children considered to be hyperactive. *American Journal of Orthopsychiatry,* 1979, *49,* 482–490.

Lapouse, R., & Monk, M. An epidemiological study of behavior characteristics in children. *American Journal of Public Health,* 1958, *48,* 1134–1144.

Lapouse, R., & Monk, M. Behavior deviations in a representative sample of children: Variation by sex, age, race, social class, and family size. *American Journal of Orthopsychiatry,* 1964, *34,* 436–446.

Lerer, R. J., Lerer, M. P., & Artner, J. The effects of methylphenidate on the handwriting of children with minimal brain dysfunction. *Journal of Pediatrics,* 1977, *91,* 127–132.

Levy, D. M. On the problem of movement restraint: Tics, stereotyped movements, hyperactivity. *American Journal of Orthopsychiatry,* 1944, *14,* 644–671.

Lipman, R. S. The use of psychopharmacological agents in residential facilities for the retarded. In F. J. Menolascino (Ed.), *Psychiatric approaches to mental retardation.* New York: Basic, 1970.

Loney, J., Kramer, J., & Milich, R. The hyperactive child grows up: Predictors of symptoms, delinquency, and achievement at follow-up. Paper presented at the meeting of the American Association for the advancement of Science, Houston, January, 1979.

Loney, J., & Milich, R. Hyperactivity, inattention, and aggression in clinical practice. In M. Wolraich & D. Routh (Eds.), *Advances in behavioral pediatrics.* Vol. 3. Greenwich, CT: JAI Press, 1982.

Milich, R., & Loney, J. The role of hyperactive and aggressive symptomatology in predicting adolescent outcome among hyperactive children. *Journal of Pediatric Psychology,* 1979, *4,* 93–112.

Morrison, J. R., & Stewart, M. A. A family study of the hyperactive child syndrome. *Biological Psychiatry,* 1971, *3,* 189–195.

Morrison, J. R., & Stewart, M. A. The psychiatric status of the legal families of adopted hyperactive children. *Archives of General Psychiatry,* 1973, *28,* 888–891.

Mulhern, T., & Baumeister, A. A. An experimental attempt to reduce stereotypy by reinforcement procedures. *American Journal of Mental Deficiency,* 1969, *74,* 69–74.

Murphy, R. J., Nunes, D. L., & Hutchings-Ruprecht, M. Reduction of stereotyped behavior in profoundly retarded individuals. *American Journal of Mental Deficiency,* 1977, *82,* 238–245.

National Institutes of Health. Consensus Development Conference statement: Defined diets and childhood hyperactivity. *Journal of the American Medical Association,* 1982, *248,* 290–292.

Needleman, H. Effects of low level lead exposure on children. In M. Wolraich & D. K. Routh (Eds.), *Advances in behavioral pediatrics.* Vol. 3. Greenwich, CT: JAI press, 1982.

Nicassio, F. J., Liberman, R. P., Patterson, R. L., Ramirez, E., & Sanders, N. The treatment of tics by negative practice. *Journal of Behavior Therapy and Experimental Psychiatry,* 1972, *3,* 281–287.

Nichols, P. L., & Chen, T.-C. *Minimal brain dysfunction: A prospective study.* Hillsdale, NJ: Erlbaum, 1981.

Patton, J. E., Routh, D. K., & Offenbach, S. I. Televised classroom events as distractors for reading disabled children. *Journal of Abnormal Child Psychology,* 1981, *9,* 355–370.

Patton, J. E., Stinard, T. A., & Routh, D. K. Where do children study? Paper presented at the meeting of the American Educational Research Association, Des Moines, Iowa, 1981.

Prinz, R. J., Roberts, W. A., & Hantman, E. Dietary correlates of hyperactive behavior in children. *Journal of Consulting and Clinical Psychology,* 1980, *48,* 760–769.

Rapoport, J. L., Buchsbaum, M. S., Weingartner, H., Zahn, T. P., Ludlow, C., & Mikkelson, E. J. Dextroamphetamine: Its cognitive and behavioral effects in normal and hyperactive boys and normal men. *Archives of General Psychiatry,* 1978, *37,* 933–943.

Reid, J. G., Tombaugh, T. N., & Van den Heuvel, K. Application of contingent physical restraint to suppress sterotyped body rocking of profoundly mentally retarded persons. *American Journal of Mental Deficiency,* 1981, *86,* 78–85.

Rie, E. D., & Rie, H. E. Recall, retention, and Ritalin. *Journal of Consulting and Clinical Psychology,* 1977, *45,* 967–972.

Rincover, A., Newsome, C. D., & Carr, E. G. Using sensory extinction procedures in the treatment of compulsivelike behavior in developmentally disabled children. *Journal of Consulting and Clinical Psychology,* 1979, *47,* 695–701.

Roberts, M. A. A behavioral method for differentiating hyperactive, aggressive, and hyperactive plus aggressive children. Unpublished Ph.D. dissertation, University of Wisconsin, Madison, 1979.

Romanczyk, R. G. Intermittent punishment of self-stimulation: Effectiveness during application and extinction. *Journal of Consulting and Clinical Psychology,* 1977, *45,* 53–60.

Routh, D. K. Hyperactivity. In P. R. Magrab (Ed.), *Psychological management of pediatric problems.* Vol. 2. *Sensorineural conditions and social concerns.* Baltimore: University Park Press, 1978.

Routh, D. K. Developmental and social aspects of hyperactivity. In C. K. Whalen & B. Henker (Eds.), *Hyperactive children: The social ecology of identification and treatment.* New York: Academic Press, 1980.

Routh, D. K., & Mesibov, G. B. Psychological and environmental interventions: Toward social competence. In H. Rie & E. D. Rie (Eds.), *Handbook of minimal brain dysfunctions.* New York: Wiley, 1980.

Routh, D. K., & Roberts, R. D. Minimal brain dysfunction in children: Failure to find evidence for a behavioral syndrome. *Psychological Reports,* 1972, *31,* 307–314.

Routh, D. K., & Schroeder, C. S. Standardized playroom measures as indices of hyperactivity. *Journal of Abnormal Child Psychology,* 1976, *4,* 199–207.

Rutter, M. Brain damage syndromes in childhood: Concepts and findings. *Journal of Child Psychology and Psychiatry,* 1977, *18,* 1–21.

Shapiro, A. K., Shapiro, E. S., Bruun, R. D., & Sweet, R. D. *Gilles de la Tourette syndrome.* New York: Raven, 1978.

Sprague, R. L., & Baxley, G. B. Drugs for behavior

management, with comment on some legal aspects. In J. Wortis (Ed.), *Mental retardation and developmental disabilities.* Vol. 10. New York: Brunner/Mazel, 1978.

Stevens, H. The syndrome of Gilles de la Tourette and its treatment: Report of a case. *Medical Annals of the District of Columbia,* 1964, *33,* 277–280.

Stewart, M. A., DeBlois, C. S., & Cummings, C. Psychiatric disorder in the parents of hyperactive boys and those with conduct disorders. *Journal of Child Psychology and Psychiatry,* 1980, *21,* 283–292.

Ter Vrugt, D., & Pederson, D. R. The effects of vertical rocking frequencies on the arousal level in two-month-old infants. *Child Development,* 1973, *44,* 205–209.

Thelen, E. Rhythmical behavior in infancy: An ethological perspective. *Developmental Psychology,* 1981, *17,* 237–257.

Varley, C. K. Effects of methylphenidate in adolescents with attention deficit disorder. *Journal of the American Academy of Child Psychiatry,* 1983, *22,* 351–354.

Varley, C. K., & Trupin, E. W. Double-blind assessment of stimulant medication for attention deficit disorder: A model for clinical application. *American Journal of Orthopsychiatry,* 1983, *53,* 542–547.

Weiss, B. Food additives and environmental chemicals as sources of childhood behavior disorders. *Journal of the American Academy of Child Psychiatry,* 1982, *21,* 144–152.

Whalen, C. K., Henker, B., & Dotemoto, S. Methylphenidate and hyperactivity: Effects on teacher behaviors. *Science,* 1980, *208,* 1280–1282.

Whalen, C. K., Henker, B., & Dotemoto, S. Teacher response to methylphenidate (Ritalin) versus placebo status of hyperactive boys in the classroom. *Child Development,* 1981, *52,* 1005–1014.

Yates, A. J. The application of learning theory to the treatment of tics. *Journal of Abnormal and Social Psychology,* 1958, *56,* 175–182.

CHAPTER 7

Sleep and Dream Disorders

Rosalind D. Cartwright and Steven M. Weber

Disturbance of sleep in infants, children, and adolescents has been an area largely overlooked by clinicians despite its potential seriousness for the child and the family (Hauri, 1982). No falser truism was ever coined than to say of someone who sleeps well, "He sleeps like a baby." Babies sleep poorly by adult standards and sometimes this persists throughout life.

Sleep disorders vary with age. Beyond the normal failure to sleep through the night of infancy which, in a few cases, can be a lasting primary insomnia, and the problems of early childhood when behaviors normal to waking (i.e., walking) can intrude into sleep, comes the hypersomnia of adolescence which, in some cases, is more than just an aggravation to those trying to get a teenager up for school and may be a seriously debilitating sleep disorder.

In DSM-III (1980), which provides an organized framework for identifying psychopathological disorders of infancy, childhood and adolescence, only two syndromes are included which occur during sleep. These are listed under the heading "Other Disorders with Physical Manifestations": sleepwalking disorder and sleep terror disorder. However, the introductory paragraph to this section is cautionary in tone concerning the role of psychological factors in these disorders. It is an accurate reflection of the present state of knowledge concerning these two patterns of bizarre behaviors to say there is divided opinion on whether emotional factors are involved in their incidence.

In addition to the two disorders listed in DSM-III, there are many other sleep disorders which are recognized in another diagnostic system. This category system, published in 1979 by the Association of Sleep Disorders Centers (ASDC), is included in the DSM-III volume as Appendix E. The ASDC system organizes the sleep and arousal disorders into four general types: (1) disorders of initiating and maintaining sleep (DIMS), commonly called the insomnias; (2) disorders of excessive somnolence (DOES), or hypersomnias; (3) disorders of sleep-wake schedule (phase-shift disorders); and (4) dysfunctions associated with sleep, sleep stages, or partial arousals (parasomnias). The two sleep problems recognized by DSM III, sleepwalking and sleep terror, fall under the last category. They are only two of a family of sleep-associated abnormal behaviors, which includes bruxism (tooth grinding), nocturnal enuresis, rocking or head banging, and sleep talking: All have several features in common, most notably a high incidence in early childhood. Children also suffer from sleep problems belonging to the other major categories as well, particularly those falling into the DIMS (insomnias) and DOES (hypersomnia) groupings. In these, too, the role of psychological factors is still controversial.

The questions for the clinical psychologist who deals with patients in the childhood through adolescence age range are these: Are those who present sleep-disordered behavior suffering from some underlying psychopathology (a primary mental disorder) which has secondary effects on sleep? Or is the sleep disorder primary with secondary psychological effects? Or is the problem a physiological disorder without any specific psychological sequelae for the child, but one that produces family anxieties needing to be addressed? All three of these possibilities appear to hold true among the various sleep disorders. Since the treatment program depends on the answers to these questions and since the answers frequently require more data than the clinician has at hand, he or she would do well to clarify matters as much as possible by a good history. The specific precipitating events and the general psychological contextual factors associated with these disturbances, the family history of similar problems, and the health and medication history all need to be reviewed. However, this will not be adequate to correctly diagnose all sleep problems. For some, a special all-night or daytime laboratory investigation is needed to differentiate among disorders which look alike. For this a referral to a sleep disorder service will be necessary.

The investigation of sleep problems requires a shift in perspective for the clinician from one of viewing the child's behavior only as it is manifest during waking hours to a twenty-four-hour model which includes the states of rapid eye movement (REM) sleep and non-rapid eye movement (NREM) sleep. The inclusion of these data in the assessment of the child has been a long-overdue development. The interaction of waking and sleep behaviors is as important to understand as are mind and body interactions. For example, it is not surprising that children who are full of anxieties during their waking life do not sleep well and have bad dreams, or that some infants who experience the waking world as abandoning and/or rejecting suffer reactive attachment disorders (anaclitic depressions) and sleep excessively (see Chapter 9, "Depressive Disorders"). On the other hand, children who suffer from some sleep disorders (such as sleep apnea syndrome) may have cognitive disturbances and appear in waking as retarded or depressed.

In this chapter we will explore three aspects of the problem of understanding and treating childhood sleep disorders. First, by addressing the normal development of sleep from birth through adolescence, a general framework will be laid for identifying deviations from norms. Second, deviations in sleep recognized in the DSM-III system will be reviewed. Last, other sleep and dream deviations which occur in infancy, childhood, and adolescence will be described and those associated with psychopathology will be differentiated from those which may be mistaken for indications of psychopathology.

The Development of Normal Sleep

Somewhere between twenty-four and thirty-six weeks after conception, the fetus in utero begins to show evidence of alternating between states of sleep and wakefulness. This lifelong pattern of alternating states emerges from a primitive undifferentiated state which is neither sleep nor wakefulness and is characteristic of premature infants born less than twenty-four weeks after conception. Some of the changes in the sleep-wake cycle of the normal human over the life cycle are a reduction in total sleep time and in the number of sleep periods per day, a change in the clock time during which the main sleep period occurs to nighttime, changes in the kind and amount of brain wave patterns, and in other physiological and behavioral variables. In order to present this development of the sleep-wake cycle from infancy through adolescence, the fully-developed sleep pattern in healthy adults will first be described.

Aserinsky and Kleitman (1953) discovered that normal adult sleep consists of the two quantitatively and qualitatively distinct states: NREM and REM sleep. Each type of sleep has its own peculiar behavioral, psychological and physiological properties and each sleep state is assessed and recognized through the application of a physiological recording technique called *polysomnography.* A polygraph (a device for recording physiological phenomena onto a long strip of paper) is used to amplify the strength of electrical signals picked up from electrodes (small metal discs which detect electrical differences) placed on the body surface. Three basic physiological parameters are always recorded on a polysomnogram: (1) the subject's brain wave pattern, the electroencephalogram (EEG); (2) the electrical activity of the muscles just below the chin, the electromyogram (EMG); and (3) the electrical signal generated by movements of the eyes, the electrooculogram (EOG). The locations on the head and face at which the electrodes are usually placed are shown in Figure 7-1, which also includes samples of the tracings of these three phenomena. It is the pattern of activity in these three signals which define the various sleep stages of NREM, REM, and wakefulness (Rechtschaffen & Kales, 1968).

Adults and children past the age of two years show two basic types of EEG patterns while they are awake: beta rhythm and alpha rhythm. The top trace of Figure 7-2 is an example of waking beta rhythm. The second trace of Figure 7-2, labeled "Drowsy," is a sample of waking alpha rhythm recorded from a drowsy but still awake adult. The EEG of wakefulness normally alternates only between alpha and beta rhythms in older children and adults. During sleep the EEG exhibits a great deal more variability.

The EMG and EOG of the waking state also exhibit variability. When muscle cell activity is high, as during active contraction, the EMG trace appears as a high amplitude, broad swath of ink laid down con-

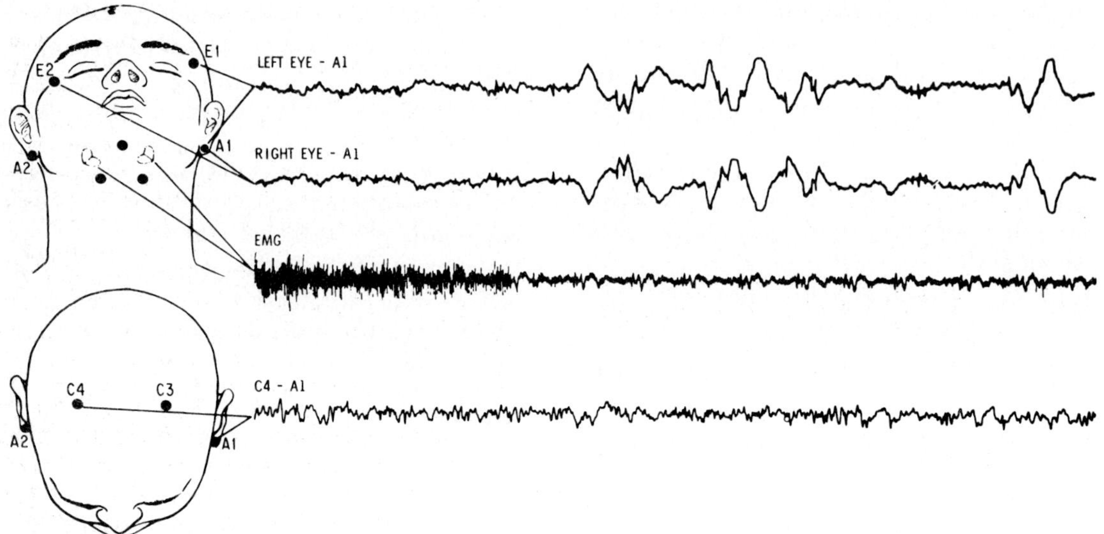

Figure 7-1. Electrodes for recording the EOG, EEG, and EMG during sleep are fixed to the scalp and face at the locations shown (from Rechtschaffen and Kales, 1968).

tinuously on the paper. When the muscle cells around the electrode are relaxed, the amplitude of the tracing decreases but never completely drops to zero in an awake subject. There is always some minimal amount of contraction, or muscle tone, present in most of the body musculature during wakefulness and it is recorded as a low amplitude, continuous EMG signal. Likewise, the EOG, or eye movement, tracing will vary with the amount and type of eye movement generated by the awake subject. Fast eye movements produce very large amplitude, sharp waves in the EOG tracing. This type of eye movement and the resulting EOG recordings are illustrated in Figure 7-1 for both the left and right eyes. Slow eye movements produce an EOG tracing which appears as a slowly undulating signal with less amplitude. An example of this slow rolling EOG signal is seen on the top trace of Figure 7-3, which is a recording of both eyes together by a single pen on the polygraph. If the eyes are not moving, the EOG shows no large deflections.

The overall pattern of activity in the EEG, EOG, and EMG recordings made in a typical sleep laboratory is used to differentiate sleep from wakefulness, NREM from REM sleep, and to distinguish the four stages of sleep within NREM.

The process of falling asleep in a healthy adult involves the rapid descent from wakefulness into NREM sleep, which is subdivided into the four sequential stages 1, 2, 3 and 4 on the basis of the EEG pattern. Figure 7-3 illustrates the pattern of eye movement, brain wave, and muscle tension activity characteristic of an awake but very drowsy person. The EEG shows the presence of waking alpha rhythm and the EMG demonstrates the presence of continuous muscle tone. In Figure 7-4, the transition from wakefulness to stage 1 of NREM has taken place. The most prominent feature of this first period of sleep is the EEG, which shows no alpha waves.

Stage 1 of NREM is a transitional phase lasting for at most ten minutes. Stage 2, which follows, is characterized by the

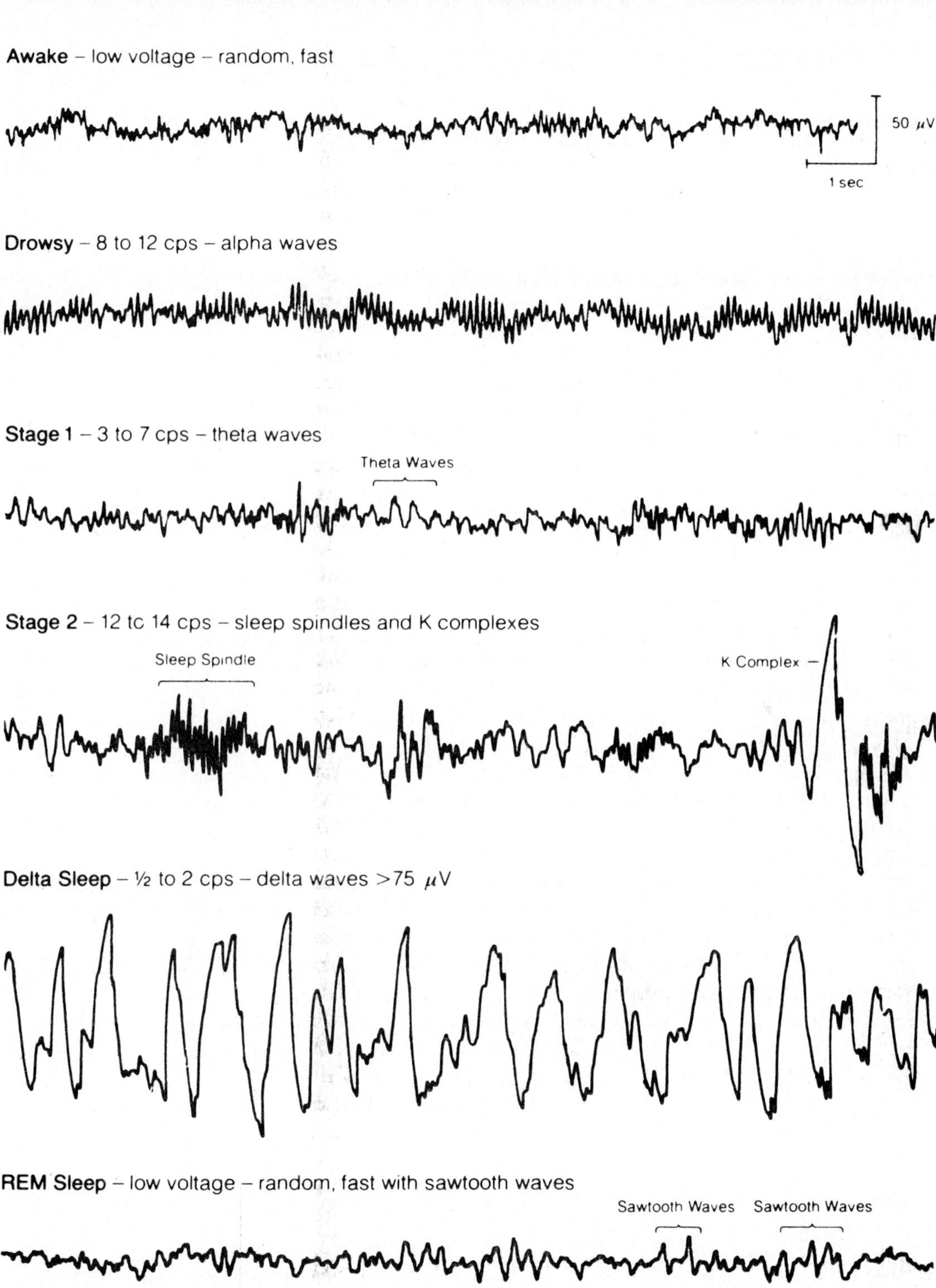

Figure 7-2. Representative EEG recordings of wakefulness, NREM, and REM sleep (from Hauri, 1977).

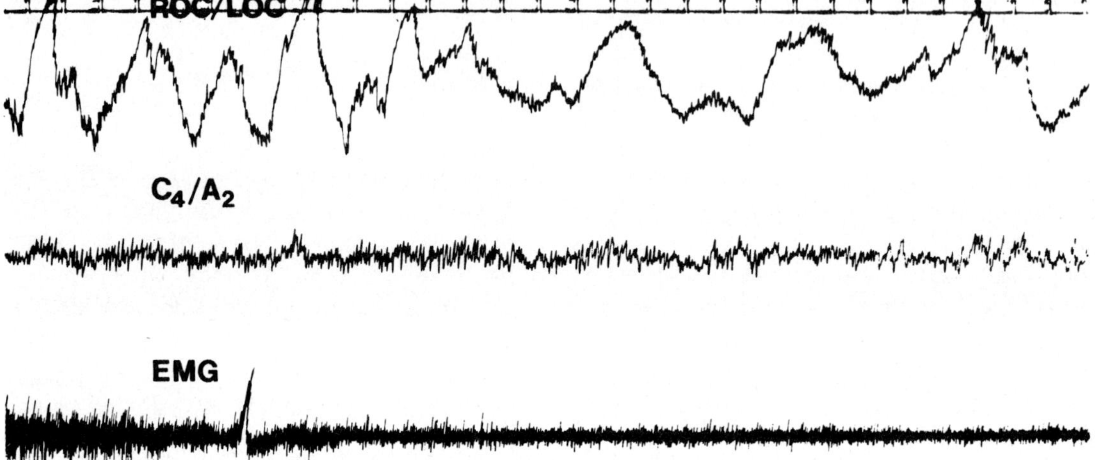

Figure 7-3. A waking polysomnogram. ROC/LOC is a single EOG tracing from both eyes. C_4/A_2 is the EEG. The EMG is recorded from the chin. The top tracing is a time line. Each interval represents one second.

presence of two new EEG events which are unique to normal sleep and do not occur during the waking state: the sleep spindle and the K-complex. An example of these brain waves is shown in Figure 7-2.

Stages 3 and 4 are often grouped together as *delta sleep* because both of these states are defined by the presence of a high amplitude, very slow waveform called delta rhythm. Stages 3 and 4 are somewhat arbitrarily differentiated by the amount of slow, high amplitude delta rhythm present. An example of almost continuous delta rhythm during Stage 4 is seen in Figure 7-2.

During the transition into sleep from wakefulness through States 1, 2, 3, and 4, the EEG changes dramatically from the

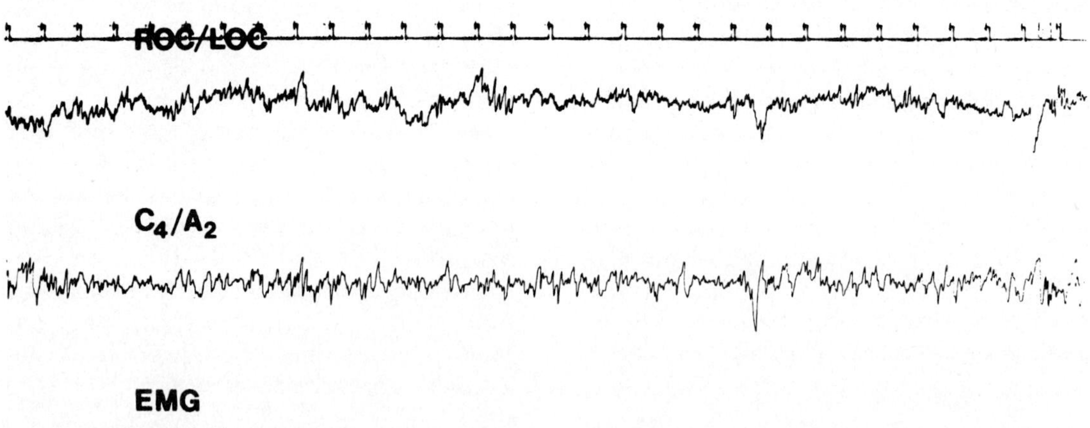

Figure 7-4. Stage 1 of NREM sleep.

rapid, irregular beta rhythm of alert wakefulness to the slower and more regular alpha rhythm of drowsiness to the still slower rhythm of stage 1 of NREM and culminates in the very slow, high amplitude waves of stage 4. The most conspicuous characteristic of NREM sleep is thus a progressive slowing of the EEG with a gradual increase in the amplitude of the waves and the appearance of many wave patterns which occur only during sleep.

The first period of NREM sleep after sleep onset lasts for approximately seventy to ninety minutes. Following this initial NREM progression, the EEG, EOG, and EMG tracings exhibit remarkable changes as the first period of REM sleep begins. REM is characterized by the sudden appearance of rapid eye movements behind the closed eyelids of the sleeper, as seen in the EOG tracing shown in Figure 7-5.

Perhaps the most unusual change in the polysomnogram during REM takes place in the EMG. The tracing in Figure 7-5 has become a pencil-thin line with only widely separated short bursts of activity. During REM sleep, the voluntary musculature of the body is paralyzed by a neurological mechanism located in the brain stem. The result is a loss of muscle tone in the various voluntary muscle groups.

Up to this point, we have discussed only electrophysiological characteristics of NREM and REM sleep. This initial concentration has been necessary in order to show how these two quite different types of sleep are defined in the normal. There is also a cognitive aspect to both NREM and REM. Soon after the discovery of REM sleep, it became apparent that *dreaming*, the surreal and highly visual narrative hallucination which we all experience during sleep, is very strongly associated with this specific sleep stage. The initial studies of the association of dreams with REM and NREM sleep stages reported that when subjects were awakened out of REM sleep they recalled a dream 72 to 94 percent of the time. In contrast, when awakened out of NREM sleep and questioned about dream content, subjects could recall dreams only 0 to 7 percent of the time. Therefore, it appeared that dreaming was an exclusive, or nearly exclusive, property of REM sleep.

Later studies reported tremendous variability in the incidence of dreams during

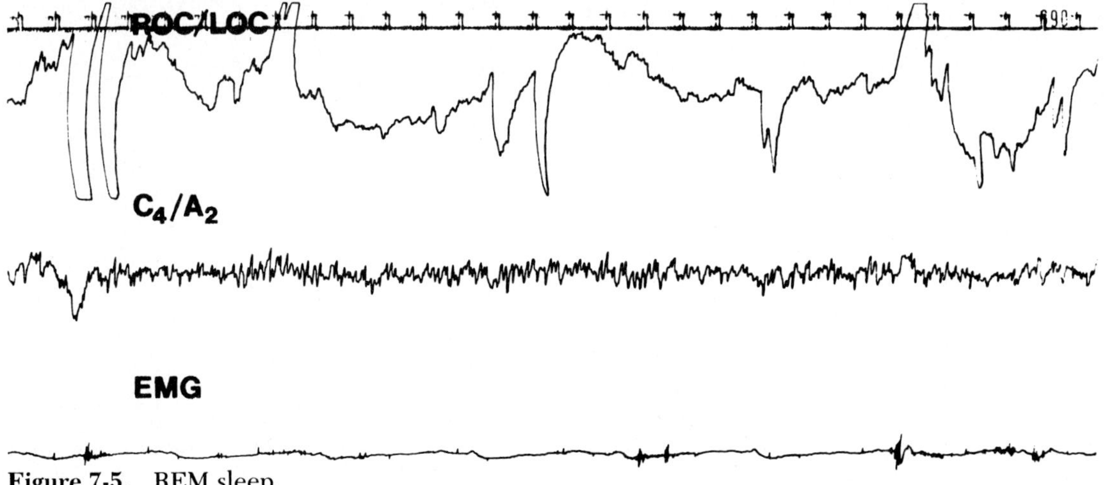

Figure 7-5. REM sleep.

NREM sleep, but consistently observed high rates of dream reports arising out of REM sleep. A review of the literature in this area (Herman, Ellman, & Roffwarg, 1978) concluded that there is cognitive activity associated with NREM, but that it is different in character from that typically elicited from REM sleep and that NREM cognition occurs much less frequently than does REM dreaming. The mentation or mental processes of NREM sleep is less bizarre, more realistic, more fragmented, less visual, and less likely to be perceived as really happening. In comparison, the cognitive component of REM sleep is more vivid, narrative in character, and visually surreal. These differences in character and in frequency of occurrence may shed some light on the function of the suppression of voluntary muscle tone during REM. There is widespread speculation that the reason for muscle tone suppression during REM sleep is to prevent overt behavioral responding to the narrative content of the dream. Given the differences in the character of cognitive activity during NREM and REM sleep, it is plausible that such a protective mechanism exists in order to protect the sleeper from potential injury while in the process of responding behaviorally to dream content (Jouvet, 1965).

The transition from wakefulness to REM sleep is called the *sleep cycle*, and the sequence of stages repeats itself during the sleep period. Figure 7-6 is a graphic presentation of several sleep cycles generated over a typical eight-hour sleep period by a healthy young adult. It reveals several interesting differences between the distribution of REM versus NREM sleep. First, the interval between the onset of successive REM periods is approximately ninety minutes. That is, REM sleep exhibits its own cycle within the overall context of sleep and tends to recur every ninety minutes. Second, REM periods become progressively longer as the sleep period continues. The first REM episode may last for only five to ten minutes. The second REM period may range between ten and twenty minutes, with subsequent periods becoming longer still. The result of this progressive lengthening is that the majority of REM sleep is concentrated within the last half of the sleep period. Unlike the distribution of REM, NREM sleep stages 3 and 4 (delta sleep) are concentrated in the first half of the sleep period. Less and less time is spent by the sleeper in delta sleep as the sleep period continues, since episodes of stages 3 and 4 gradually shorten in duration over successive sleep cycles and eventually disappear from the polysomnogram. Therefore, not only do REM and NREM sleep differ in terms of their behavioral, psychological, and physiological characteristics, they also demonstrate sharp differences in the way in which they are distributed in time. The total distribution of the sleep stages over the sleep period, as illustrated in Figure 7-6, is termed *sleep architecture* to convey the notion that, in the healthy young adult, sleep is an orderly and predictable structure. Sleep architecture exhibits developmental changes from birth to old age and is very important in the definition and diagnosis of many child and adult sleep disorders.

The brain wave patterns, sleep stages, and sleep architecture of the neonate are very different from those of a young adult. All of these features gradually evolve over infancy, childhood, and adolescence in a roughly predictable manner to produce the adult sleep pattern, which then remains relatively stable in character until old age. Rather than classify sleep into the two general adult categories of NREM and REM, neonatal sleep is described in a three-part system: quiet sleep (QS), active

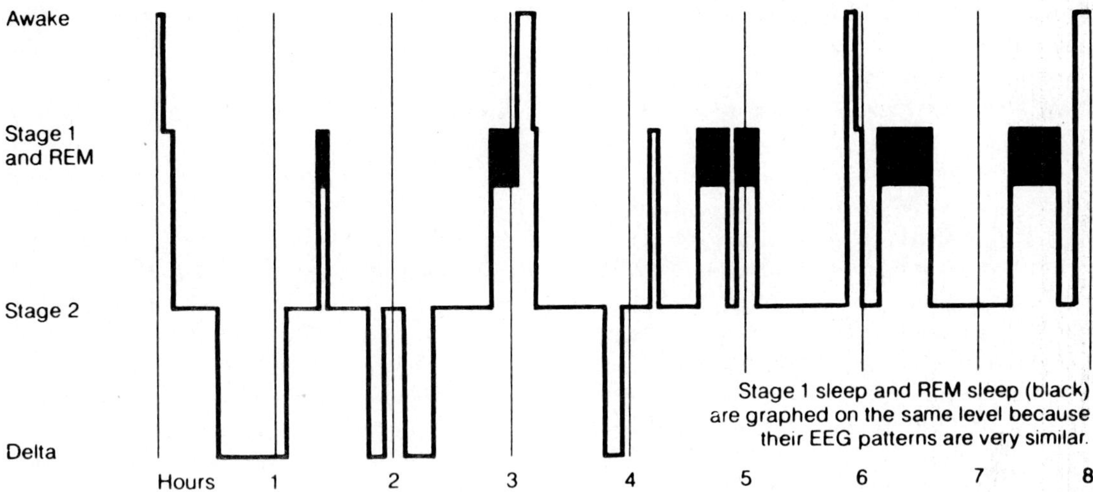

Figure 7-6. Sleep architecture of a young adult. Periods of REM sleep are shaded (from Hauri, 1977).

sleep (AS), and indeterminate sleep (IS) (Anders, Emde, & Parmalee, 1971).

QS is the infant analog of NREM sleep. It is not divided into substages. The definition of QS requires the evaluation of more parameters than that of NREM, and is defined by a variety of EEG patterns, along with the absence of observable behaviors and body movements.

AS is the infant analog of REM sleep in the adult, in that rapid eye movements occur singly or in bursts and frequently, but not always, the EMG is suppressed. There are three possible EEG patterns which may occur. During AS respiration is often irregular in rate and depth and a wide variety of stereotypical behaviors may be present. Facial movements are common and may consist of smiles, grimaces, and frowns. Episodic sucking movements of the cheeks and lips may occur, along with gross body writhing and occasional vocalization.

The third category of infant sleep in the neonatal period, indeterminate sleep, is relatively easy to define. Any 30-second portion of the polysomnogram which does not meet the criteria for AS or QS is dubbed indeterminate. It is used when it is not possible to determine whether the neonate is awake or asleep—a situation which is very common.

Given that the sleep stages of the full-term neonate and their defining features are so different from those of the young adult, it is not surprising that major differences exist in other aspects of sleep. The neonate will sleep an average of sixteen to eighteen hours a day, distributed over six to nine periods. Fifty percent of this total sleep time will consist of AS (adults spend approximately 20 to 25 percent of total sleep time in REM), with a sleep cycle ranging between thirty to forty minutes. Periods of AS tend to occur at much shorter intervals than periods of REM sleep in the adult. Another difference is that normal neonates have the ability to enter AS directly from wakefulness, without any transition through QS (Ellingson, 1979). Normal adults usually require approximately ninety minutes of NREM before the first episode of REM sleep occurs.

Between four and ten weeks after birth,

the neonatal sleep pattern begins to resemble the adult sleep pattern. The transition occurs over a period ranging between two to four weeks and consists of three major changes. First, the direct passage from wakefulness to AS no longer occurs. A thirty to forty minute episode of mandatory QS is necessary before AS appears in the polysomnogram. Second, the beginning seeds of stages 3 and 4 of NREM appear. Third, sleep spindles appear during QS. Thus, the sleep architecture of the older infant approximates that of the adult in terms of the wake-sleep transition and the EEG pattern of QS contains features of NREM in the form of sleep spindles and periods of high voltage slow activity.

At three to four months of age, the waking alpha rhythm appears in the EEG at a relatively low frequency, allowing a more accurate index of the onset of sleep. The frequency of the alpha rhythm increases gradually, attaining 5 to 6 Hz by twelve months of age, until it stabilizes between 9 and 11 Hz close to eight years of age (Shagass, 1972). The individual's adult frequency is usually present by age fifteen.

At the same time of life that the waking EEG assumes more mature characteristics (three to four months of age), sleep stages become classifiable as NREM and REM. The stages of QS, AS, and IS are no longer applicable. NREM can be split into two substages, which are termed Stage 1–2 and Stage 3–4. By six months of age, stages 1 and 2 of NREM sleep are separable, and after one year stages 3 and 4 can be discriminated. Thus, the sleep stages of the adult appear rather rapidly during the first year of life (Guilleminault & Souquet, 1979). However, several other features of sleep in young adulthood require considerably more time to mature.

The sixteen to eighteen hours per day spent by the neonate in sleep drops to approximately twelve hours per day at one year of age. Total sleep time is further reduced to around ten hours per day by age ten and does not approximate the average adult duration of eight hours per day until between thirteen and sixteen years. Likewise, the number of sleep periods per day exhibits a fairly long and variable decline. Around three-and-one-half months after birth, the sleep of the infant begins to consolidate into the nocturnal phase of the 24-hour day. This is seen as a gradual lengthening of periods of nocturnal sleep accompanied by a progressive shortening of daytime naps. During the first through the second year, the number of sleep periods is reduced to two or three per day with a single sustained period of nocturnal sleep accompanied by one or two short daytime naps. The single nocturnal sleep period characteristic of North American culture emerges usually by the fifth, but can be as late as the tenth, year of life. Similarly, the high proportion of total sleep time occupied by the REM sleep in early infancy undergoes a steady decline until it assumes the adult value of approximately 20 to 25 percent between the third and fifth year of age. Also, the neonatal forty-minute sleep cycle begins to lengthen after one year of age and achieves a duration of ninety minutes in the early teenage years (Kleitman, 1963; Roffwarg, Munzio, & Dement, 1966).

The proportions of total sleep time spent in NREM stages 1 through 4 approximate young adult values between three and five years of age, and the cyclic progression of NREM and REM is now well established. The main difference between children and young adults in sleep architecture is seen in delta sleep. Children from the ages of three to early adolescence have higher proportions of delta sleep early in the sleep period, and the delta waves present in these stages are much higher in amplitude and are much more abundant in the EEG tracing than those of the young adult. This predominance of delta is implicated in one class of childhood sleep disorders, the disorders of partial arousal. Between the ages of three through twelve, there occur some gradual and subtle changes in sleep architecture. As already described, total sleep time decreases. Accompanying this reduction are slight increases in the proportion of total sleep time spent in stages 1, 3, and wakefulness, apparently at the expense of a slight reduction in the proportion of REM sleep.

One of the more important developmental features of the sleep-wake cycle from infancy through adolescence and early adulthood is the increasing social control of the sleep period as the child matures. During the neonatal period and through early infancy, the sleep period is more or less biologically dictated. It is very difficult to keep a sleepy infant awake without heroic measures and parents are generally content, and often grateful, to allow the child to sleep at any time of the day. As the socialization process ensues, particularly with the onset of the school years, the sleep period becomes increasingly under the control of social constraints.

A recent review of sleep during the second decade of life (Carskadon, 1982) has suggested that the enforcement of a fixed wake-up time in the absence of a fixed bedtime in order to meet educational obligations may affect the quantity of nocturnal sleep and the level of daytime alertness in older (twelve and thirteen year olds) versus younger (ten and eleven year olds) adolescents. A survey of sleep patterns in the older group indicated that, in general, total sleep time on school nights was approximately forty minutes to one hour less than that reported on the weekends. These older adolescents had fixed wake times on school days but no fixed bedtime; i.e., they went to bed at a time chosen by themselves. It appears that the increase in weekend sleep time was compensatory in nature. This difference was not seen in the younger group, who tended to have parentally-enforced bedtimes. It was further reported that complaints of increased daytime sleepiness and disturbed nocturnal sleep increase with age in adolescence. This increase in daytime sleepiness may be due to a socially-induced decrease in nocturnal sleep which was reported during puberty. It may also reflect an intrinsic maturational increase in sleepiness due to metabolic changes.

This review of the developmental changes leading to the normal sleep of the adult is a necessary background for interpreting sleep complaints in the child. When should a child be expected to sleep through? How long should the total sleep period be? When should children be able to confine sleep to the night period? Is sleepwalking a normal phenomenon? As more of these questions are investigated by laboratory tests it is important to understand how these data are recorded and what the normative values are for sleep duration, cycle length, and sleep stage percentages. These norms are now available for boys and girls, ages three through nineteen (Williams, Karacan & Hursch, 1974).

Sleep Disorders

In this section the diagnosis and treatment of the two disorders identified as part of the DSM-III classification, sleepwalking and sleep terrors, are considered. Both are grouped in the ASDC nosology as parasomnias: dysfunctions associated with sleep, sleep stages, or partial arousals. More particularly, they are both identified as partial arousal disorders (Broughton, 1968). Sleepwalking and sleep terrors are closely related to each other, often occurring in the same individual and loading strongly within family members (Kales et al., 1980a). Both occur during the transition from delta to REM sleep early in the night's sleep activity.

Sleepwalking

Clinically, *sleepwalking*, or somnambulism, is described as repeated episodes of arising from bed during sleep and walking about, for several minutes up to forty minutes. During these episodes, which typically occur during the first third of the night's sleep, the individual gets out of bed and moves about in a confused and clumsy manner. The person may then show more complicated and purposeful behaviors. Usually it is difficult to awaken the child fully. Although most often the child returns to bed without help, occasionally he or she may terminate an episode by lying down elsewhere and only become aware that a walk took place upon awakening in a strange place. For the most part, the sleepwalker is completely amnesic for the episode, although the child may have mumbled semicoherent answers to questions posed at the time. Contrary to belief, the sleepwalker can be hurt. Sleepwalkers have been known to wander out of doors in pajamas and bare feet on winter nights and be found a block or more from home.

Sleepwalking behaviors are not overtly different from other automatisms that occur in states of incomplete alertness, such as may occur after head injuries, in some drug intoxication states, or in "status absence" (Broughton, 1980). The main difference between sleepwalking and these other disorders is that sleepwalking is typically initiated during the transition from the deepest stage of NREM sleep (delta) to REM sleep. Ordinarily this transition, which takes place at the end of the first or second cycle, takes several minutes to accomplish. During this period the sleeper shifts from the deeply relaxed physiological and psychological state characterized by the high amplitude, slow waves of delta sleep to a situation which is the reverse of this in REM sleep. In delta sleep, there is a slow, even respiratory rate; reduced blood pressure; slow, even heart rate, along with a high auditory threshold and only a little vague, spontaneous mental activity. In REM sleep, the state is one of high cerebral arousal; a low voltage, random EEG; irregular pulse and respiratory rate; the characteristic rapid eye movements, accompanied by a loss of muscle tonus and the hallucinations of dreaming. At the end of a delta period, instead of arousing into this activated sleep state, the sleepwalker arouses motorically. The sleepwalker is not acting out a dream; the child has aborted a dream. During the walk itself the EEG is desynchronized, looking like a stage 1 sleep or wakefulness with alpha activity (Jacobson et al., 1965; Jacobson & Kales, 1967), but this is not accompanied by either the rapid eye movements or the mental content typical of dreaming.

The incidence of sleepwalking is unknown, but is reported by Jacobson, Kales, and Kales (1969) to occur at least once in approximately 15 percent of all children in the five- to twelve-year age range, equally in both sexes. An occasional walker is not as much a clinical problem as is the child with frequent attacks in which bizarre or dangerous behaviors occur or who disrupts the sleep of the household repeatedly. Especially of concern are those who do not "outgrow" these behaviors as the length of the delta sleep in the first cycle reduces with the further maturation of adolescence. Children who continue to sleepwalk into adulthood do become problems of note. The frequency of this latter group is estimated at 2.5 percent by Bixler et al. (1979).

Sleepwalking is found among the relatives of somnambulistic patients much more commonly than it is in the family histories of children without such incidents. Monozygotic twins are concordant for the disorder six times more frequently than dizygotic twins (Bakwin, 1970), and near relatives are more likely to have a history of sleepwalking than distant relatives. Kales et al. (1980a) traced the families of twenty-five sleepwalkers and reported 80 percent had one or more relatives who were also affected. They conclude that the prevalence is ten times greater in first-degree relatives than in the general population, and that heritable factors predispose an individual to this disorder. These authors feel that the high degree of psychopathology in adult sleepwalkers (Kales et al., 1978) argues that the expression of this trait is multiply determined.

Sleep laboratory studies attempting to discover differences between nights when an episode occurs from nights when the child sleeps through have been unsuccessful. Jacobson and Kales (1967) felt that the importance of psychological factors as precipitants is relatively low since an attack can be initiated simply by standing a known sleepwalker on his feet while he is in a delta sleep state. Broughton (1980) argues that the precipitants for an arousal in a confusional state from delta sleep may be any one of a number of types: exteroceptive or external stimuli; interoceptive or internal stimuli; arousal due to normal cyclic processes inherent in sleep structure, including an early onset of some REM-based arousal; or some deeply unconscious disturbing mental activity associated with delta sleep. Since any of these might trigger an episode in a prone individual, what was involved in a particular child on a particular night would be difficult to determine. Some children may have more psychogenic and others more physiological triggers for these attacks.

Aside from the genetic loading, a prone person also seems to be a pathologically deep sleeper, as indicated by difficulty awakening to full arousal in response to either a meaningful stimulus, such as being called by name, or a meaningless stimulus, such as loud noise. Sleep recordings have shown the presence of distinctive rhythmic, paroxysmal, high voltage, slow delta bursts just before episodes of sleepwalking (Kales et al., 1966). These bursts, while common in infants prior to a year of age, decrease markedly as the child matures. Only 3 percent or normal seven- to nine-year-olds show such bursting. The presence of this activity in sleepwalkers has been interpreted as a sign of CNS (central nervous system) immaturity. Actually, during the teenage years, both sleepwalking and this EEG anomaly gradually reduce in frequency of occurrence so that most prone persons are free of these symptoms by age twenty. Other factors related to occurrences of these arousal episodes are any of those which contribute to a deepening or prolonging of the early night delta sleep. Kales et al. (1979) report that a number of cases had their first sleepwalking episode during or following an illness with high fever. Their interpretation of this correlation is that since fever causes a fragmentation of sleep and lightening of stage 4, once the fever abates there will be a compensatory deepening and prolonging of the delta sleep, and it is this abnormally deep delta that can then cause an abnormal, partial arousal during the transition from NREM to REM sleep.

Other factors which act similarly to deepen or lengthen stage 4 sleep also increase the probability of an attack. Sleep deprivation and unusually heavy physical exercise are two such factors, and both should be avoided for the child who is prone to these episodes.

What to do for the sleepwalker who is severely affected, that is, who has one or more episodes per week, who engages in behavior dangerous to self or others, or whose walking limits normal waking activities such as attendance at camp, sleeping over with friends, or trips away from home?

Reassurance, nighttime safety precautions, adequate rest, and avoidance of strenuous physical exercise may on occasion be supplemented by a nighttime dose of diazepam. This medication provides symptom relief by lightening stages 3 and 4 sleep. The transition from delta to REM is less abrupt (Glick, Schulman, & Turecki, 1971).

A psychological approach was reported by Reid, Ahmed, and Levie (1981), who have had good success with hypnotherapy for adult walkers. For six sessions these patients were given the suggestion to arouse fully from their trance state when their feet hit the floor. This presumably then generalized to prevent sleepwalking by causing them to wake up from their "trance-like" state as they got out of bed.

Generally, the consensus is that sleepwalking behaviors can be interpreted for their underlying motivational component and therefore addressed in psychological treatment. One young adult patient treated in our service had not had any sleepwalking episodes for a number of years until he left home to attend college. There he began sleepwalking from the dorm. This was considered dangerous and, as a consequence, he had to return to living at home, which he experienced as a failure. At home he continued sleepwalking. During one episode he displayed his hostility to his younger brother by throwing his brother's stereo out the window. His conflict about dependency and independence manifested when he left the house and wandered several blocks away. Treatment consisted of both diazepam and confidence-building to develop independent behaviors.

Another patient, who was eight years old, developed a sleep jumping behavior. He would get out of bed and jump in place straight up and down with open, glazed eyes. This began when his divorced parents both remarried and started trading him back and forth, a week with one family and a week with the other. This was too much "jumping around" for him, and he only slept through on the nights when he stayed with his grandmother. In this case, there was a genetic propensity for an arousal disorder in that the father had been a sleepwalker as a child. His two sets of parents were so at odds they were not able to coordinate their efforts to bring the child in to treatment, unfortunately.

The clinician dealing with sleepwalking needs to listen for those factors which precipitate the episodes in prone persons, for despite the general rule that these will wane in most persons as maturation continues, those who continue to sleepwalk into their twenties are those with a disorder needing some intervention. In a recent study, Kales et al. (1980b) report that adult sleepwalkers differ on MMPI patterns from nonwalking controls and from a group who had previously walked as children. The adult walkers showed more underlying anger in reaction to frustration, to failure, and to loss of self-esteem. These are issues which can be addressed in psychotherapeutic treatment.

The evaluation of the complaint of sleepwalking in the child or adolescent, then, requires a careful history, including the presence of other sleepwalkers in the family history, age of onset, frequency of episodes, clock time of the occurrence, how long after sleep onset, behaviors during the episode, general life adjustment, and general as well as specific stresses around the time of occurrences. This will help to sort out those who appear to be more functional from those who are more organic in nature and guide the treatment into either a wait-it-out or an intervention choice.

Sleep Terrors

Sleep terrors, also called night terrors and, in the child, pavor nocturnus, is another one of the disorders of partial arousal occurring in young children in the first third of the night during the transition from delta sleep to REM sleep. These episodes are described as very abrupt arousals, usually involving a sit-up, with wide, staring eyes and a blood-curdling scream. The child appears to be in a panic state both behaviorally and by the intensity of the autonomic activation. The heart races, often doubling or even tripling in rate, respiratory rate increases, and skin resistance drops. Yet the child is usually amnesic for any mental content accompanying these episodes. If any reasons for the panic are given, they tend to be of a single image, such as an attacking or smothering animal, rather than of an elaborated dream story. Seventy-five percent of these attacks occur at the end of the first NREM sleep cycle, although some individuals have multiple episodes per night. Only in those with multiple attacks is an episode likely to initiate during stage 2 sleep. Many individuals who have sleep terror episodes also sleepwalk. In fact, after the sit-up and scream, lasting only a few minutes, many will then get out of bed and walk about for a while without awareness before returning to bed.

This blending of sleep terror and sleepwalking occurred in a patient who called these his "flyswatter" experiences. He would arise in terror, feeling a gigantic flyswatter was about to come down on him. This propelled him out of the bed to escape. On the last occasion before his hospitalization he was propelled out of his bedroom window. He only became conscious when he was outside looking into his bedroom which, luckily, was in a basement apartment.

The prevalence of sleep terrors is unknown. It is thought to be much less common than sleepwalking, with the prevalence per thousand children estimated at between 1.5 and 2.9. As with sleepwalking, recall for these activities next day is poor, which helps to differentiate sleep terrors from nightmares.

Nightmares is a term reserved for frightening dreams which occur during REM sleep. Nightmares are not accompanied by the extreme autonomic arousal associated with sleep terror episodes, although the nightmare sufferer will give an account of a very terrifying dream that preceded the awaking. Since they occur during, rather than prior to, REM sleep, a nightmare is more likely to occur in the last third of the night when REM sleep is more prevalent.

The sleep of those suffering from sleep terrors shows no disturbance of REM sleep. In fact, the only EEG phenomenon associated with these episodes is that the intensity of the attack appears to correlate to the length of the preceding delta sleep: the longer the preceding delta, the higher the heart rate, and the more intense the anxiety in the episode (Fisher, et al., 1974).

Both diazepam and imipramine have been used to treat sleep terrors pharmacologically (Kahn, et al., 1971; Pesikoff & Davis, 1971). The positive effect of these drugs for this condition appears to be not so much in suppressing delta sleep as in their tranquilizing effect on the physiological arousal.

Agrell and Axelsson (1972) have approached treatment another way. They report that of twenty-three children with sleep terrors and enlarged adenoids, twenty-two became symptom-free following adenoidectomy. This suggests that the smothering imagery and panic associated with sleep terrors in some children may be related to an obstruction of the nasal/oral airway. This then results in some hypoxia leading to a fearful arousal. This possibility should certainly be checked in patients prone to these attacks.

The high frequency of sleepwalking in the family histories of sleep terror patients led Kales et al. (1980a) to suggest that these two have a common genetic and neurophysiological substrate. There is some indication that the adult who continues to have sleep terror attacks is characterized by high anxiety, depression, and inhibition in outward aggression. Psychotherapy for these patients is, therefore, directed to helping them express their angers and fears of failure during waking hours and to develop more active coping mechanisms.

The problem for the clinician dealing with children and adolescents with sleep terror attacks is to determine whether or not sufficient psychopathology is present to make psychological treatment a reasonable approach. Again, as with sleepwalking, the first step is a good history, including the incidence of both these disorders in the family, the life events surrounding the initiation of this complaint, the frequency of attacks, the degree of disruption to the family at large, and the degree to which the patient's own life is limited. To differentiate sleep terrors from the more common REM nightmares, information on the time of night when these occur and the degree of recall for the fantasy material accompanying them is important. If they occur in the early night with little or no recall, and if a parent or bed partner can describe the wide-eyed horror and scream, unarousability, and profuse sweating and palpitation, the diagnosis can be made fairly confidently.

A confirmatory evaluation by clinical polysomnography is rarely indicated for either sleepwalking or sleep terrors since it might take many all-night recordings before an episode occurs. This would be prohibitively expensive. The only justification for such a diagnostic procedure would be if there were doubt about whether the episode was one of a nocturnal seizure of a temporal lobe type or if the sleepwalking was actually a fugue state or some other manifestation of a hysterical personality. Even when there is a question of differential diagnosis, tests performed during waking, such as a clinical EEG with nasopharyngeal leads or psychological testing, might provide a faster and more economical answer. Persons being monitored while sleeping in the laboratory for the first time are apt to sleep somewhat more lightly than they do at home and so not show the deep, prolonged, early delta sleep, following which the disorder of arousal behavior is likely to appear.

The usefulness of suppressing these symptoms with diazepam must be weighed against the problems associated with long-term use and withdrawal from this class of drugs in the young. Parents and children need to be reassured that these disorders diminish in frequency and only rarely persist into adulthood. If family inheritance appears absent and psychological factors are present, if the occurrences are frequent and disturbing to the family and potentially dangerous, psychotherapy can be suggested along with recommendations to the parents to keep the factors associated with especially deep delta sleep at a minimum—heavy physical exercise late in the day and late nights leading to sleep deprivation. Another approach is to use a sleepwalking alarm. One such instrument developed at our laboratory rings if the patient attempts to leave the bed without first turning it off, and this act takes a high degree of conscious coordination. This has had some success in retraining persistent walkers.

Other Sleep and Dream Disorders

Disorders of Initiating or Maintaining Sleep

Perhaps the most troublesome sleep disorder is insufficient sleep. The sympton of *insomnia* may occur as a delayed onset to sleep, a difficulty maintaining sleep throughout the night, an early offset of sleep, or any combination of these. In the discussion of the normal ontogeny of sleep it was noted that the consolidation of sleep into the night and the ability to sleep through takes several months to accomplish. Seventy percent of babies are quiet throughout the night by age three months and 83 percent by six months, but there are 10 percent who have still not "settled" by their first birthday. Among these the distinction has been made between the child who won't sleep—who refuses to go to bed or stay in bed—and the child who can't sleep. Night waking has been reported to be related to a variety of organic and functional factors. Organic problems such as night seizures and medical disorders which induce pain, such as middle ear infections, are obvious, but suboptimal conditions, such as inadequate nourishment, have also been implicated in night waking (Jones et al., 1978).

There are other organic factors that can account for poor sleep in the young child, such as nocturnal myoclonus. This repetitive jerking of one or both legs that occurs only in sleep is found in 10–20 percent of those with chronic insomnia. This disorder is presently little understood and treated only symptomatically with medication.

In the functional realm, inconsistent sleep-wake schedules imposed by parents, nighttime fears of separation from parents, real separations due to hospitalizations, anxieties associated with a move to a strange bedroom, the introduction of a new sibling, and the presence of marital disharmony can all contribute to poor sleep. As with adult insomnia, this may be transient or become chronic.

Chronic insomnia in the young child is strongly associated with psychological distrubances, particularly chronic anxiety. If a child is frightened of falling asleep or wakes with anxiety during the night, perhaps with a bad dream or a fear of loss of bladder of bowel control, this pattern may be reinforced if the child is punished for these "accidents." Many such factors may start a pattern of needing nocturnal parental reassurance. The problem can be exacerbated if treatment consists of excessive and frequent nighttime feedings or the misuse of medication. Both can produce a chronic dependency. Reassurance is better when given during waking, and security is induced by regularizing the child's expectations that he or she will be able to sleep.

Among adolescents attending a clinic for some emotional disturbance, sleep disturbances are prevalent. Marks and Monroe (1976) report 33 percent of a large national sample of such cases either referred to the service because of a sleep problem or with sleep difficulties. These patients had symptoms of anxiety, tension, depression, and somatic concerns. These findings contrast with those who were emotionally disturbed but good sleepers. These latter patients were more often "acting out" types.

In general, insomnia is most likely to begin when more stressful life events occur. The question is: Why does the poor sleep not remit when the events are long past? This question has been addressed by Healey et al. (1981). Their data, based on a comparison of matched good and poor sleeping groups, showed poor sleepers were more emotionally upset as children, less content with their parents and family lives, and not able to express this overtly. The chronic insomniac is one who internalizes and somaticizes stress. This patient suffers from feelings of inadequacy and is preoccupied with his or her health. The difficulty such patients have in expressing strong emotion and in coping with stress-producing events results in chronic psychological, cognitive, and physiological arousal. This high arousal state is incompatible with good sleep.

A higher rectal temperature, increased number of body movements, and higher levels of adrenocortical activity have been reported in several studies to differentiate the poor from the good sleeper (Monroe, 1967; Johns et al., 1971). The poor sleeper is more physiologically aroused both in waking and sleep. That this pattern can be set up in childhood and persist is clear from the histories of adult insomniacs. Psychotherapy, which actively engages the patient in learning more direct coping skills and trains out bedtime rumination and fears of not sleeping, can be very helpful. This is particularly true when patients realize that while they may not have had much power to deal with the events they experienced as stressful when the insomnia first began, they can now change their own response patterns.

Again, with insomnias, taking a good sleep history to determine important variables is critical. Not only should psychological factors be included, but also medical conditions that might contribute to nighttime disruption, such as pain. It is particularly important to note any medications being taken which have an adverse effect on sleep. Stimulants, such as amphetamines, bronchodilators, or caffeinated soft drinks and coffee, should certainly be inquired into and reduced or removed near bedtime.

A patient who had persistent insomnia reported that he was given coffee as an infant in order to delay his sleep onset so that he would sleep later in the morning. This pattern suited the parents' preferred sleep routine; however, it set up a delayed sleep phase problem that became chronic. The patient was not able to fall asleep until very late at night and would awaken late in the morning. When this pattern was coupled with the need to get up early for school, an inadequate amount of sleep, or insomnia, was reported. This was not technically the correct diagnosis since the patient was able to sleep a full eight hours, —whenever he was allowed his delayed sleep phase schedule. This problem required a special rescheduling of the time of sleep. This treatment, called *chronotherapy*, delays sleep onset progressively three hours a night for eight nights until the desired sleep onset time is reached.

Not only stimulants, but also some pharmacological agents used to induce sleep, even when used only for a short time, can produce a rebound insomnia on their withdrawal. Even the short-acting benzodiazepine hypnotics can have this effect and should be used cautiously and for limited periods of time only, such as during a crisis.

Instead of medication, the more psychologically based insomnias of childhood can be approached behaviorally. Kellerman (1980) reports three cases in which operant reinforcement of appropriate nighttime behaviors was used to overcome the anxiety associated with sleep. In all three cases very rapid control of nighttime anxiety was achieved. Within three sessions one five-year-old boy who was experiencing frequent night awakenings was trained to express anger toward the Dracula monster of his nightmares, as this response is incompatible with fear. This training was coupled with prohibiting him from sleeping with his parents but permitting sleep in places other than his own bed at first. He was also given a monetary reinforcement for sleeping through the night. All of this was effective within three weeks.

Anderson (1979) reports similar rapid success in controlling a more chronic insomnia of a thirteen-year-old boy through a combination of relaxation training and a reduction of parental attention. In this case, the mother had been sitting up late to comfort her son and going with him to the living room when he awakened during the night. By teaching the child relaxation techniques and having him do these prior to sleep and whenever he awakened, and prohibiting the mother from joining him at night, the disrupted sleep pattern disappeared rapidly.

In general, the therapeutic rules for gaining control over an insomnia are the same as those for good health. Taking some physical exercise on a daily basis but not close to bedtime or avoiding overstimulation of a psychological nature close to bedtime, such as hard studying, are two such rules. Other helpful conditions include having a quietly relaxing, wind-down period, with comforting bedtime routines: a storytime for the young, a regular bedtime hour, and reassurance from parents that they are there and will see their child in the morning.

The worst problem in treating the insomnia patient is the induced anxiety that each night will be worse than the last. This loss of confidence that sleep will come leads to increasing tension around bedtime. Under these circumstances it is important to use some stimulus control procedures to associate the bedroom with pleasant, rather than unpleasant, activity and the bed itself only with sleep. When not sleeping, the child should be required to leave the bed and quietly do something pleasantly distracting, such as looking at pictures for a short while, then go back to bed when drowsy and try again. If daytime napping is also prohibited, this usually results in a rapid resumption of sleeping through.

Persistent insomnia, like persistent sleepwalking and sleep terrors, appears to be a manifestation of underlying psychopathology. Not so the next category of disorders where a sleep disturbance is primary, though this usually results in many secondary emotional difficulties.

Disorders of Excessive Somnolence

Aside from insomnia, the next most frequent sleep disorder is that of *excessive sleepiness.* In the adult the most prevalent diagnoses falling into this class are narcolepsy, sleep apnea syndrome, and depression. In the child, these disorders also occur but they are frequently overlooked. Typically, it is in infancy and early childhood when the problem of sleep maintenance begins. The disorders of partial arousal are at their peak in the young and mid-childhood age range (three to ten years). The hypersomnias, however, are initiated more frequently in adolescence. It is then that parents may note a change in sleep habits. Children who previously were up early and eager to start the day are now sleeping late and are hard to arouse in the morning. Some may even resume taking afternoon naps. This may bring on parental concerns of laziness or suspicion of indulgence in drugs or alcohol. However, this is a time when discrepancy has been noted to occur between the length of sleep on school nights and weekends, with school nights typically averaging one hour less of sleep. By making up sleep on weekends, adolescents behave as if they are chronically sleep-deprived, and there is evidence that this may, in fact, be accurate.

Anders, Carskadon, and Dement (1978) prevented this extra sleep by controlling the sleep length to a constant ten hours on both weekdays and weekends for a group of adolescents who had been followed from the time they were healthy preadolescents. They found when subjects were held to this constant amount that they increased in daytime sleepiness. This was established in the laboratory by the Multiple Sleep Latency Test, which is designed to measure the need for sleep by providing five opportunities throughout the day to take a twenty-minute nap. These periods are spaced two hours apart. The amount of time taken to achieve sleep (sleep latency) on EEG criteria is then totaled across the five naps. On this measure the adolescents increased in daytime sleepiness and fell asleep more rapidly as adolescence progressed. It appears that two factors are involved: This age group needs more sleep than preadolescents and also they usually get up earlier on weekdays and go to bed later on weekend nights. Thus they accumulate a sleep deficit.

One adolescent patient had difficulty remaining awake during classes and difficulty falling asleep at night unless he exhausted himself physically. After he kept a sleep log for a two-week period, it became clear that his sleep cycle was highly disrupted. He had periods when he could not fall asleep until later and later each night, followed by a very early afternoon sleep onset. This patient liked to sit up very late with his grandmother and watch old movies on TV. After her death, some eight months before he was first seen, he continued this practice on weekends. This caused a profound sleep deprivation and disrupted his natural rhythm of sleep. The patient, an only child of two working parents, was a friendless and lonely boy. The grandmother had done a good deal of the mothering and he missed her nighttime companionship. He was reluctant to promise to give up the weekend late, late shows until a substitute reinforcement was worked out: an opportunity to play cards with his father and mother. This worked to keep him to a sleep schedule.

Narcolepsy

In addition to their kind of social-activity-induced daytime sleepiness and general increased sleep need, adolescents are also at risk for two other disorders of excessive somnolence: narcolepsy and sleep apnea syndrome. The peak age of onset for narcolepsy is the second decade of life. Actually, the ages fifteen to twenty-five are the years in which an adult patient most often traces the onset of symptoms. Although adolescence is when this disorder typically starts, this is rarely the age at which it is diagnosed and treated unless the patient was also hyperactive as a child. Since Ritalin (methylphenidate) is typically used to help counteract the sleepiness of narcolepsy and is also prescribed to control hyperactivity, some patients have been given this medication fortuitously prior to their being diagnosed as narcoleptic. Actually, hyperactivity has been diagnosed in the early history of many narcoleptic patients. This may represent a behavioral restlessness adapted by the patient to counteract overpowering sleepiness. Inattentiveness is also characteristic of both disorders, as is distractibility. In the narcoleptic, these cognitive signs are due to the overwhelming urge to sleep, but this causes some real confusions across these two diagnoses in children.

There are four symptoms which make up the narcolepsy tetrad: two intrude during waking and two on the transition between waking and sleep. The *two daytime symptoms* are short attacks of irresistible sleepiness occurring during passive activity, such as riding the bus, sitting in class or watching TV; and cataplexy, episodes of sudden complete or partial loss of muscle tonus occurring in response to strong emotion, such as laughter, anger, or surprise. The *two sleep-related symptoms* are episodes of sleep paralysis, which are short periods at sleep onset or on morning awakening when the person is awake but there is an inability to move voluntarily; and, lastly, hypnogogic hallucinations, which are complex, sensory experiences, occurring just prior to sleep onset, often frightening in character as they appear real. All four of these symptoms implicate a dysfunction of the REM-sleep mechanism. The daytime sleep attacks are typically attacks of REM sleep; the cataplexy and sleep paralysis symptoms are manifestations of the loss of muscle tone of the REM state; and the hypnogogic hallucinations are dissociated dream content phenomena. Somehow REM sleep is not confined to sleep but intrudes into the waking state and into the transition from waking to sleep or sleep to waking.

There is a fifth symptom which is less common than the other four, but tends to confuse the diagnosis when it does occur. This is *automatism.* When narcoleptic patients attempt to carry on normal activity while in a sleepy period, they may find themselves talking or writing nonsense, or wandering aimlessly on foot or by car far from their intended destination. These experiences have sometimes been confused with temporal lobe epilepsy or fugue states. By far the commonest symptoms are the daytime sleepiness and cataplexy. These two are frequently missed or mistaken, leading to a long delay in treatment. Typically, patients will have seen four or five physicians and been given a variety of medications, such an antidepressants or anticonvulsants, before receiving a correct diagnosis. During the fifteen to twenty years it takes the typical patient to be correctly treated, he or she—for this disorder occurs equally in the two sexes—may well have suffered extensive psychological and social damage. Patients report problems with teachers, parents and employers.

In a recent study of fifty narcoleptic patients (eighteen to seventy-two years of age) who had both sleep attacks and cataplexy, Kales et al. (1982) found more psychopathology than in a control group of age and sex matched subjects without sleep disorders. This psychopathology is an effect rather than a cause of the narcolepsy. Sixty-two percent of this group had psychosocial problems associated with being narcoleptic as early as their childhood or adolescence.

One common theme expressed by these patients is the constant struggle to maintain control over their emotions in order to avoid the embarrassment of a cataplectic attack. This frequently results in an intentional avoidance of contacts with others and a rather bland life style which may be misjudged as schizoid. The Minnesota Multiphasic Personality Inventory (MMPI) profiles of narcoleptic patients are significantly more elevated, with the three highest scales being those resembling schizophrenia, depression, and hysteria. The typical narcoleptic, because of such an early onset and such a long and lonely struggle before getting a diagnosis and appropriate treatment, suffers internalized distress, a reduction of pleasure, confusion, and a negative self-image.

Narcolepsy affects somewhere between .02 to .10 percent of the general population. It is a life-long disorder which is not progressive. There appears to be a genetic component based on the strong family histories of other first-degree relatives having excessive daytime sleepiness. It is best diagnosed in the sleep laboratory by means of the Multiple Sleep Latency Test. Not only should the patient prove to be pathologically sleepy on this test, by having a summed sleep latency (how long it takes to fall asleep) across the five naps of less than twenty-five minutes, but, like the infant, he or she should also show a strong tendency to have a REM-sleep episode close to the onset of any sleep period. Typically, a positive diagnosis for narcolepsy is made if REM sleep occurs on two or more of these short naps.

The treatment of narcolepsy involves medication for its two components—the excessive sleepiness and the loss of muscle tone—and counseling for the problems of living with this disorder. The tendency to sleep is combated with an alerting medication, such as Dexedrine, Ritalin, or a more recent addition which is nonaddictive, Cylert. The cataplexy, which is as troublesome as the sleepiness, is treated with one of the tricyclic antidepressants, such as imipramine. The narcoleptic patient and family should also be counseled that if the patient will take short, planned naps at least once, and preferably twice, daily, medication levels and the degree of overwhelming sleepiness can be kept at lower levels. Most important is counseling of the patient, the family, and school personnel on the nature of this disorder. This should help to reduce secondary psychopathology and thereby permit the patient to enjoy a fuller emotional life. Patients need to be warned of the possibility of genetic transmission and of the dangers associated with escalating medication and of driving. They should also have some career counseling to avoid repetitive, monotonous, sedentary jobs, and, if possible, to seek active, interesting work.

Narcolepsy is a specific disorder of REM sleep which is underdiagnosed at the time it usually develops, probably because so many adolescents have an increase in sleepiness. Since so much life-long distress can follow from the need to struggle to remain awake, clinicians should be alert to the presence of cataplexy and the other narcoleptic symptoms in any sleepy adolescent patient. Although there is no cure, the symptoms of narcolepsy can be managed with understanding, support, and medication, including regular drug holidays, thus avoiding much of the dangers of drug toxicity and secondary psychopathology.

Sleep Apnea Syndrome

The other major sleep disorder which produces excessive daytime sleepiness is sleep apnea syndrome. *Sleep apnea* is a respiratory problem involving repetitive pauses in breathing associated with sleep. One form of this disorder involves a repeated cessation of respiratory effort, called *central sleep apnea.* This has been implicated as a possible cause of sudden infant death syndrome. If children prone to this disorder survive the first year of life, they appear to mature out of this unstable respiratory pattern of sleep.

Much more common is sleep apnea due to an obstruction. Such children are, like the narcoleptics, excessively sleepy during wakefulness, but the pattern of their complaint is very different. The sleep attacks are longer in duration, more resistible, and less refreshing than the brief narcoleptic attacks. These are not attacks of REM sleep but are more likely to be of light NREM sleep, stages 1 or 2.

This disorder is found predominantly in males, in about an 85 to 15 percent ratio. The night sleep is accompanied by loud snoring and interrupted by repetitive pauses in respiration lasting from 10 seconds up to one minute or more. These pauses are typically followed by a reduction in the level of oxygen saturation in the blood. Both these changes in blood gas concentration and the disruption of normal sleep by the need to arouse to resume respiration appear to result in daytime sleepiness and in some cognitive difficulties. Many children with severe obstructive sleep apnea have been thought to be mentally retarded. They also typically show elevated blood pressure, enuresis, and morning headache. Many are overweight; some show failure to thrive. The chronic airway obstruction is sometimes secondary to micrognathia or hypertrophy of the tonsils and adenoids.

Despite the seriousness of their difficulties in sleep as they struggle to breathe at night and their waking problems, apneic patients tend not to come to the attention of a health care specialist until there is some severe learning or behavioral difficulty. It is estimated that approximately 15 to 20 percent of those with symptoms of excessive daytime sleepiness have obstructive sleep apnea.

The diagnosis can sometimes be made in the office with the aid of a cassette tape recording made at home by the bedside of the patient. If there is loud snoring followed by silences of over ten seconds' duration, broken by gasping or snorting sounds, the diagnosis is highly likely. Confirmation in a sleep laboratory should be done to determine the type, frequency, and duration of the pauses and the extent of the oxygen desaturation. Untreated sleep apnea is typically progressive. The picture is of increasingly severe respiratory difficulties in sleep accompanied by hypoxemia and cardiovascular changes with essential hypertension, pulmonary hypertension, cor pulmonale, and right-sided cardiac failure. This produces a light, broken sleep with little or no delta sleep. Since delta sleep is associated with growth hormone release, it is suspected that the loss of this sleep may be implicated in the growth failure of some of these patients when this problem starts at an early age. To diagnose sleep apnea in a laboratory, the regularity of air flow is monitored by means of a temperature transducer which records changes in temperature at the nose and mouth level. A strain gauge or chest impedance technique is used to measure respiratory effort. These along with an ear oximeter for recording oxygen saturation and the usual EEG, eye movement, and chin EMG recordings complete the monitors needed to determine when the episodes are occurring in REM and NREM sleep, and the degree of concomitant loss of oxygen to the brain.

Studies of the apneic young child by cinefluoroscopy (Felmann, et al., 1979) found that during inspiration the tongue and hypopharyngeal soft tissues collapse and completely, or almost completely, obstruct the air flow. The need for a sleep laboratory examination in suspected cases must be emphasized, as waking pulmonary function tests and radiographic examinations are usually normal. The consequences of this condition for intellectual, physical, and emotional functioning are grave and their reversibility with treatment at this point variable.

Treatment of sleep apnea often involves surgery: tonsillectomy, adenoidectomy, tracheostomy, or cranial facial surgery to correct the micrognathia when an anatomical obstruction is involved. Other treatments are weight control for the obese, treatment of allergies by medication, or the use of a mouth prosthesis during sleep to hold the tongue forward and away from the top of the airway (Cartwright & Samelson, 1982). These patients also need some support and counseling to understand the reasons for their psychological and intellectual difficulties. With treatment that corrects the respiratory problem in sleep the patient becomes more alert in waking time. Then the other difficulties also show improvement: Social activity returns and the mind seems to clear from its sleepy fog.

There are at this time no figures on the prevalence of sleep apnea in childhood. Surveys of fifteen- to eighteen-year olds report that 50 percent admit to feeling tired most of the time (Price, Coates, & Thoresen, 1978). Some of this may well be due to sleep apnea. A careful nose and throat examination is important if the history shows loud snoring, obesity, or some of the other ancillary symptoms.

Hypersomnia can also be psychogenic. In these cases, it is more often of the extended night sleep variety rather than of sleepiness intruding into daytime. This is often related to an underlying depression. Adolescent depression can be difficult to diagnose. It may be bipolar (manic-depressive) or unipolar (depressive only) in character. Both have some characteristic sleep features when evaluated in the laboratory. A decreased latency to the first rapid eye movement sleep period is one such marker.

The sleepy adolescent can then be normal, narcoleptic, sleep apneic, or depressed. Each has characteristic differences in the kind, amount, and distribution of sleep in the 24-hour period. The normal extends the nighttime sleep until late morning and is hard to arouse; the narcoleptic has REM onset sleep at night and sleep attacks with early REM during the day; the sleep apneic has little or no delta and very light sleep due to repetitive arousals to resume respiration and sleepy periods during the day of NREM sleep; the depressed adolescent has a prolonged sleep and an early first REM period at about half normal latency. Since each requires unique treatment, a careful differential sleep diagnosis is important.

Dream Disturbances

Since REM sleep occurs periodically throughout the night, children can have as many as six or nine REM periods per night. Most children experience some of these as bad dreams which frighten them at some time during their growing years. When this is an occasional phenomenon it is of little consequence. The parent should be encouraged to listen to the dream content, rather than ignore it, to reassure the child that the dream was one of his or her own construction, and to tell the child he or she can learn to understand and to stop a bad dream when it is unpleasant. The child who has frequent nightmares and is awakened from sleep in fear one or more times per week may need to be seen: first, to reassure the parent; and, second, to determine if anything else is wrong, to differentiate whether these are sleep terrors (a delta sleep phenomenon) or nightmares (REM sleep phenomenon). Judicious questioning of both parents and child must be done to establish the time of night dreams occur and whether or not there is any content associated with the fearful awaking. If these are nightmares, they are usually related to immediate psychological stressors and will remit with reassurance and a little help from some nighttime protective rituals—never underestimate the power of a stuffed animal or blanket. If nightmares persist after the age of six, the child can be taught first to pop his or her eyes open to stop it. Once control is established the child can then be taught to take charge in the dream itself, to be more powerful and able to cope with the dreamed trouble.

A group of adult nightmare sufferers who have been studied by Hartmann et al. (1981) reported they had suffered for as long as they could remember, since age five or earlier. Like the sleepwalker and sleep terror adult, those whose nightmaring has not waned with maturity tend to have more psychopathology. Their reports of their childhood indicate they were sensitive, easily hurt, and unhappy despite relatively good family situations. However, for many there was considerable family history of schizophrenia, alcoholism, and suicide.

Typically, the first nightmare content is of being chased and about to be hurt by a large animal or monster. This changes later to being pursued by a person. These adults reported that their nightmares increased during times of stress and that they increased during adolescence, when sleep time is prolonged. The study concluded that the nightmare sufferer whose difficulty persists into the adult years is probably biologically vulnerable for schizophrenia but has avoided chronic mental illness. Those who still are having nightmares into early adolescence may be a group at some risk.

Many of the sleep disorders occurring during the childhood years are self-limiting if not treated and do not implicate psychopathology, although they can cause much disruption. Once understood, they can be helped a good deal with supportive treatment, behavioral management programs, and some parental guidance. However, there are others which are indicators of serious organic or psychological disturbances. These need to be identified and treated swiftly to avoid, if possible, their becoming chronic. As clinicians become more familiar with these disorders, differential diagnosis among those that share similar symptom pictures will improve. This will enhance the chance that the sleep patient and the family will receive help. Most narcoleptic patients have gone undiagnosed or been misdiagnosed as epileptics for years before receiving an appropriate treatment, although their problem typically began in adolescence. No one knows how many infants who survived a near miss episode of sudden infant death syndrome are later diagnosed in middle age as having sleep apnea. It is known that roughly 94 percent of adult apneic patients snored loudly before the age of twenty one, but it is usually another twenty years before this is recognized as contributing to daytime sleepiness by a health care professional.

When a childhood sleep problem persists and affects waking functioning it may be useful for the clinician to consult a sleep disorder service for help in clarifying the nature of the problem. Research in the area of childhood sleep pathology has lagged behind the study of adult disorders. The clinician who deals with children can exert some influence on this process by documenting the waking symptoms of such cases and bringing these to the attention of sleep experts. They, in turn, can study the sleep behaviors and recommend appropriate treatments. This partnership should greatly improve the care of children in this area.

REFERENCES

Agrell, I. G., & Axelsson, A. The relationship between pavor nocturnus and adenoids. *Acta Paedopsychiatrica,* 1972, *39,* 46–53.

Anders, T., Carskadon, M., Dement, W., & Harvey, K. Sleep habits of children and identification of pathologically sleepy children. *Child Psychiatry and Human Development,* 1978, *9,* 56–62.

Anders, T., Emde, R., & Parmalee, A. (Eds.). *A manual of standardized terminology, techniques, and criteria for scoring states of sleep and wakefulness in newborn infants.* Los Angeles: UCLA Brain Information Service/Brain Research Institute, 1971.

Anderson, D. Treatment of insomnia in a 13-year-old boy by relaxation training and reduction of parental attention. *Journal of Behavior Therapy and Experimental Psychiatry,* 1979, *10,* 263–265.

Aserinsky, E., & Kleitman, N. Regularly occurring periods of eye motility, and concomitant phenomena, during sleep. *Science,* 1953, *118,* 273–274.

Bakwin, H. Sleepwalking in twins. *Lancet,* 1970, 446–447.

Bixler, E., Kales, A., Soldatos, D., Kales, J., and Healey, S. Prevalence of sleep disorders in the Los Angeles metropolitan area. *American Journal of Psychiatry,* 1979, *136,* 1257–1262.

Broughton, R. Sleep disorders: Disorders of arousal. *Science,* 1968, *159,* 1070–1078.

Broughton, R. Childhood sleepwalking, sleep terrors and enuresis nocturna: Their pathophysiology and differentiation from nocturnal epileptic seizures. In *Sleep,* 1978, Fourth European Congress on Sleep Research, S. Karger. Basel: 1980, 103–111.

Carskadon, M. A. The second decade. In C. Guilleminault (Ed.), *Sleeping and waking disorders: Indications and techniques.* Menlo Park: Addison-Wesley, 1982.

Cartwright, R., & Samelson, C. The effects of a nonsurgical treatment for obstructive sleep apnea. *Journal of American Medical Association,* 1982, *248,* 705–709.

Diagnostic and statistical manual of mental disorders (3d Ed.). Washington, DC: American Psychiatric Association, 1980, 82–86.

Ellingson, R. J. EEGs of premature and full-term newborns. In D. W. Klass & D. D. Daly (Eds.), *Current practice of clinical electroencephalography.* New York: Raven, 1979.

Felman, A., Loughlin, G., Leftridge, C., & Cassisi, N. Upper airway obstruction during sleep in children. *American Journal of Radiology,* 1979, *133,* 213–216.

Fisher, C., Kahn, E., Edwards, A., & Davis, D. A psychophysiological study of nightmares and night terrors. *Psychoanalysis and Contemporary Science,* 1974, *3,* 317–398.

Glick, B., Schulman, D., & Turecki, S. Diazepam (Valium) treatment in childhood sleep disorders: A preliminary investigation. *Diseases of the Nervous System,* 1971, *32,* 565–566.

Guilleminault, C., & Souquet, M. Sleep states and related pathology. In R. Korobkin & C. Guilleminault (Eds.), *Advances in perinatal neurology* (Vol. 1). New York: Spectrum, 1979.

Hartmann, E., Russ, D., Van der Kolk, B., Falke, R., & Oldfield, M. A preliminary study of the personality of the nightmare sufferer: Relationship to schizophrenia and creativity. *American Journal of Psychiatry,* 1981, *138,* 794–797.

Hauri, P. *The sleep disorders,* 2nd Ed., *Current concepts.* Kalamazoo, MI: The Upjohn Company, 1982.

Healey, S., Kales, A., Monroe, L., Bixler, E., Chamberlin, K., & Soldatos, C. Onset of insomnia: Role of life-stress events. *Psychosomatic Medicine,* 1981, *43,* 439–451.

Herman, J. H., Ellman, S. J., & Roffwarg, H. P. The problem of NREM dream recall reexamined. In A. M. Arkin, J. S. Antrobus, & S. J. Ellman (Eds.), *The mind in sleep: Psychology and psychophisiology.* New York: Wiley, 1978.

Jacobson, A., & Kales, A. Somnambulism: All night EEG and related studies. In S. Kety, E. Evarts, & H. Williams (Eds.), *Sleep and altered states of consciousness.* Baltimore: Williams & Watkins, 1967, 424–455.

Jacobson, A., Kales, A., Lehmann, D., & Zweizig, J. Somnambulism: All night electroencephalographic studies. *Science,* 1965, *148,* 975–977.

Jacobson, A., Kales, J., & Kales, A. Clinical and electrophysiological correlates of sleep disorders in children. In A. Kales (Ed.), *Sleep: Physiology and pathology.* Philadelphia: Lippincott, 1969, 109–118.

Johns, M., Gay, T., Masterson, J., & Bruce, D. Relationship between sleep habits, adrenocortical activity, and personality. *Psychosomatic Medicine,* 1971, *33,* 499–508.

Jones, B., Ferreira, R., Brown, F., & Macdonald, L. The association between perinatal factors and late night awakening. *Developmental Medicine and Child Neurology,* 1978, *20,* 427–434.

Jouvet, M. Behavioral and EEG effects of paradoxical sleep deprivation in the cat. In *Proceedings of the 23rd International Congress of Physiological Sciences* (Vol. 4). Excerpta Medica, No. 87, Tokyo, 1965.

Kahn, E., Fisher, C., Byrne, J., Edwards, A., & Frosch, A. The influence of Valium, Thorazine and Dilantin on Stage 4 nightmares. *Psychophysiology,* 1971, *7,* 350.

Kales, A., Jacobson, A., Paulson, M., Kales, J., & Walter, R. Somnambulism: Psychophysiological correlates. I. All night EEG studies. *Archives of General Psychiatry,* 1966, *14,* 586–594.

Kales, A., Soldatos, C., Bixler, E., Caldwell, A., Cadieux, R., Verrechio, J., & Kales, J. Narcolepsy-cataplexy. II. Psychosocial consequences and associated psychopathology. *Archives of Neurology,* 1982, *39,* 169–171.

Kales, A., Soldatos, C., Bixler, E., Ladda, R., Charney, D., Weber, G., & Schweitzer, P. Hereditary factors in sleepwalking and night terrors. *British Journal of Psychiatry,* 1980, *137,* 111–118. (a)

Kales, A., Soldatos, C., Caldwell, A., Kales, J., Humphrey, F., Charney, D., & Schweitzer, P. Somnambulism: Clinical characteristics and personality patterns. *Archives of General Psychiatry,* 1980, *37,* 1406–1410. (b)

Kales, J., Humphrey, F., Martin, E., Russek, E., Kuhn, W., Pelicci, I., & Kales, A. Clinical characteristics of patients with sleepwalking: Further studies. *Sleep Research,* 1978, *7,* 192.

Kales, J., Kales, A., Soldatos, C., Chamberlin, K., & Martin, E. Sleepwalking and night terrors related to febrile illness. *American Journal of Psychiatry,* 1979, *136,* 1214–1215.

Kellerman, J. Rapid treatment of nocturnal anxiety in children. *Journal of Behavior Therapy and Experimental Psychiatry,* 1980, *11,* 9–11.

Kleitman N. *Sleep and wakefulness* (Rev. Ed.) Chicago: University of Chicago, 1963.

Marks, P., & Monroe, L. Correlates of adolescent poor sleepers. *Journal of Abnormal Psychology,* 1976, *85,* 243–246.

Monroe, L. Psychological and physiological differences between good and poor sleepers. *Journal of Abnormal Psychology,* 1967, *72,* 255–264.

Pesikoff, R., & Davis, P. Treatment of pavor nocturnus and somnambulism in children. *American Journal of Psychiatry,* 1971, *128,* 778–781.

Price, V., Coates, T., & Thoresen, C. Prevalence and correlates of poor sleep among adolescents. *American Journal of Diseases of Child,* 1978, *132,* 583–586.

Rechtschaffen, A., & Kales, A. (Eds.). *A manual of standardized terminology, techniques and scoring system for sleep stages of human subjects.* Washington DC: Public Health Service, U.S. Government Printing Office, 1968.

Reid, W., Ahmed, I., & Levie, C. Treatment of sleepwalking: A controlled study. *American Journal of Psychotherapy,* 1981, *35,* 27–37.

Roffwarg, H. P., Munzio, J. N., & Dement, W. C. Ontogenetic development of the human sleep-dream cycle. *Science,* 1966, *152,* 604–619.

Shagass, C. Electrical activity of the brain. In N. S. Greenfield & R. A. Sternbach (Eds.), *Handbook of psychophysiology.* New York: Holt, Rinehart, & Winston, 1972.

Williams, R., Karacan, I., & Hursch, C. *Electroencephalography of human sleep: Clinical applications.* New York: Wiley, 1974.

CHAPTER 8

Eating and Elimination Disorders

Bryan D. Carter and C. Eugene Walker

At first glance, the unifying theme of the present chapter may seem somewhat obscure. Eating and elimination are, however, biologically complementary, being associated with opposite ends of the alimentary canal. This tubular passageway through the body with openings at the mouth and the anus frequently evokes great concern. Children's problems associated with elimination are second only to school related problems among parents who seek advice from child development specialists (Ilg & Ames, 1962). In a study of psychologists working in a private pediatric practice, toileting problems were second only to "negative behaviors" in frequency of referrals, while food and eating problems appeared tenth on the list (Mesibov, Schroeder, & Wesson, 1977; Schroeder, 1979).

The primary elimination disorders, enuresis and encopresis, and the associated area of toilet training have been the subject of a great deal of popular and professional literature. An extensive review of popular parent guide books on toileting found a relative scarcity of even the most rudimentary factual information on the subject (Shaw, 1976). Additionally, the "experts" were found to differ considerably in their recommendations to parents. Advice regarding toilet training ranges from the relatively laissez-faire approach of Brazelton (1962) to the highly structured and relatively complex program developed by Azrin and Foxx (1974).

In a number of studies, consummatory problems in children have been found to affect up to approximately 25 percent of the pediatric population (Linscheid, 1978). In younger children these problems are manifested in a variety of ways:

refusal to accept solid foods or oral medication, multiple food dislikes, pica, mealtime tantrums, delayed development in self-feeding, rumination disorder of infancy, and a variety of related difficulties. In older children, eating disturbances such as childhood and adolescent obesity, anorexia nervosa, and bulimia nervosa present themselves to the professional.

Since these disorders may have an organic etiology, a collaborative relationship between the pediatrician and psychologist is important for successful evaluation and treatment. However, since most studies indicate that the etiology in well over 90 percent of the cases is psychological, the pediatrician will generally have to rule out organic etiology while the psychologist will be called upon for a more major intervention to deal with the problem.

Enuresis

DSM-III criteria for functional enuresis are: (a) repeated involuntary voiding of urine by day or at night; (b) at least two such events per month for children between the ages of five and six, and at least one event per month for older children; and (c) not due to a physical disorder such as diabetes or seizure disorder.

Developmental Physiology of Micturition

A brief review of the physiology of urination is necessary to understand the possible causes of enuresis. In the neonate, voiding is an automatic process, i.e., it is basically reflexive. During infancy the bladder holds a very small amount of urine and the child is unable to initiate or stop the urinary stream. Instead, when the bladder becomes sufficiently filled, the sphincter muscles relax and the detrusor muscle contracts. This process continues until the bladder empties. By the second year of life, the child becomes able to detect bladder fullness and develops the ability to voluntarily contract the sphincter muscles, thus holding urine for brief periods of time. This retention ability builds until daytime control of voiding is obtained, usually between the ages of two and three; by the age of four or five, almost 80 percent of children have also developed night control.

It is obvious from this very brief overview that normal physiological function of the bladder is mandatory for the proper acquisition of control of micturition. However, since in a purely statistical sense, organic factors seldom account for inadequate control of micturition, the basic problem in the vast majority of cases appears to be one of learning to voluntarily control the sphincters in order to delay the reflexive emptying of the bladder (Walker, 1978). The developing child must learn to postpone the urination process, as well as to initiate and complete the emptying of the bladder at the appropriate time and in the appropriate setting. This learning task can be difficult and complex for many children.

Etiology

One major distinction with enuretics is that made between nocturnal and diurnal enuresis. *Nocturnal enuresis* refers to nighttime bedwetting, while *diurnal enuresis* refers to wetting that occurs during the day. Studies have shown that nighttime bladder control is generally achieved at least a year or two later than the acquisition of daytime control. Thus, children who are still wetting during the day beyond the three- to four-year age range are frequently considered enuretic (Walker, 1978).

Another distinction is that between primary and secondary enuresis. *Primary enuresis* refers to incontinence that has existed since birth, while *secondary*, or onset, *enuresis* refers to the loss of previously acquired continence. Operational definitions of secondary enuresis have generally accepted a period of at least six months bladder control before the loss of proper voiding performance.

Studies of sexual differences in occurrence indicate that boys are almost twice as likely to have the problem as girls (Doleys, 1977). Predictably, Doleys found the proportion of enuretics decreases until the later teenage and adult years when a 1 to 2 percent prevalence is found.

Etiological factors for urinary incontinence fall into three major categories: organic disorder, emotional disturbance, and learning problems (Walker, 1978). Strictly speaking, of course, functional enuresis refers only to those cases where there is no organic basis. Still it is important for us to be aware of the multitude of organic disorders which may result in voiding dysfunction in children (Kaplan & Brock, 1980). Among the many conditions which can cause urinary incontinence in children are allergic reactions, urinary tract infections, and structural disorders, such as distal urinary obstruction. The presence of disease or infection may be signaled by such symptoms as pain, fever, burning sensation while urinating, dribbling, increased frequency or urgency of voiding, small or irregular urine stream, or the passage of blood in the urine. Diseases known to be associated with enuresis are diabetes and sickle cell anemia.

In the past several decades, perhaps the most widely accepted etiological theory of enuresis has been the psychodynamic formulation. Basically, this model suggests that enuresis is a symptom indicating some underlying emotional dysfunction, psychological conflict, or anxiety (Pierce, 1972). Psychoanalysts have frequently related enuresis to sexual conflicts, with the process of urination being symbolic of suppressed masturbation, ejaculation, or sexual identity confusion (Fenichel, 1946). Others have interpreted enuresis as a regressive behavior, a plea for attention and help, a repressed display of resentment or anger toward parents, a clinging to infancy, or even a form of weeping. However, several studies (Hallgren, 1956; Werry, 1965; and Tapia, Jeckel, & Demke, 1960) have found little or no relation between emotional disturbance and enuresis in children. In those cases where enuresis was associated with emotional problems, the emotional problems may have been the result of enuresis rather than the cause (Werry, 1967).

Enuresis has also been conceptualized as the consequence of a developmental delay or maturational lag in neural development. Evidence of a mild developmental disorder has been suggested by findings of EEG abnormalities in enuretics (Lovibond & Coote, 1969). In one series of studies, enuretics were found to spend significantly more time in REM sleep (stage 4) than nonenuretics (Finley & Besserman, 1973), which was interpreted as a sign of central nervous system immaturity. Many studies relate EEG findings to disturbances in sleep patterns (Finley & Besserman, 1973; Gastout & Broughton, 1964). The finding by some researchers of irregularities in the sleep patterns of enuretic children and the frequent complaint by their parents that these children are "deep sleepers" add support to the developmental delay etiological theory. However, the findings from studies of both depth of sleep and arousability are inconsistent (Doleys, 1979; Salmon, Taylor, & Lee, 1973). Somewhat related to this line of investigation is the finding by Oppel, Harper, and Rider (1968) that low birth weight of subjects in their study was associated with a delayed development of bladder control compared to subjects with normal birth weights.

Another body of evidence believed by some researchers to support a maturational lag etiology comes from studies that have shown that many enuretic children have a smaller functional bladder capacity than nonenuretic children. This is manifested by increased frequency of voiding and an urgency to void once they become aware of the need (Wright, Schaefer, & Solomoans, 1979). This characteristic refers to the functional ability of the bladder to retain a given volume of urine, rather than the actual physical size, which is generally normal for the age of the child. Such children have been observed to pass the same amount or volume of urine as nonenuretics, but to do so in smaller quantities and at more frequent intervals, both during the day and at night (Esperana & Gerrard, 1969). Doleys (1978) has noted that a smaller functional bladder capacity appears to be more frequently observed in primary enuretics than in secondary enuretics.

A positive history of enuresis among family members of enuretic children also has been noted, suggesting a genetic basis for the symptom (McLain, 1979). In a review of twin data (Bakwin, 1973), monozygotic twins had a 68 percent concordance rate for enuresis, while dyzygotic twins had a 36 percent rate. In a study of six families in which both parents had been enuretic, Bakwin found that 77 percent of their children were enuretic; where only one parent was enuretic, 44 percent of the children were enuretic. Only 15 percent of the children were enuretic when neither parent had a history of enuresis. However, it could be argued that the effects of faulty family training habits or parental expectations influenced proper bladder control and toileting behaviors in these families (Walker, 1978). At present, it is safe to say only that a hereditary component to this symptom is strongly suspected.

From the perspective of the behavioral model, enuresis is viewed as arising from inadequate learning experiences or inappropriate reinforcement contingencies (Jay & Wright, 1982). A wide range of prerequisite skills and discriminative tasks must be learned by the child before adequate control can be attained (Azrin & Foxx, 1974; Brazelton, 1962). When the child fails to learn these behaviors, the result is enuresis. Simply stated, this view is that (1) urination is a reflex; (2) control over this reflex can be learned, and (3) successful treatment, therefore, may be based on principles of conditioning and learning. Support for this point of view comes from the fact that treatment strategies based on a learning formulation of the problem routinely result in very high success rates. These data will be reviewed later in this chapter.

Treatment of Enuresis

Medication. A variety of pharmacological agents have been employed as treatments for enuresis. Imipramine, a tricyclic antidepressant, is the medication most commonly employed. While results show this drug significantly decreases wetting in 40 to 50 percent of enuretic children, with another 10 to 20 percent showing some improvement, the relapse rate is high (Perimutter, 1976). Many children on drug treatment decrease, but do not cease wetting, and as many as two-thirds of enuretics resume wetting after the drug is discontinued. (Bindelglas, 1975; Marshall & Marshall, 1973; McKendry & Stewart, 1974). While the mechanism of action of tricyclic antidepressants in the treatment of enuresis is not understood, several theories have been proposed. The anticholinergic side effects of these drugs are thought to produce urinary retention by Greenberg and Stephans (1977). Other proposed mechanisms of action are in decreasing the depth of sleep in certain subjects, the placebo effects of giving the drug, and the antidepressant effect of the medication. It should be noted that the FDA has recommended that imipramine be used only as a "temporary adjunctive therapy" for enuretic children six years of age and older (Physician's Desk Reference, 1980). The tricyclic antidepressants have potentially serious side effects and a number of deaths due to overdose have been reported. Due to these dangers and to the very modest success rate for drug treatment, it has been suggested that these medications be reserved for those cases where other therapies are not practical or effective (Gaultieri, 1977).

Psychotherapy. Verbal psychotherapy is an often recommended treatment for enuresis (Nelson, Vaughan, & McKay, 1969). This is no doubt due to the general acceptance by professionals and the lay public of psychodynamic etiological theories (Werry, 1979). Nonetheless, a number of studies have shown verbal psychotherapy, including family therapy, to be no more effective than no treatment at all (DeLeon & Mandell, 1969; Friedman, 1968; Novick, 1966; Werry & Cohrssen, 1965). The data available do not support the use of verbal psychotherapy for the treatment of enuresis, especially when compared to the demonstrated effectiveness of the behavioral-learning approaches.

Awakening and Reinforcement Methods. One relatively simple technique for the treatment of enuresis involves having the parent periodically wake the child throughout the night to go to the bathroom. Schedules of awakening can be randomized, but also include awakening the child at those times when the child generally urinates (Walker, 1978). Young (1964) applied "staggered" awakening procedures with fifty-eight enuretic children over a four-week period. During this treatment, ten of the children became completely dry, with a total of 67 percent showing some improvement. Young's method was also employed in a study of nine subjects in an institutional setting (Creer & Davis, 1975), where four of the subjects became completely continent and the remainder had significant decreases in the frequency of bedwetting. It has been noted that this procedure is most effective when carried out over a period of several weeks (Walker, 1978). Another variation of the waking procedure involves having the child awaken himself or herself with the use of an alarm clock (Singh, Phillips, & Fischer, 1976).

Bladder Retention and Sphincter Control Exercises. Kimmel and Kimmel (1970) developed a *bladder retention training technique* designed to increase the functional bladder capacity of enuretics. Basically, this procedure involves having the child go to the toilet when the urge to urinate is first detected. Then the child is instructed to hold back or refrain from urinating as long as possible. Initially the child retains urine for only a few seconds. However, the child is challenged to increase the retention time with each succeeding episode of voiding. A chart is kept and rewards are given for success. When the child is able to retain urine for twenty or thirty minutes, the child leaves the bathroom and returns later to urinate. This procedure may also be combined with sphincter control exercises to be discussed below. The child is typically started on such a program on the weekend or during a vacation period so that proper initiation of the program and accurate recording are possible.

The results on the effectiveness of bladder retention control training are conflicting. Kimmel and Kimmel (1970) and Miller (1973) reported the method to be highly successful based on the treatment of a number of cases ranging in age from four to ten years. However, Doleys et al. (1977), in comparing retention control training to an operant conditioning program, found no change in functional bladder capacity in their subjects during a six-week treatment period. Another study (Paschalis, Kimmel, & Kimmel, 1972) found that less than half of a sample of thirty-five children were dry for seven consecutive days following a fifteen- to twenty-day treatment program (Paschalis, Kimmel, & Kimmel, 1972; see also Rocklin & Tilker, 1973). Harris and Purohit (1977) applied a retention control program for thirty-five days to nine enuretic children. While they did find an increase in bladder capacity, there was no reduction in bedwetting. Thus, support for this method is somewhat tentative and further research is required.

Other clinicians have recommended the adjunctive use of *sphincter control exercises* with bladder retention control training (Miller, 1973). In this procedure, the child practices starting and stopping the stream of urine while urinating in the toilet, thus developing improved control over the internal and external sphincter muscles. Often these exercises are applied after three to four weeks of bladder retention training, when the child is able to retain urine for twenty to thirty minutes. An increase in fluid intake, generally a cup or two of fluid per hour, is often used to facilitate the frequency of urination and therefore the number of opportunities for training as well as to produce some degree of overlearning. However, caution should be taken not to force excessive amounts of fluid or to attempt to have the child retain urine for an unusually long period of time (Walker, 1978). We have also found it useful to reinforce children with a small toy or money for breaking their record of time urine is retained on each successive trial as well as for successfully accomplishing the starting and stopping exercises.

Urine Alarm Training. Variously known as the urine alarm system, pad and bell, and bed buzzer system, this method for treating enuresis has been demonstrated to be highly effective over many years of careful research. The *urine alarm system* employs an apparatus consisting of a pad sensitive to urine. This pad is placed in the bed of the child and attached to a device which triggers a bell, buzzer, and/or light when the child urinates on the pad. The alarm awakens the child who then goes to the bathroom to complete urinating. Typically, a parent assists the child by wiping his or her face with a wet washcloth to insure that the child is awake and can carry out the rest of the procedure. The child is then responsible for changing the sheets and resetting the alarm before returning to sleep.

Studies with the urine alarm system have shown that this method initially eliminates the symptom in approximately 75 to 90 percent of the subjects. Treatment duration generally ranges from five to twelve weeks (Doleys, 1977). However, relapse rates are generally high, occurring in between 15 to 46 percent of the cases. Reinstatement of the urine alarm procedure usually brings cessation of bedwetting and treatment time is shorter. The clinician can generally expect a quarter of all children with nocturnal enuresis to become dry in two to six weeks with the urine alarm method; half will be dry in three months; nearly 90 percent will be dry within four to six months (Dische, 1973).

In response to the high relapse rate problem, Young and Morgan (1972a,b) found that relapses could be cut from 35 to 13 percent if children were conditioned with the urine alarm device until dry and then given increased fluids prior to going to bed. Morgan (1978) found a relatively low 12.8 percent relapse rate with the inclusion of this overlearning procedure.

Other attempts to reduce the relapse rate with the urine alarm method have involved the application of an intermittent rather than continuous reinforcement schedule. Studies by Finley & Besserman (1973) employed a nightly intermittent schedule of 70 percent reinforcement and found significantly fewer relapses.

Another study (Wagner et al., 1982) assessed the change in frequency of enuresis using the urine alarm, drug therapy (imipramine), and a control group. The urine alarm was found to be significantly more effective than medication or no treatment at all.

In sum, the urine alarm device continues to be regarded as one of the most effective methods for treatment of nocturnal enuresis. A major problem with this method is the high relapse rate. However, newer variations of apparatus and approach appear to significantly reduce this difficulty (Hansen, 1979; Schmitt, 1982).

Dry-Bed Training. Azrin, Sneed, and Foxx (1974) have developed a highly effective and rapid treatment program for enuresis based on operant conditioning principles. Referred to as "dry-bed training," this somewhat complex program consists of one day of intensive training by behavioral technicians. It involves reinforcement for inhibiting urination, practice of appropriate urination, bladder awareness training, copious drinking, self-correction and positive practice for accidents, awakening training, use of a pad and bell device, and family encouragement. A number of modifications of this program have been made since the original study, including the omission of the urine alarm and having parents conduct the training with minimal direct supervision (Azrin & Thienes, 1978; Azrin & Besalel, 1979; Christophersen & Rapoff, 1978). Early studies with this method suggested that it might be superior to others in rapidity of improvement and relapse rate (Azrin, Sneed, & Foxx, 1974; Azrin & Thienes, 1978; Bollard and Woodrofe, 1977; Doleys et al., 1977). However, studies that omitted the pad and bell (Nettelbeck & Langeluddecke, 1979) or that employed parents rather than behavioral technicians to administer the program had more limited success (Bollard & Woodrofe, 1977). Thus, while this approach appears promising, much more research is needed to establish the actual success rate of the program and to determine the key effective components of this rather elaborate and multifaceted intervention package.

Encopresis

Functional encopresis is described by DSM-III as (a) repeated involuntary or voluntary passage of feces into places not appropriate (usually the clothing) for that purpose; (b) at least one such event per month after the age of four; and (c) not due to a physical disorder such as aganglionic megacolon or anal fissure (APA, 1980).

The ability to control defecation is dependent upon adequate innervation of the colon and anus as well as the ability to purposively relax and contract the external sphincter. The toilet training process is designed to teach the child to recognize the proprioceptive stimuli from the colon and to coordinate these with the relaxing of the external anal sphincters while being properly seated over a toilet or potty chair.

Among the organic conditions which may cause fecal incontinence are: dietary factors; allergic reactions to food and other substances; infectious diseases of the large intestine; and anomalies of the intestinal tract and/or of the nerve supply to the tract (Vaughan, McKay, & Nelson, 1975). A careful history and appropriate medical diagnostic procedures should reveal such organic conditions. When such factors are present, suitable medical treatment should be pursued. The diagnosis of functional encopresis is made only in the absence of an organic cause. The term *primary encopresis* (or continuous encopresis) is used to refer to the child who has never achieved bowel control. *Secondary* (or noncontinuous) *encopresis* refers to the child who has been known to be continent for at least six months prior to the onset of soiling (Anthony, 1957). While most encopretics soil during the day, some cases of nocturnal soiling have been reported in the literature (Jay & Wright, 1982).

Prevalence

Walker (1978) distinguished three subtypes of encopresis. The first, *manipulative soiling,* is postulated to occur in children as either a conscious or unconscious behavior intended to manipulate the family or other aspects of the child's environment (e.g., expressing hostility toward a parent, school avoidance, as an attention-getting device, etc.). While numerous references in the literature seem to imply that this is the most common form of encopresis (Hilburn, 1968; Lifschitz & Chovers, 1972; Ringdahl, 1980), most studies have found relatively few cases of encopresis to fall into this category (Fitzgerald, 1975; Wright, 1973; Wright & Walker, 1978).

The second type of encopresis is a result of emotional upset and reaction to stressful life situations. This form has been referred to in the literature as *chronic diarrhea or irritable bowel syndrome* (Davidson, 1973). Children in this category react somatically to stress, with resultant periods of incontinence or diarrhea.

Anywhere from 80 to 95 percent of children brought to pediatricians for fecal incontinence present a history of fecal retention and/or constipation (Christophersen & Rapoff, 1978; Fitzgerald, 1975; Levine, 1975). This third type, which Walker (1978) refers to as *chronic constipation,* obviously comprises the largest number of cases. A host of factors can result in the child developing constipation, such as an inherited tendency toward becoming constipated, poor dietary choices, emotional factors, painful bowel movements, and so forth.

When constipation is chronic, there is an impaction of accumulated fecal material. The buildup of fecal material stretches the colon and decreases normal muscle tone, further inhibiting bowel activity. Eventually, severe impaction and megacolon (a greatly enlarged colon) result. Liquid material from the stomach and small intestines may passively seep out around the impaction, resulting in stains on the child's underclothing. This is usually of a pasty-watery consistency and the child often states that he/she was not aware of the need to defecate when the soiling occurred. This report is generally accurate because the passive leaking of material does not produce the normal sensations associated with active defecation. Large bowel movements occur occasionally both in the child's clothing or in the toilet when large quantities of the impacted feces suddenly loosen. Severe impactions can result in an extended abdomen, tearing of the colon, and infection. In such cases, surgical intervention may be required. It is obvious that chronic megacolon poses a potentially serious health hazard (Jay & Wright, 1982; Walker, 1978).

Estimates of prevalence of this disorder are from 1.5 to 7.5 percent of children (Doleys, Schwartz, & Ciminero, 1981). In relation to age differences, Bellman (1966) found that 8.1 percent of 3-year-olds were still soiling their clothing, with 2.8 percent of the four-year-olds in his study and 2.2 percent of the five-year-olds manifesting fecal incontinence. In Levine's (1975) study of 102 encopretics, eighty-seven were in the four-to-thirteen-year age group and 85 percent of the total were males. It is generally agreed that encopresis is a very underreported disorder. Careful interviewing turns up many cases that otherwise would go undiscovered.

Etiology

In general, psychodynamic theories have conceptualized encopresis to result from either anal erotic gratification obtained through retaining the feces or as the unconscious expression of hostile and aggressive impulses (through soiling) toward parental figures (Shane, 1967; Lifschitz & Chovers, 1972). Doleys, Schwartz, and Ciminero (1981) summarized the host of psychoanalytic formulations as follows: encopresis can be viewed as a symptom of an unconscious conflict due to the "lack of parental love, guilt value of feces, separation anxiety, fear of loss of the feces, pregnancy wishes, aggression against a hostile world, response to familial dysfunction, and traumatic separation from the mother between the oral and anal stages of psychosexual development" (p. 696). Not surprisingly, the mother-child relationship during the toilet training period has been implicated by a number of analytic writers (Bemporad, 1978; Hersov, 1977). It is postulated that mother-child conflict, often elicited during the toilet training process, results in coercive methods being imposed that lead to the development of retentive encopresis (Anthony, 1957). While inappropriate toilet training methods may play a role in the development of encopresis, it is not generally accepted that this symptom is the result of unconscious psychic conflicts (Doleys, Schwartz, & Ciminero, 1981). Indeed, most encopretic children do not seem to manifest severe emotional disturbance (Walker, 1978).

The medical model of encopresis often assumes such possibilities as an obstruction of the colon, neurodevelopmental defects, immaturity, dietary factors, and constitutional variables (Davidson, 1958; Doleys, Schwartz, & Ciminero, 1981). While a genetic or constitutional predisposition to constipation has been proposed (Bell & Levine, 1954), there are few empirical data to support this (Walker, 1978; Wolters & Wauters, 1975). Undeniably, some cases of fecal incontinence are organically based, though 90 percent or more are probably psychogenic in origin. However, even when organic pathology is present, behavioral procedures may be of value in the treatment process (Doleys, Schwartz, & Ciminero, 1981; Epstein & McCoy, 1977). Medical correction of underlying organic conditions does not always result in proper toileting behavior and such skills must be taught to the child following medical interventions.

Within a behavioral or learning model, encopresis is conceptualized as being due to a breakdown in the process of learning cognitive control of the bowels. This model has something in common with the organic theories of etiology. In this model, it is assumed that failure to learn proper control of the bowel (or loss of such control once learned) occurs due to the fact that the constipation and resulting megacolon significantly compromise the normal functioning of the colon.

Treatment

Medical Treatment. Hein and Beerends (1978) described a program consisting of dietary control, enemas, bowel training, and parent consultation in which fourteen of eighteen encopretic children were completely cured of soiling, with three more showing significant improvement.

An 80 percent success rate was found by Davidson, Kugler, and Bauer (1963) in their treatment of ninety encopretics. Their three-phase program consisted of initial enemas to eliminate impaction, regular oral ingestion of mineral oil to induce consistent bowel movements, a second three-month phase in which mineral oil was faded out while bowel habit training was conducted, and a third phase where parent counseling and followup were employed to maintain the gains made during treatment. While the data are impressive, there were many methodological problems in this study. These include inadequate documentation of pretreatment soiling behavior, vague descriptions of treatment procedures and subject responses, erratic follow-up data collection, lack of frequency data regarding proper toileting behavior, and the absence of control subjects (Doleys, 1979).

When parental cooperation and resistance to other forms of treatment become a problem, a number of authors recommend hospitalization of the encopretic child (Doleys, Schwartz, & Ciminero, 1981; Ravitch, 1958; Ringdahl, 1980).

Other than the application of laxatives, mineral oil, and stool softeners, there has not been extensive investigation into the usefulness of pharmacological agents in the treatment of encopresis. In one study by Gavanski (1971), imipramine (Tofranil) was administered in conjunction with psychotherapy in the treatment of three nonretentive secondary encopretics. While the form of psychotherapy in this study was not specified, and the effects of the psychotherapy could not be distinguished from the effects of the medication, the author did find this combined approach successful in all three cases.

Psychotherapy. Perhaps even more so than with enuresis, verbal psychotherapy is a frequent recommendation for the treatment of encopresis. Usually treatment focuses on encopresis conceptualized as a refusal to defecate or as defiant soiling (Pinkerton, 1958).

While there has been very little research on psychotherapy for encopresis, Pinkerton (1958) treated thirty encopretic children through parent consultation designed to remove parental fear and prejudices along with play therapy for the encopretic child to remove the pathological defenses and provide insight into the source of the problem. Seventeen of the thirty children improved, with a followup period of up to three and a half years. A combination of play therapy, clay modeling and finger painting, along with conjoint parental counseling, was employed by McTaggert and Scott (1959) in the treatment of twelve encopretic children. Of the twelve children, seven were judged to be cured and three as significantly improved. However, in reviewing the records of seventy encopretics treated with verbal psychotherapy, Berg and Jones (1964) found that the remission rate for those receiving therapy was not significantly different from those who did not. Doleys (1979) has noted that the absence of studies employing a control group, the vague and generic use of the term *verbal psychotherapy*, and inadequate descriptions of treatment procedures have made it impossible to accurately evaluate the effectiveness of verbal psychotherapy and play therapy in the treatment of encopresis.

Behavioral-Learning and Combined Treatment Programs. Studies of the behavioral treatment of encopresis have manipulated reinforcement and punishment contingencies for soiling and proper toileting. Doleys (1978) divided operant conditioning studies into the following categories: (1) those employing positive reinforcement only, with no consequences for soiling; (2) those programs relying solely on punishment for soiling; (3) programs combining the use of positive reinforcement for appropriate toileting and nonsoiling, with use of punishment or aversive consequences for soiling episodes; (4) combined programs which include medical or physical forms of treatment (e.g., enemas and suppositories) with behavioral conditioning procedures; and (5) treatment programs which employ additional behavioral procedures such as full cleanliness training, positive practice, and the use of mechanical devices. One shortcoming of research on behavioral treatment approaches is that the majority are based on single case reports rather than large group studies (Walker, 1978; Wells & Forehand, 1981).

The combined use of positive reinforcement for appropriate elimination and punishment for soiling episodes has been reported. In one study, sixteen out of eighteen encopretics ceased soiling after two months of treatment with no relapse reported during followup (Ashkenazi, 1975). This program consisted of having the child sit on the toilet after eating; use of positive reinforcement for nonsoiling and elimination; and the application of suppositories if defecation did not take place during the appropriate period.

A number of treatment programs have been developed which combine the use of operant learning techniques as well as certain medical or pediatric treatment approaches into a fairly comprehensive intervention package. One such program was developed by Wright (1973) and further described by Wright and Walker (1977, 1978). This treatment approach combines both cathartics and contingency management. Wright (1973) successfully treated fourteen patients with this method with a mean time of treatment of seventeen weeks. Walker (1978) found this method to be virtually 100 percent successful with over 200 encopretic children when given proper follow-up. Parental compliance is of the utmost importance with this approach, and 10 to 15 percent of the families drop out early in the course of treatment.

Two techniques developed by Azrin and Foxx (1971) and Foxx and Azrin (1973) are full cleanliness training and positive practice. *Full cleanliness training* requires children to overcorrect the results of soiling by thoroughly cleaning themselves and their clothes. This theoretically serves as training in responsible behavior as well as a negative consequence. *Positive practice* requires the child to practice required toileting behaviors (going to the bathroom, removing clothing, and sitting on the toilet). Doleys and Arnold (1975) and Doleys et al. (1977) reported success with several cases using this method combined with positive reinforcement for clean pants and proper toileting. Butler (1977) employed overcorrection methods successfully with three encopretic children, while Freeman and Pribble (1974) found these methods effective with a five-and-a-half-year-old autistic child who evacuated in inappropriate places on an inpatient unit.

Breunlin (1980) has described the use of multimodal behavioral treatment in the successful treatment of an enuretic and encopretic preschooler. Paradoxical instruction techniques were employed successfully in the treatment of a nine-year-old male retentive encopretic using an *ABAB reversal design* (Bernstein, et al., 1981). In this case the child was instructed to sit on the toilet every hour for five minutes and act as if "you have to make a bowel movement but do not allow that to occur." The authors proposed that instructing the child to not perform the behavior reduced his anxiety and facilitated the occurrence of proper defecation.

As mentioned previously, Walker (1978) has delineated three types of encopresis: manipulative soiling; the irritable bowel syndrome; and retentive encopresis. Manipulative soiling is viewed as the child's attempt to control his/or parents or environment through inappropriate elimination. These cases are felt to be most responsive to family oriented treatment which focuses on teaching the child to express himself/herself in a more appropriate manner, as well as guiding family members in methods of extinguishing soiling behavior while reinforcing proper toileting behavior. Thus, family therapy and/or a straightforward behavior modification program are viewed as the most appropriate treatment for this type of soiling (Walker, 1978).

With the irritable bowel syndrome encopretic (or nonretentive encopretic), frequent soiling is the result of diarrhea caused by tension, anxiety, and stress. Walker (1978) suggests that environmental manipulation, supportive therapy, and possibly medication be utilized to reduce the sources of stress and anxiety along with teaching the child coping strategies to deal more effectively with stress. Such methods as systematic desensitization (Cohen & Reed, 1968; Hedberg, 1973), hypnosis (Byrne, 1973), relaxation training (Bernstein & Borkovec, 1973; Walker et al., 1981), and assertive training (Alberti and Emmons, 1974; Walker et al., 1981) have been effectively employed with this form of encopresis.

Eating Disorders

For the newborn, feeding is the first significant interaction with his or her mother. While the feeding response is initially a reflexive behavior, it involves the mutual contribution of both the feeder and the infant in such a way that they reciprocally influence one another's responses. The outcome of this mutual interaction is instrumental in setting the stage for subsequent more or less adaptive patterns of interaction outside of, as well as within, the realm of feeding (Linscheid, 1978).

While the prevalence of eating problems has been estimated at between 25 and 35 percent of children in the general population (Palmer & Horn, 1978), this is probably an underestimation. The prevalence of some childhood eating disturbances are likely to be higher than 35 percent, since most figures are based on cases where the parents sought professional assistance.

Linscheid (1983) has expanded the proposed classification by Palmer, Thompson, and Linscheid (1975) into what is perhaps the most comprehensive classification system of eating disorders available (see Table 8-1). In Linscheid's system, all possible etiologies and classifications according to the DSM-III eating disorder subsystem are accounted for.

Anorexia Nervosa

DSM-III criteria for anorexia nervosa:

A. Intense fear of becoming obese

B. Disturbance of body image, e.g., claiming to "feel fat" even when emaciated

C. Weight loss or projected weight loss of at least 25 percent (loss from original body weight plus projected weight gain expected from growth charts may be combined to make the 25 percent)

D. Refusal to maintain normal body weight

E. No known physical illness that would account for the weight loss

Prevalence, Etiology, and Behavioral Correlates. While the prevalence of anorexia nervosa in the general population has been estimated to be relatively low, recent studies have shown that reported cases are on the increase, and the condition may have been much under-reported in the past. A survey of several school systems in England found the prevalence to be one in every 200 girls, with a rate of one in about every 100 girls in those aged sixteen and over (Crisp, Palmer, & Kalacy, 1976). While these rates seem to be overestimates, the alarming increase in this

TABLE 8-1

An Expansion of the Palmer, Thompson, and Linscheid Classification System for Childhood Feeding Problems

	Behavioral Mismanagement	Neuromotor Dysfunction	Mechanical Obstruction	Medical or Genetic Abnormalities
Major Problems		*Possible Causes*		
Mealtime tantrums	X			
Bizarre food habits	X			X
Multiple food dislikes	X			X
Prolonged subsistance on pureed foods	X	X	X	
Delay or difficulty in chewing, sucking or swallowing		X	X	
Delay in self-feeding	X	X	X	
Pica	X			X
Excessive overeating	X			X
Excessive underintake of food	X	X	X	X
Rumination	X	X		X

disorder, which occurs predominately in females (only 4–6 percent are males), has been attributed to several factors. Crisp, Palmer, and Kalacy (1976) summarize these as:

> (a) Our affluent and overnourished society; (b) the rapid biological growth through puberty which the latter promotes, especially amongst females who thereby especially come to associate their mounting fatness with their adolescent self-consciousness and turmoil; (c) the associated propensity for almost universal attempts at dieting among female adolescents, in which respect they are singularly different from the majority of adolescent males; (d) the particular psychological problems of an existential kind for adolescents, which are of a different order from those which confronted previous generations (p. 553).

The anorexic accomplishes weight loss through one or more means. These include a drastic reduction in the total intake of food (usually with disproportionate decrease in high fat- and carbohydrate-containing foods); self-induced vomiting, which often occurs after binge-eating (bulimic) episodes; the abuse of laxatives and/or diuretics; and paradoxical hyperactivity or overactivity, often involving prolonged periods of exercise without regard to malaise or the patient's debilitated condition (Halmi, 1978). Obviously, such practices can seriously endanger physical health and, accordingly, anorexia nervosa has the highest mortality rate of perhaps any psychiatric condition. Mortality rates range from 5 to 21 percent (Bruch, 1971; Crisp, 1965; Halmi, Brodland, & Rigas, 1975).

Differential diagnosis of anorexia nervosa must rule out the possibility that the symptoms are primarily due to schizophrenia, hysterical disorders, or depression (of which the last is a frequent accompaniment in anorexics who are prone toward bulimic episodes and self-induced vomiting). Anorexia nervosa must also be distinguished from organic disorders in which severe weight loss occurs, e.g., certain malignant tumors. However, in most organic conditions there is no evidence of an intense fear of obesity or disturbed body image as seen with the anorexic.

In the large majority of cases, onset occurs in puberty and adolescence. This observation has led a number of contemporary writers to suggest that, "Anorexia nervosa is rooted in various constellations of pre-existent psychological vunerability and as such represents a compensatory adaptation set in motion to suppress pubertal changes in body weight and shape and attenuate maturational anxieties triggered by adolescent growth and development" (Strober, 1981a, p. 286). From this perspective, the refusal to eat is regarded as an unconscious attempt to stop growing up and an avoidance of anxieties associated with adolescent sexual development and the beginning of heterosexual relationships (Bruch, 1980).

Studies have shown that a variety of physiological abnormalities are evident in the actively starving phase of the anorexia nervosa syndrome (Agras & Werne, 1981). A total cessation of menses or a delay in the onset of menses occurs in most patients, often even before weight loss is reported.

Disordered interpersonal relationships and cognitive disturbance in the early life experiences of anorexics have been postulated to account for distortions of body image and perception (Agras & Werne, 1981; Bruch, 1978). This has led to a wealth of research. For example, several studies using a visual size estimation apparatus and markings of indicated body points on a sheet of paper have shown anorexics overestimate their body size (Garfinkle, Moldofsky, & Garner, 1979; Pierloot & Houben, 1978; Strober et al., 1979). Nevertheless, one study (Casper et al., 1979) failed to replicate these findings with a sample of seventy-nine female anorexia nervosa patients and a control group. In this investigation both groups tended to overestimate their body widths. Among the anorexic patients, the extent of overestimation was found to be associated with less weight gain during treatment and greater denial of illness. Likewise, Strober et al. (1979) did not find size estimation differences between hospitalized adolescent anorexia nervosa patients and controls.

Strober (1980, 1981a, 1981b) conducted an extensive comparative analysis of fifty anorexia nervosa patients with equal-sized matched groups of depressed and antisocial adolescent females using a variety of personality assessment instruments. On Cattell's High School Personality Questionnaire, he found that anorexics were more regulating of their emotional behavior; more conscious of and attentive to social and ethical norms of behavior; experienced more pronounced anxiety and self-doubt; demonstrated a higher degree of social conformity; were less assertive; less demonstrative in the affective domain; and more inhibited interpersonally (Strober, 1981*a*). Thus, the anorexics were readily distinguished from two nonanorexic clinical populations and the characteristics found were generally in accord with previous anecdotal clinical reports of personality factors in anorexia nervosa (e.g., Bruch, 1973; Selvini-Palazzoli, 1978; Sours, 1980).

A number of investigators have emphasized the influence of family variables on the behavior of the anorexic and see the patient as simply the symptom bearer for a dysfunctional family system (Minuchin et al., 1975; Minuchin, Rosman, & Baker, 1978; Selvini-Palazzoli, 1978). The anorexic's symptoms are conceptualized as having the effect of detouring family conflicts and thus temporarily stabilizing the family system. Therapeutic change requires disengaging the patient from the parental conflict in order to allow the family system to become more flexible.

To the clinician, perhaps the most striking feature of the anorexia nervosa syndrome is the bizarreness of the extreme weight loss contrasted with the patient's sense of benignness or innocence. While some authors have viewed anorexia as a variant of borderline personality or even schizophrenia, many anorexics seem to function in a superior manner in a number of life areas. Indeed, they seem to do exceptionally well at accomplishing something that defeats many people for a lifetime, i.e., losing weight. Yet, it is readily apparent that their fear of weight gain and distorted sense of physical self border on the delusional in spite of the fact that they are in generally good contact with reality.

Prognosis. While research into the treatment of anorexia nervosa continues, the overall prognosis is not especially optimistic. In their review of data from twelve major outcome investigations, Schwartz and Thompson (1981) found that at followup more than half the adolescents continued to manifest eating difficulties in adulthood and an additional 46 percent demonstrated serious psychiatric symptoms in areas that were not directly related to food or weight. In the total of 478 patients included in the study there was also evidence of continued poor social and marital adjustment. Halmi et al. (1979) studied the pretreatment characteristics of eighty-one anorexia nervosa patients and found that positive outcome (in terms of weight gain) was related to an absence of previous hospitalization for the condition, evidence of overactivity before treatment, a lower degree of denial of illness, less psychosexual immaturity, and an admission of feelings of hunger.

Treatment. The potentially serious medical complications of this condition usually require ongoing medical management along with psychological treatment. In the acute phases of the illness, hospitalization is frequently necessary in order to stabilize weight loss and initiate nutritional and weight increase programs.

White and Schnaultz (1977) found imipramine to be effective in improving depressive symptomatology in two cases of secondary anorexia nervosa, i.e., those patients where the age of onset is later in puberty than the primary group and where the patient has an awareness of his or her emaciated appearance and odd eating habits (Bruch, 1976). The tricyclic antidepressant was believed to have led to improved affect with concomitant weight gain and improvement in physical condition.

Cyproheptadine, a relatively safe weight-inducing drug, was found to be effective in producing significant weight gain in a subgroup of more severe anorexics characterized by a history of birth delivery complications, loss of gross body weight between 41 and 52 percent from the norm, and prior outpatient treatment failure (Halmi et al., 1979). Hyperalimentation and intravenous feeding have been shown to be effective, but serious medical complications were frequent with the use of these techniques (Pertschuk et al., 1981).

Family system theorists, such as Minuchin, Rosman, and Baker (1978), have developed a treatment program that entails hospitalization, frequent family therapy sessions while the patient is hospitalized, and followup after discharge. They reported an 86 percent recovery rate for the anorexic patients treated in their family therapy program, based upon data from fifty-three cases. However, family therapy studies suffer from insufficient standardization of treatment methodology, making treatment replication most difficult.

There is comparatively little in the analytic literature regarding the individual psychotherapy of the anorexic patient. In fact, one analytic perspective holds that traditional psychoanalysis is inadvisable with these patients, as it is more likely to elicit negativism and mistrust rather than enhance their body image and correct their perceptual disturbances (Sours, 1979). Bruch (1973) advocates confronting the patient with the abnormality of her eating behavior by interpreting it as a metabolic device for both decreasing her anxiety-arousing sexual feelings as well as increasing the emotional attachment with the mother.

The majority of reports on the behavioral treatment of anorexia nervosa have detailed specific programs applied during hospitalization for the reinforcement of weight gain and increase in caloric intake. After a baseline is established, a daily weight gain (typically 0.5 pounds per day) is required for access to activities, social interaction, and privileges in the hospital milieu (Garfinkle, Kline, & Stancer, 1975). Important components in such programs are the provision of regular feedback to the patient regarding caloric intake and weight gain, regular reinforcement for increases in weight, and the established contingency of weight gain leading to hospital discharge (Linscheid, 1978).

Blinder, Freeman, and Stunkard (1970) successfully made access to physical activity contingent upon weight gain with three highly active anorexics. Agras et al.

(1974) noted that their patients continued to gain weight on an inpatient program even after the removal of external reinforcement. Further investigation revealed that the patients realized that continued weight gain would lead to discharge from the hospital, and weight decreased if the length of stay and other reinforcers were not contingent on weight gain.

Agras and Werne's (1981) inpatient behavioral treatment program includes operant conditioning principles combined with patient responsibility, mandatory group and individual therapy sessions, as well as couple and family sessions. Follow-up data on this program has revealed that since its inception, forty-five percent of the patients demonstrated marked improvement, with 16 percent showing no appreciable improvement (Agras & Werne, 1978).

Bruch (1978) criticized the behavior modification approach for treating only the superficial symptoms of anorexia nervosa and has cited cases where patients experienced rapid weight loss following discharge from an operant treatment program. In addition, she indicated that patients treated through behavior modification alone are more likely to experience residual feelings of depression, guilt, and a lack of trust because they have been "tricked" into eating. Bruch implied that this may then make the anorexic at greater risk for suicide. In response, Kellerman (1977a) reviewed eleven studies employing operant conditioning principles and found that follow-up indicated the majority of patients maintained full or partial weight gain and showed positive concommitant changes in social functioning and self-esteem. None of the patients had died or committed suicide.

Poole and Sanson (1978) reported the highly successful treatment of five female patients with a comprehensive behavioral program. Unique to this study was the inclusion of a follow-up contract in which the patient agreed to readmission should weight fall below a certain level. Follow-up appointments were arranged on a random schedule so that short-term manipulation of weight was more difficult, a component to this program which seems particularly effective.

Bulimia

DSM-III criteria for diagnosing bulimia are as follows:

A. Recurrent episodes of binge eating (rapid consumption of a large amount of food in a discrete period of time, usually less than two hours)

B. At least three of the following:
   (1) Consumption of high caloric, easily ingested food during a binge
   (2) Inconspicuous eating during a binge
   (3) Termination of such eating episodes by abdominal pain, sleep, social interruption, or self-induced vomiting
   (4) Repeated attempts to lose weight by use of severely restrictive diets, self-induced vomiting, cathartics, or diuretics
   (5) Frequent weight fluctuations greater than ten pounds due to alternating binges and fasts

C. Awareness that the eating pattern is abnormal and fear of not being able to stop eating voluntarily

D. Depressed mood and self-deprecating thoughts following eating binges

E. Bulimic episodes not due to anorexia nervosa or any known physical disorder.

While the presence of bulimia—variously referred to as bulimia nervosa (Russell, 1979), bulimarexia (Boskind-Lodahl, 1977), dysorexia (Guiora, 1967), and dietary chaos syndrome (Palmer, 1979)—has been reported in 47 percent of a series of 105 patients with anorexia nervosa (Casper et al., 1980), no data exist as to the incidence of this disorder in the general population. And, while the presence of bulimic behavior in anorexics has been shown to be a poor prognostic indicator, no data have been collected which would allow a prognostic prediction for nonanorexic bulimia patients. Patients who suffer from bulimia nervosa have been known to vomit as much as several times a day every day of the week (Rosen & Leitenberg, 1982).

As opposed to the denial found in many anorexics, the bulimic often demonstrates considerable insight into the disorder and typically expresses feelings of guilt and self-disgust. The bulimic experiences eating as a compulsion that is overwhelming and which is at odds with his/her great concern regarding weight and personal appearance. In contrast to anorexics, bulimics have been found to be only slightly underweight, while some are of normal or even excessive weight. Amenorrhea is a relatively rare accompaniment of bulimia, with the large majority of patients maintaining regular menstruation. In common with anorexics, though, bulimics demonstrate a classic pathological perception of body size as well as a morbid fear of fatness and weight gain beyond normal standards. And, while patients with anorexia nervosa may engage in vomiting and purging, such behavior has been found to be generally less frequent and habitual in these patients than in bulimics (Russell, 1979).

From the psychoanalytic perspective Guiora (1967) conceptualized bulimia as an arrest in psychological development at the oral stage. It is the symptomatic manifestation of hostility toward, and lack of identification with, the mother figure. Emotional deprivation in the early mother-child relationship is experienced in the process of food intake and the pubertal onset of bulimia results in the direct expression of an "all destroying rage," with the act of binge eating being a direct expression of repressed oral aggression. However intriguing this interpretation may seem, there is no empirical evidence to support it.

As with anorexia nervosa, the eating habits associated with bulimia can lead to serious physical complications, e.g., potassium loss and cardiac problems. However, some of the more severe accompaniments of extreme starvation associated with anorexia nervosa are not likely to be manifest in the bulimic.

From the behavioral perspective, the binge eating and self-induced vomiting cycle of bulimia nervosa have been conceptualized as a learned habit pattern than leads to anxiety reduction. Rosen and Leitenberg (1982) state: "Once an individual has learned that vomiting following food intake leads to anxiety reduction, rational fears no longer inhibit overeating. Thus, the driving force of this disorder may be vomiting, not binging; binging might not occur if the person could not vomit afterwards" (p. 118).

While bulimia has been treated with Dilantin (Wermuth et al., 1977), analytically-oriented psychotherapy, and family therapy, at present no treatment outcome data from controlled studies exists regarding the effectiveness of these procedures (Rosen & Leitenberg, 1982). Russell (1979), in his study of thirty bulimia nervosa patients, recommended a comprehensive treatment program which involved hospitalization to interrupt the cycle of overeating and self-induced vomiting, skilled nursing care, encouragement of regular eating habits in the company of others, supervision after eating whereby the patient was encouraged to lie on her bed to relax until the temptation to vomit subsided, and persuading the patient to accept a higher weight. Follow-up outpatient psychotherapy of an interpretive nature was suggested, yet no data were provided regarding its application in this program. While there is a consensus that the prognosis for bulimia nervosa is less favorable than that for anorexia nervosa (Guioria, 1967; Pyle, Mitchell & Eckert, 1981; Russell, 1979), more large scale studies need to be conducted with a variety of treatment modalities to evaluate the response of this syndrome to various treatments.

Pica

Pica refers to repeated eating of a nonnutritive substance for at least one month which is not due to another mental disorder, such as infantile autism or schizophrenia, or to a physical disorder such as Klein-Levin syndrome (APA, 1980).

While all children occasionally mouth or swallow nonfood items, this practice typically declines and is discontinued around the time the child begins to walk. As pica persists after that time, it has been found to become particularly resistant to change (Bakwin & Bakwin, 1972). A higher incidence is found in Blacks, in women during pregnancy, and in children between the ages of eighteen and twenty-four months of age (De la Burde & Reames, 1973). Pica becomes a problem of grave concern when it involves the ingestion of substances which are toxic. The most common substance in this regard is lead-based paint, which children often gnaw from the woodwork and windowsills of older housing. Serious central nervous system damage and mental retardation often are the result.

Proposed causes of pica include iron deficiency (especially in pregnancy), inadequate hemoglobin, a buccal mucosal enzyme deficiency, calcium deficiency and specific nutritional needs that occur in pregnant women (Wright et al., 1979). Other physiological factors suspected of being involved include toxicosis, genetic predisposition, and gastrointestinal malaise (Mitchell, Winter, & Morisaki, 1977).

Psychological factors proposed have included mental retardation, cultural tradition, habit, emotional deprivation, and the persistence of infantile hand/mouth behavior (Mitchell, Winter, & Morisaki, 1977). There is evidence that in certain cultures the prevalence of pica is responsive to complex social forces, e.g., changes due to urbanization in more primitive societies (Eastwell, 1979). Pica has also been proposed as a learned habit acquired through the inadvertent reinforcement of parental attention, or perhaps as a form of drive-reduction wherein a decrease in tension is associated with chewing behavior (Wright, Schaefer, & Solomoans, 1979).

Treatment. Medical treatments for pica vary according to the nature of the substance ingested and the implication this has for the child's unmet biochemical needs. For example, in cases of geophagia (dirt eating), the provision of iron supplements and a diet high in protein may be recommended (Ziai, Janeway, & Cooke, 1975). If a biochemical deficit exists, provision of the substance lacking is obviously necessary.

However, in some cases, the most obvious solution to the problem of the ingestion of inappropriate material is the elimination of that material from the child's environment (Linscheid, 1983). Community groups in urban areas have organized to seek out sources of toxins (e.g., lead based paint) and alert the community to their danger. Thus, primary prevention is the favored approach with some forms of pica.

In those situations where removal of the ingested object is impractical or perhaps impossible, the focus has been on decreasing the frequency of ingestion of the substance. In the case of lead ingestion, an association between the emotional and intellectual stimulation available in the child's environment and the prevalence of lead ingestion has been found. Madden, Russo, and Cataldo (1980) reduced the overall frequency of pica in children by providing access to toys and adult interaction. Thus environmental enrichment may be the treatment of choice in such situations.

Pica is often a severe problem among the mentally retarded in institutional situations. These patients often ingest such materials as feces, stones, grass, paint and unclean food. Bucher, Reykdal, and Albin (1976) reported the treatment of two profoundly retarded children who ingested inappropriate food and small objects. Brief physical restraint was employed as a form of mild punishment. Training took place in several settings in order to facilitate generalization. While one subject demonstrated suppression of the pica behavior in the trained setting, no generalization to other settings was observed. A significant decrease in the inappropriate eating was obtained with the second subject, but again no generalization was observed. Complete suppression of the behavior in the trained settings was obtained only when restraint was applied at the earliest detectable sequence of the pica response.

Foxx and Martin (1975) have employed an overcorrection procedure in the treatment of a number of retarded children who suffered from intestinal blockages and parasites due to the ingestion of inappropriate objects, including feces and cigarette butts. In the case of ingestion of feces, the children are required to spit them out, engage in an oral hygiene procedure wherein they brush their teeth and gums with an antiseptic saturated toothbrush, wipe their lips with an antiseptic cloth, and then wash their hands, fingernails, and anal areas. The final procedure is for the children to disinfect the area where the feces had been eaten. The authors reported this procedure was extremely effective in eliminating the pica as well as eradicating the presence of intestinal parasites in all subjects treated.

Finney, Russo, and Cataldo (1982) developed a behavioral treatment package designed to eliminate pica in a group of children hospitalized due to high blood lead levels. Four young children (age two to five years) participated in the study. The initial phase consisted of discrimination training in which the children were taught to differentiate edible from nonedible objects. If this procedure alone proved ineffective, the child entered a DRO (Differentive Reinforcement for Behavior Other than Pica) training, in which increased periods of no pica were reinforced with verbal praise and treats. A final DRO plus overcorrection (brushing the mouth and teeth for one minute with a toothbrush dipped in Listerine, contingent upon pica behavior) phase was added for those children who persisted in pica behavior in the training room setting. In addition, parents were trained in the use of the procedures in the home. All four children showed significant reduction in pica, with the discrimination and DRO procedures being sufficient for two children, and the addition of the overcorrection procedure being necessary in the treatment of the other two children.

Rumination Disorder Of Infancy

Rumination disorder is defined as repeated regurgitation without nausea or associated gastrointestinal illness for at least one month following a period of normal functioning and which results in weight loss or failure to make expected weight gain (APA, 1980). The regurgitation or vomiting typically occurs at the end of a behavior chain of abdominal muscular contractions, tongue movements, and stimulation of the mouth and throat with the hands. Due to this sequence it is regarded as a voluntary and pleasurable behavior (O'Neil, et al., 1979).

While there are no exact incidence data available on this disorder, it is believed to be rare and declining in frequency. If the regurgitated food is of substantial volume and is not reingested, malnutrition and dehydration may ensue, creating a life-threatening condition. Mortality rates have ranged from 12 to 21 percent (O'Neil et al., 1979).

Psychoanalytic theory considers infantile vomiting to be a manifestation of prolonged psychological and body tension (Ferholt & Provence, 1976). The source of this disturbance is believed due to severe deficiencies in the nurturing aspects of the mother-infant relationship. Concomitant psychological disturbances include delays and distortions in object relations, drive development, and early ego functions. However, not all cases of psychogenic vomiting in children have shown evidence of demonstrable psychopathology.

While behavioral theory has not attempted to develop an etiological formulation regarding this disturbance, a variety of stimuli can cause psychogenic vomiting, even those conditions postulated by psychoanalytic theory (Wright, Schaefer, & Solomoans, 1979). Yet, once the behavior has been initiated, a variety of reinforcement contingencies may come into play, thus maintaining the behavior in the absence of the original stimulus. Rumination may occur when the infant's perceptual focus is directed toward internal somatic cues rather than the external environment. That is, vomiting and regurgitation become a means of self-stimulation to the exclusion of external stimulation (Wright & Thalassinos, 1973) when the external environment is painful or significantly lacking in pleasurable stimuli.

The mothers of ruminating infants have been described as having difficulty relating to their babies, being fearful of the possible death of their infant, and demonstrating immaturity in the form of an incapacity to want, accept, and give to their infants. However, Linscheid (1983) has cautioned that when analyzing the mother-infant interaction it is important not to confuse cause and effect. In other words, it may be just as likely that the mother's characteristics are due to the chronic ruminating of her infant as the reverse.

Treatment. A number of physical causes for vomiting exist and these need to be ruled out by medical examination. However, by definition, rumination disorder involves a functional cause.

Psychoanalytic treatment consists in providing the child with a warm, supportive, and stimulating environment, often through the use of a mother substitute (Ferholt & Provence, 1976). Supportive and insight-oriented psychotherapy for the mother or primary caretaker are also recommended. While the outcome of this approach has been generally favorable (in terms of decreasing rumination and increasing infant weight), weight attainment has been found to be relatively slow (O'Neil et al., 1979).

One of the more frequently employed behavioral treatment procedures utilized with infant rumination has been the application of aversive procedures for regurgitating along with attention and positive reinforcement for not regurgitating. The use of a mild electric shock has proven effective in eliminating rumination in a number of studies (Cunninghman & Linscheid, 1976; Linscheid & Cunningham, 1977; Toister et al., 1975).

Linscheid and Cunningham (1977) administered a series of 0.5-sec shocks at 0.5-sec intervals when a ruminating sequence was observed and terminated the shock when it ceased. Ruminative vomiting in a nine-month-old infant dropped from a five-day baseline mean of 114 to a single instance of vomiting on treatment day three. Removal of the treatment condition resulted in an increase in rumination. Treatment was then reinstituted for ten more days and ruminating again decreased. After ten days treatment was terminated. While the infant did ruminate several times during the first two weeks posttreatment, this decreased rapidly and a nine-month follow-up found no recurrence. Sajwaj, Libet, and Agras (1974) successfully employed the use of lemon juice squirted into the child's mouth as an alternative aversive stimulus in the treatment of infant rumination, but this can have harmful side effects, such as mouth ulceration and tooth decay.

Atypical Eating Disorder

Included in this category are such conditions as food refusal, refusal to eat special types or classes of food, unwillingness to accept foods of certain textures, and improper eating practices.

In order to assess the existence of feeding disturbances in children, it is mandatory that the clinician have a working knowledge of developmental patterns in eating behavior (Linscheid, 1983). Careful education of parents on the part of pediatricians may serve to reduce the chances of parent-child conflict over inappropriate expectations for the child's eating practices (Christophersen & Hall, 1978). Such conditions as infant cholic, if it becomes chronic, may result in feelings of guilt and self-doubt on the part of inexperienced parents who are unsuccessful in their efforts to comfort their distressed child. Employing a developmentally appropriate transition from breast feeding to pureed and eventually solid foods can prevent difficulties which may arise if a more abrupt transition is attempted at a more developmentally inopportune time. Linscheid (1978) and Schwartz (1958) have suggested guidelines for the pediatrician to follow in discussing feeding patterns and stages with new parents so as to prevent feeding disturbances in children.

Feeding problems have been found to be generally responsive to the application of behavioral principles (Linscheid, 1983). Positive reinforcement, time out from positive reinforcement, extinction, successive approximations in teaching new behaviors, fading of manual guidance, and a variety of other procedures may be successfully employed once an adequate functional analysis of the feeding environment and consumatory response has been performed (Wright, 1971).

Holmes (1982) successfully increased the oral intake of a five-and-one-half-year-old severely retarded boy by having the parents collect data regarding daily feedings: lists of the types and amounts of food consumed and ratings of each feeding session. During the three-week baseline data period, the parents began to alter their expectations and interactions with their child during feedings, based solely on the information they gained as a result of their data collection experiences. Their new understanding of their child's feeding patterns was conceptualized by Holmes as the major contributor to the change in their child. No other treatment was required. Six- and twelve-month follow-ups indicated that the improvement in eating behavior was maintained. Additionally, since the parents monitored the eating behavior of the child, this study reflected the reciprocal intertwining of child and parent behavior in the feeding process.

A case of food refusal by a two-year-old girl was successfully treated by Hatcher (1979) during a thirteen-week inpatient program. This child had a long history of poor eating with recent weight loss, complicated by an involved medical history. The behavior modification program employed was based on the Premack principle. This child was observed to readily accept fluids but to refuse solid foods. Therefore, the high frequency behavior (ingestion of liquids) was made contingent upon the low frequency behavior (ingestion of solid foods). As anticipated, the patient's initial response was to refuse both liquids and solids, which resulted in a significant weight loss. However, following this initial phase, the child began to accept increasing amounts of solid foods. Her weight went from 12 lb 5 oz to 14 lb 10 oz at time of discharge. Monthly follow-ups for two years after treatment revealed that the patient continued to gain weight and to accept solid foods in her diet. A similar procedure was successfully employed by Wright (1971) in his treatment of a five-and-one-half-year-old retarded child who had refused solid food since age two. Additionally, Wright successfully used social praise and contingent access to toys and other play objects to increase the fluid intake of a mongoloid child aged three years and nine months suffering from diabetes who refused to accept oral fluids.

Food refusal is perhaps one of the most dramatic psychological disturbances in that it can often result in death. Obviously, disorders of food intake are deserving of considerably more research attention than they have received in the professional literature.

Childhood Obesity

While not classified as a disorder in DSM-III, obesity is one of the nation's major health-related problems (Stunkard & Mahoney, 1976). Both the high prevalence of this problem and the indirect role it plays in impaired health and reduced life expectancy (Ross, 1981) have led to a gradual increase in the attention that childhood obesity has received from child practitioners and researchers. The prevalence of childhood obesity is estimated to be 25 percent of all children (Johnson, Burke, & Mayer, 1956).

In a society as health- and appearance-conscious as America, the obese child often suffers the psychological and emotional consequences of abuse by his or her peers, discrimination on the part of adults, poor self-concept, a disturbed body image, and a greater frequency of disturbed family interactions (Linscheid, 1983).

While not confirming a genetic basis for obesity, it has been shown that obesity in parents is related to the incidence of obesity in their offspring (Schultz & Parra, 1970). If both parents are of normal weight, the probability of one of their children being obese is 7 percent. The probability rises to 40 percent in the case where one parent is obese and increases to 80 percent when both parents are obese. Support for a genetic basis for obesity was found in a study by Mayer (1975). In this study, no significant correlation was found between the weight of a given child and his or her adoptive parents. However, very high correlations were found between the weight of children and their natural parents. Additionally, identical twins reared apart were more similar in their weights than fraternal twins (Mayer, 1975). Other physiological causation theories have implicated possible lesions in the hypothalamus as being the source of specific characteristics which lead to overeating and obesity, e.g., an increased sensitivity to food stimuli, an increased propensity toward eating more food when it is readily available and less when it is not, and a lack of responsiveness to internal hunger and satiation cues (Schachter, 1971). Eid (1970) found the best single predictor of obesity in later life was weight gain during infancy. In his study, weight gain in infancy predicted future weight gain more accurately than either birth weight or the weight of the parents. Hirsch (1975) carried this further by postulating that the practice of overfeeding in infancy can lead to an increase in the number and size of fat cells. This supposedly results in an increased need to eat more food in order to provide nourishment to these additional fat cells and so leads to obesity. However, this theory still lacks empirical substantiation.

Psychoanalytic theory focuses on obesity as a manifestation of oral fixation and dependency, as the result of a symbolic fear of sex and pregnancy in adolescence (which is avoided by becoming obese and unattractive), and on the notion of rejection of gender role. From this perspective, obesity, like anorexia, becomes a strategy for avoiding heterosexual contacts and issues associated with adolescence (Wright, 1979).

From a behavioral perspective, two factors—an excessive intake of food and a relative lack of adequate physical exercise—are conceptualized as the main contributors to childhood obesity. While remaining cognizant of the potential for a genetic predisposition toward obesity, the behavior theorist conceptualizes excessive intake and lack of exercise as learned habit patterns which are subject to modification through the application of behavioral principles and techniques (Linscheid, 1983).

Treatment. Perhaps the most popular treatment approach to obesity is diet. Yet, despite the claims of proponents, few diet programs have gained widespread acceptance by medical or nutrition experts and the overall effectiveness of any has not been clearly demonstrated (Wright, Schaefer, & Solomoans, 1979).

While dynamic clinicians have speculated that childhood obesity is the symptomatic manifestation of individual intrapsychic and/or intrafamilial conflicts, there are no data in the literature that have clearly demonstrated the effectiveness of traditional individual or family psychotherapy in treating childhood obesity (Linscheid, 1983). Indeed, emotional problems in the obese child may be as much the effect of the obesity as the cause and there is no assurance that indirect treatment of the emotional or family difficulties will necessarily lead to weight loss. Childhood obesity has just begun to receive behavioral attention (Kingsley & Shapiro, 1977). Agras and Werne (1981) have grouped behavioral treatment techniques and strategies into the following categories: self-monitoring of consumption patterns; stimulus control of eating; alteration of eating style; caloric modification and nutritional education; exercise; reinforcement for behavior change and weight loss; and miscellaneous procedures. To this list Linscheid (1983) would add cognitive restructuring and family intervention (parental involvement in arranging stimulus control factors and behavioral contingencies).

Perhaps the earliest behavioral treatment program was developed by Rivinus, Drummond, and Combrinck-Graham (1976). Seven females and three male lower-class children were seen for ten weekly meetings with their mothers. Each meeting lasted two hours. Parents were instructed in the use of rewards, behavioral contracts, and modeling of appropriate behavior. A unique component to this program was the employment of a group supper at which the children and parents, while sitting at different tables, were supervised in the selection of low-calorie, nutritionally balanced meals and reinforced for appropriate eating behaviors. Target behaviors included slowing down in eating, putting down utensils between bites, and self-monitoring of consumption.

The children maintained daily records of caloric intake and behavioral changes in eating patterns. The children began at an average of 71 percent overweight and attained an average weight loss of 2.8 kg (6.21 lb). Follow-up at one month indicated that four of the children continued to lose weight, two maintained the loss acquired during treatment, and the remaining two gained more weight than they had lost during the treatment program. One child dropped out of the treatment program and was not included in the data. Among the four children who had mothers of normal weight there was an average of 5.0 kg (11.4 lb) lost while the five children in the study who had obese mothers lost an average of only 1.2 kg (2.64 lb).

Kingsley and Shapiro (1977) saw forty ten- and eleven-year-olds who were above the 90th percentile in weight for their ages. Three groups were formed: a child-only group, a group of mother-child pairs, and a mother-only group. A no-treatment control group was also included. In the mother-only group the mothers were instructed in methods of helping their children overcome weight problems through the application of the same behavioral techniques employed in the other two groups. The treatment consisted of eight weekly one-hour group meetings built around a modification of Stuart and Davis's (1972) behaviorally oriented weight reduction program. Weight loss was encouraged through reduction in food consumption and increase in physical exercise. While the children in the treatment groups lost a combined average of 3.5 lb during the eight-week treatment program, those in the control group gained an average of 2 lb during the same period. While the mother's weight was not a specific focus of the treatment groups, the authors noted that the women in the mother-only group lost an average of 6.25 lb which was significantly more than the mothers in any of the other groups. Six- and twenty-week follow-ups indicated that all three groups tended to maintain their improvement and that weight gain continued at an age-appropriate level. Follow-up data were not available for the control group. The mothers who had lost weight in the mother-only group could not be distinguished from the other group of mothers at the twenty-week follow-up. Also of interest is the fact that of the three groups, the mothers in the mother-child group expressed the greatest satisfaction with how the groups were composed.

Although behavioral treatment is credited with producing the weight loss observed in such programs, few studies have actually measured changes in the behavioral variables and correlated these with weight change (Brownell & Stunkard,

1980). However, Coates (1977) conducted a ten-week behavioral treatment program with two severely obese adolescent girls and demonstrated, through observation of eating behavior, the relationship between alteration in these patterns and weight loss. His ten-week treatment package included stimulus control, self-monitoring, modification of eating behavior, and the use of reinforcement contingencies. Additionally, a cognitive restructuring procedure was included which focused on the patients' self-critical and self-defeating thought patterns that reinforced their continued weight gain. During the ten-week treatment period, the two patients lost 9.5 lb (4.3 kg) and 5.2 lb (2.3 kg), respectively. A third subject was placed in a treatment regimen that was not specific in its methodology and this subject gained 3.97 lb (1.8 kg) during the corresponding period. Behavioral observations of all three subjects indicated that the third patient did not change her eating behavior patterns and gained weight while the behavior change in the two treatment subjects showed a clear correlation with actual weight loss.

Epstein et al. (1980) compared a family-based behavior modification and nutrition education program to a nutrition education program alone in the treatment of thirteen obese children ranging in age from six to twelve. All children were greater than 20 percent above their ideal weight and had at least one parent willing to participate. Both treatment groups included dietary recommendations with limits of 1200 to 1500 calories per day, the use of color-coded schemes to indicate the caloric and nutritional values of specific food items, and exercise instruction which included aerobics and stretching exercises. In addition, the behavior modification group included self-monitoring, training in social reinforcement and modeling, procedures aimed at slowing down the rate of eating, and frequent follow-up phone contacts. A response-cost contract was also included for self-monitoring, not eating high caloric and low nutritional value foods, and for weight loss (a $65.00 deposit was required). The subjects in the nutrition education group continued to receive additional lectures regarding food selection and preparation procedures while the subjects in the behavior modification group received the behavioral treatment package.

Results indicated that the subjects participating in the behavior modification program demonstrated a significantly lower average percent overweight during treatment and follow-up than the participants in the nutrition education group. However, Lavigne and Daruna (1982) have criticized Epstein and his colleagues' (1980) conclusions on the basis of their data analysis procedure.

While it is apparent that the application of behavioral principles holds much promise in the treatment of childhood obesity, it is also obvious that significantly more attention needs to be given to those procedures which will maintain the treatment effect over longer periods of time. The final outcome after several months or years of followup does not present a bright picture. Most patients achieve a modest weight loss during treatment (though a significant number fail to do even this); however, most gain this weight back and often exceed pretreatment levels of weight.

Compliance with weight reduction treatment is a significant problem, especially with children and teen-agers who are often brought for treatment rather than volunteering. One of the authors of this chapter has developed a strategy to cope with this problem which involves making a highly desired reinforcer (e.g., use of the family car, dating, tickets to rock concerts) contingent on weight loss.

With the patient thus motivated, the therapist becomes his or her ally in obtaining the desired reward. The therapist can then proceed to instruct the patient in nutrition, behavioral strategies for controlling eating, and similar components of good weight reduction. Changes in lifestyle are needed to maintain weight loss, and preventive measures may ultimately be a preferable answer to the problem of obesity than remediation.

POLYDYPSIA

Polydypsia, or psychogenic water drinking, is another consummatory abnormality which is not classified as a specific childhood disorder in DSM-III. The symptom of frequent water consumption is usually indicative of one of a variety of diseases affecting the renal concentrating mechanism. Disorders of this nature would include intrinsic renal and genitourinary pathology, sickle-cell anemia, and diabetes insipidus and diabetes mellitus (Linshaw, Hipp, & Gruskin, 1974). Excessive water consumption is also necessary to maintain water balance due to abnormal renal losses in cases of hypokalemic nephropathy and hypercalciuria.

Polydypsia involves the ingestion of greater amounts of water than is needed to maintain normal water balance. While the most frequent etiological factors are organic, this symptom can also have a psychogenic origin. One conceptualization is that psychogenic polydypsia represents an obsessive-compulsive behavior in which frequent fluid consumption serves to reduce anxiety, much like thumb sucking or nail biting (Wright, Schaefer, & Solomoans, 1979). In a study of four psychogenic polydypsia cases, ranging in age from one-and-one-half months to two-and-one-half years, Linshaw, Hipp, and Gruskin (1974) observed the presence of a disturbed parent-child interaction which they believed resulted in continuous drinking as a mechanism for compensating for the feelings of deprivation and emptiness the child experienced. An analogy between water drinking and nursing was viewed by the authors as supportive evidence for their formulation.

From a behavioral perspective polydypsia can be viewed as learned behavior that is reinforced due to its association with anxiety reduction. Once polydypsia is initiated, the patient may obtain other rewards which perpetuate this pattern of behavior. An example seen by one of the authors was a seven-year-old male who manifested considerable anxiety over parental expectations regarding academic performance. His frequent water consumption (there was a water fountain in the classroom) resulted in a need to make frequent trips to the bathroom (polyuria) which removed him from the anxiety-producing classroom situation. In addition, the symptoms became the cause of much parental concern and attention.

Treatment. Polydypsia is most frequently seen in the medical setting by the pediatrician. It is obviously important that the referring physician rule out the presence of any organic condition which may be causing the increased water consumption.

In their treatment of the study described above, Linshaw, Hipp and Gruskin relied primarily on parent consultation to decrease the fluid intake of their patients. They provided no information regarding their intervention other than the fact that they directly advised the parents to restrict their child's fluid intake. Follow-up of their cases up to two years later revealed normal development and no resumption of increased fluid intake.

A seemingly drastic measure, electroconvulsive therapy, was employed by Barlow and de Wardener (1959) in their treatment of nine patients with severe psychogenic polydypsia. Four of the nine patients reportedly improved; the remaining five demonstrated no change in their water consumption. Both electroconvulsive therapy and dynamically oriented individual psychotherapy were ineffective in a case of psychogenic polydypsia treated by Resnick and Patterson (1969). Electroconvulsive therapy was justified by the authors on the grounds that severe water intoxication was life threatening if the water consumption was not halted. Wright, Schaefer, and Solomoans (1979) have recommended the use of a behavioral approach involving both aversive conditioning for water drinking as well as reinforcement of incompatible behavioral responses in the treatment of this disorder. With older patients and adolescents they recommend reciprocal inhibition and implosive therapy. However, they present no empirical or case study data in support of their position.

As is the case with many of the functional disorders discussed in this chapter, polydypsia is often only one symptom in a matrix of difficulties representing an emotional disturbance. Accordingly, specific interventions may be necessary to assist with the more pervasive difficulties of which polydypsia may be only one symptom.

REFERENCES

Agras, W. S., Barlow, D. H., Chapin, N. H., Abel, G. G., & Leitenberg, H. Behavior modification of anorexia nervosa. *Archives of General Psychiatry,* 1974, *30,* 279–286.

Agras, S., & Werne, J. Disorders of eating. In S. M. Turner, K. S. Calhoun, & H. F. Adams (Eds.), *Handbook of clinical behavior therapy.* New York: Wiley, 1981.

Agras, W. S., & Werne, J. Behavior therapy in anorexia nervosa: A data-based approach to the question. In J. P. Brady & K. Brochie (Eds.), *Controversy in psychiatry.* Philadelphia: Saunders, 1978.

Alberti, R. E., & Emmons, M. L. *Your perfect right* (2d. Ed.). San Luis Obispo, CA: Impact, 1974.

American Psychiatric Association. *Diagnostic and statistical manual of mental disorders* (3d. Ed.). Washington, DC: American Psychiatric Association, 1980.

Anthony, E. J. An experimental approach to the psychopathology of childhood encopresis. *British Journal of Medical Psychology,* 1957, *30,* 146–175.

Ashkenazi, Z. The treatment of encopresis using a discriminative stimulus and positive reinforcement. *Journal of Behavior Therapy and Experimental Psychiatry,* 1975, *6,* 155–157.

Azrin, N. H., & Besalel, V. A. *A parent's guide to bedwetting control: A step-by-step method.* New York: Simon & Schuster, 1979.

Azrin, N. H., & Foxx, R. M. *Toilet training in less than a day.* New York: Simon & Schuster, 1974.

Azrin, N. H., Sneed, T. J., & Foxx, R. M. Dry bed: a rapid method of eliminating bedwetting (enuresis) of the retarded. *Behavior Research and Therapy,* 1973, *11,* 427–434.

Azrin, N. H., Sneed, T. J., & Foxx, R. M. Dry-bed: Rapid elimination of childhood enuresis. *Behavior Research and Therapy,* 1974, 12, 147–156.

Azrin, N. H., & Thienes, P. M. Rapid elimination of enuresis by intensive learning without a conditioning apparatus. *Behavior Therapy,* 1978, 9, 342–354.

Bakwin, H. The genetics of enuresis. In I. Kolvin, R. C. Mackeith, & S. R. Meadow (Eds.), *Bladder control and enuresis.* Philadelphia: Lippincott, 1973.

Bakwin, H., & Bakwin, R. M. *Behavior disorders in children.* Philadelphia: Saunders, 1972.

Barlow, E. D., & de Wardener, H. E. Compulsive water drinking. *Quarterly Journal of Medicine,* 1959, *28,* 235–258.

Bell, A. L., & Levine, M. I. Course and treatment of chronic constipation. *Pediatrics,* 1954, *14,* 259–266.

Bellman, M. Studies on encopresis. *Acta Pediatrics Scandinavia* (Supplement) 1966, *170,* 1–137.

Bemporad, J. R. Encopresis. In. B. B. Wolman, J. Egan, and A. O. Ross (Eds.). *Handbook of treatment of mental disorders in childhood and adolescence.* Englewood Cliffs: Prentice-Hall, 1978.

Berg, I., & Jones, K. V. Functional fecal incontinence in children. *Archives of Diseases in Children,* 1964, *39,* 465–472.

Bernstein, D. A., & Borkovec, T. D. *Progressive relaxation training: A manual for the helping professions.* Champaign, IL: Research Press, 1973.

Bernstein, P. H., Sturm, C. A., Retzlaff, P. D., Kirby, K. L., & Chong, H. Paradoxical instruction in the treatment of encopresis and chronic constipation: An experimental analysis. *Journal of Behavior Therapy and Experimental Psychiatry,* 1981, *12,* 167–170.

Bindelglas, P. M. The enuretic child. *The Journal of Family Practice,* October 1975, 375–380.

Blinder, B. J., Freeman, D. M. A., & Stunkard, A. J. Behavior therapy of anorexia nervosa: Effectiveness of activity as a reinforcer of weight gain. *American Journal of Psychiatry,* 1970, *126,* 77–82.

Bollard, R. J., & Woodrofe, P. The effects of parent-administered dry-bed training on nocturnal enuresis in children. *Behavior Research and Therapy,* 1977, *15,* 159–165.

Boskind-Lodahl, M. The definition and treatment of bulimarexia: The gorging purging syndrome of young women. Unpublished doctoral dissertation, Cornell University, 1977.

Brazelton, T. B. A child-oriented approach to toilet training. *Pediatrics,* 1962, *29,* 121–128.

Breunlin, D. C. Multimodal behavioral treatment of a child's eliminative disturbance. *Psychotherapy: Theory, Research and Practice,* 1980, *17,* 17–23.

Brownell, K. D., & Stunkard, A. J. Behavioral treatment of obesity in children. In P. J. Platon (Ed.), *Childhood obesity* (2d. Ed.) Littleton, MA: PSG, 1980.

Bruch, H. Preconditions for the development of anorexia nervosa. *The American Journal of Psychoanalysis,* 1980, *40,* 169–172.

Bruch, H. *The golden cage: The enigma of anorexia nervosa.* Cambridge: Harvard University, 1978.

Bruch, H. The enigma of anorexia nervosa. *Medical Times,* 1976, *104,* 108–118.

Bruch, H. Anorexia nervosa. In A. E. Lindner (Ed.), *Emotional factors in gastrointestinal illness.* The Netherlands: Excerpta Medical, 1973.

Bruch, H. Death in anorexia nervosa. *Psychosomatic Medicine,* 1971, 33, 135–144.

Bucher, B., Reykdal, B., & Albin, J. Brief physical restraint to control pica in retarded children. *Journal of Behavior Therapy & Experimental Psychiatry,* 1976, *7,* 137–140.

Butler, J. F. Treatment of encopresis by overcorrection. *Psychological Reports,* 1977, *40,* 639–646.

Byrne, S. Hypnosis and the irritable bowel: Case histories, methods, and speculations. *American Journal of Clinical Hypnosis,* 1973, 15, 263–265.

Casper, R. C., Eckert, E. D., Halmi, K. A., Goldberg, S. C., & Davis, J. M. Bulimia: Its incidence and clinical importance in patients with anorexia nervosa. *Archives of General Psychiatry,* 1980, *37,* 1030–1035.

Casper, R. A., Halmi, K. A., Goldberg, S. C., Eckert, E. D., & Davis, J. M. Disturbances of body image estimation as related to other characteristics and outcome in anorexia nervosa. *British Journal of Psychiatry,* 1979, *134,* 60–68.

Christophersen, E. R., & Hall, C. L. Eating patterns and associated problems encountered in normal children. *Issues in Comprehensive Pediatric Nursing,* 1978, *3,* 1–16.

Christophersen, E. R., & Rapoff, M. A., Enuresis treatment. *Issues in Comprehensive Pediatric Nursing,* 1978, *2,* 35–52.

Coates, T. J. The efficacy of multicomponent self-control program in modifying the eating habits and weight of three obese adolescents. Unpublished thesis, Stanford University, Stanford, Calif., 1977.

Cohen, S. I., & Reed, J. L. The treatment of nervous diarrhea and other conditioned autonomics disorders by desensitization. *British Journal of Psychiatry,* 1968, *114,* 1275–1280.

Creer, T. L., & Davis, M. H. Using a staggered-wakening procedure with enuretic children in an institutional setting. *Journal of Behavior Therapy and Experimental Psychiatry,* 1975, *6,* 23–25.

Crisp, A. H. Some aspects of the evaluation, presentation, and follow-up of anorexia nervosa. *Proceeding of the Royal Society of Medicine,* 1965, *58,* 814–820.

Crisp, A. H., Palmer, R. L., & Kalacy, R. S. How common is anorexia nervosa? A prevalence study, *British Journal of Psychiatry,* 1976, *128,* 549–554.

Cunningham, C. E., & Linscheid, T. R. Elimination of chronic infant ruminating by electric shock. *Behavior Therapy,* 1976, *7,* 231–234.

Davidson, M. Chronic nonspecific diarrhea syndrome: The irritable colon of childhood. In S. S. Gellis and B. M. Kagan (Eds.) *Current pediatric therapy.* Philadelphia: Saunders, 1973.

Davidson, M. Constipation and fecal incontinence. In H. Bakwin (Ed.) *Pediatric clinics of North America.* Philadelphia: Saunders, 1958.

Davidson, M. D., Kugler, M. M., & Bauer, C. H. Diagnosis and management in children with severe and protracted constipation and obstipation. *Journal of Pediatrics,* 1963, *62,* 261–275.

De la Burde, B., & Reames, B. Prevention of pica, the major cause of lead poisoning in children. *American Journal of Public Health,* 1973, *63,* 737–743.

DeLeon, G., & Mandell, W. A comparison of conditioning and psychotherapy in the treatment of functional enuresis. *Journal of Clinical Psychology,* 1966, *22,* 326–330.

Dische, S. Treatment of enuresis with an enuresis alarm. In I. Kolvin, R. C. MacKeith, & S. R. Meadow (Eds.) *Bladder control and enuresis.* Philadelphia: Lippincott, 1973.

Doleys, D. M. Assessment and treatment of childhood enuresis. In A. J. Finch & P. C. Kendall (Eds.), *Treatment and research in child psychopathology.* New York: Spectrum, 1979.

Doleys, D. M. Assessment and treatment of enuresis and encopresis in children. In M. Hersen, R. Eisler, & P. Miller (Eds.), *Progressive behavior modification* (Vol. 5). New York: Academic, 1978.

Doleys, D. M. Behavioral treatment of nocturnal enuresis in children: A review of the recent literature. *Psychological Bulletin,* 1977, *84,* 30–54.

Doleys, D. M. Enuresis. In J. Ferguson & C. B. Taylor (Eds.), *Advances in behavioral medicine,* New York: Spectrum, 1980.

Doleys, D. M., & Arnold, S. Treatment of childhood encopresis: Full cleanliness training. *Mental Retardation,* 1975, *13,* 14–16.

Doleys, D. M., Ciminero, A. R., Tollison, J. W., Williams, C. L., & Wells, K. C. Dry bed training and retention control training: A comparison. *Behavior Therapy,* 1977, *8,* 541–548.

Doleys, D. M., McWhorter, A. O., Williams, S. C., & Gentry, W. R. Encopresis: Its treatment and relation to nocturnal enuresis. *Behavior Therapy,* 1977, *8,* 77–82.

Doleys, D. M., Schwartz, M. S., & Ciminero, A. R. Elimination problems: Enuresis and encopresis. In E. J. Mash & L. G. Terdal (Eds.), *Behavioral assessment of childhood disorders.* New York: Guilford, 1981.

Eastwell, H. D. A pica epidemic: A price for sedentarism among Australian ex-hunter-gatherers. *Psychiatry,* 1979, *42,* 264–273.

Eid, E. E. Follow-up study of physical growth of children who had excessive weight gain in first six months of life. *British Medical Journal,* 1970, *2,* 74–76.

Epstein, L. H., Masek, B. J., & Marshall, W. R. A nutritionally-based school program for control of eating in obese children. *Behavior Therapy,* 1978, *9,* 766–778.

Epstein, L. H., & McCoy, J. F. Bladder and bowel control in Hirschsprungs disease. *Journal of Behavior Therapy and Experimental Psychiatry,* 1977, *8,* 197–199.

Epstein, L. H., Wing, R. R., Steranchak, L., Dickson, B., & Michelson, J. Comparison of family-based behavior modification and nutrition education for childhood obesity. *Journal of Pediatric Psychology,* 1980, *5,* 25–36.

Esperana, M., & Gerrard, J. W. Nocturnal enuresis: Studies in bladder function in normal children and enuretics. *Canadian Medical Association Journal,* 1969, *101,* 324–327.

Fenichel, O. *The psychoanalytic theory of neurosis.* London: Routledge and Kegan, 1946.

Ferholt, J., & Provence, S. Diagnosis and treatment of an infant with psychophysiological vomiting. *The Psychoanalytic Study of the Child.* 1976, *31,* 439–459.

Finley, W. W., & Besserman, R. L. Differential effects of three reinforcement schedules on the effectiveness of the conditioning treatment for enuresis nocturna. *Proceedings of the American Psychological Association,* 1973, *8,* 923–924.

Finney, J. W., Russo, D. C., & Cataldo, M. F. Reduction of pica in young children with lead poisoning. *Journal of Pediatric Psychology,* 1982, *7,* 197–208.

Fitzgerald, J. F. Encopresis, soiling, constipation: What's to be done? *Pediatrics,* 1975, *56,* 348–349.

Foxx, R. M., & Azrin, N. H. *Toilet training the retarded.* Champaign, IL: Research Press, 1973.

Foxx, R. M., & Martin, E. D. Treatment of scavenging behavior (coprophagy and pica) by overcorrection. *Behavior Research and Therapy,* 1975, *13,* 153–162.

Freeman, B. J., & Pribble, W. Elimination of inappropriate toileting behavior by overcorrection. *Psychological Reports,* 1974, *35,* 802.

Friedman, A. R. Behavior training in a case of enuresis. *Journal of Individual Psychology,* 1968, *24,* 86–87.

Garfinkle, P. E., Kline, S. A., & Stancer, H. C. Treatment of anorexia nervosa using operant conditioning techniques. In A. P. Goldstein & L. Krasner (Ed.) *Behavior therapy and health care.* New York: Pergamon, 1975.

Garfinkle, P. E., Moldofsky, H., & Garner, D. M. The stability of perceptual disturbances in anorexia nervosa. *Psychological Medicine,* 1979, *9,* 703–708.

Gastout, H., & Broughton, R. J. Conclusions concerning the mechanisms of enuresis nocturna. *Electroencephalography and Clinical Neurophysiology,* 1964, *16,* 625–629.

Gaultieri, C. T. Imipramine and children: A review and some speculations about the mechanisms of drug action. *Diseases of the Nervous System,* 1977, *38,* 368–375.

Gavanski, M. Treatment of non-retentive secondary encopresis with imipramine and psychotherapy.

Canadian Medical Association Journal, 1971, *104*, 46–48.

Greenberg, L. M., & Stephans, J. H. Use of drugs in special syndromes: Enuresis, tics, school refusal, and anorexia nervosa. In J. M. Weiner (Ed.) *Psychopharmacology in childhood and adolescence.* New York: Basic, 1977.

Guiora, A. Z. Dysorexia: A psychopathological study of anorexia nervosa and bulimia. *American Journal of Psychiatry*, 1967, *124*, 147–149.

Hallgren, B. Enuresis II: A study with references to certain physical, mental, and social factors possibly associated with enuresis. *Acta Psychiatrica Neurologia Scandinavia*, 1956, *81*, 405.

Halmi, K. A. Anorexia nervosa: Recent investigations. *Annual Review of Medicine*, 1978, *29*, 137–148.

Halmi, K. A. Anorexia nervosa: Demographic and clinical features in 94 cases. *Psychosomatic Medicine*, 1974, *36*, 18–25.

Halmi, K. A., Brodland, G., & Rigas, C. A followup study of 79 patients with anorexia nervosa: An evaluation of prognostic factors and diagnostic criteria. *Life History Research in Psychopathology*, 1975, *4*, 290–301.

Halmi, K. A., Goldberg, S. C., Casper, R. C., Eckert, E. D., & Davis, J. M. Pretreatment predictors of outcome in anorexia nervosa. *British Journal of Psychiatry*, 1979, *134*, 71–78.

Hansen, G. D. Enuresis control through fading, escape, and avoidance training. *Journal of Applied Behavior Analysis*, 1979, *12*, 303–307.

Harris, L. S., & Purohit, A. P. Bladder training and enuresis: A controlled trial. *Behavior Research and Therapy*, 1977, *15*, 485–490.

Hatcher, R. P. Treatment of food refusal in a two-year old child. *Journal of Behavior Therapy and Experimental Psychiatry*, 1979, 10, 363–367.

Hedberg, A. G. The treatment of chronic diarrhea by systematic desensitization: A case report. *Journal of Behavior Therapy and Experimental Psychiatry*, 1973, *4*, 67–68.

Hein, H. A., & Beerends, J. J. Who should accept primary responsibility for the encopretic child? A successful pediatric program based on dietary control, bowel training, and family counseling. *Clinical Pediatrics*, 1978, *17*, 67–70.

Hersov, L. Fecal soiling. In M. Rutter and L. Hersov (Eds.) *Child psychiatry: Modern approaches.* Philadelphia: Blackwell, 1977.

Hilburn, W. B. Encopresis in childhood. *Journal of the Kentucky Medical Association*, 1968, *66*, 978–982.

Hirsch, J. Cell number and size as a determinant of subsequent obesity. In M. Winnick (Ed.), *Childhood obesity.* New York: Wiley, 1975.

Holmes, C. S. Self-monitoring reactivity and a severe feeding problem. *Journal of Clinical Child Psychology*, 1982, *11*, 66–71.

Ilg, F. L., & Ames, L. B. *Child behavior.* New York: Harper & Row, 1962.

Jay, S. M., & Wright, L. V. Behavioral treatment of enuresis and encopresis in children. In F. Masur (Ed.), *Psychological techniques in primary care.* New York: Plenum, 1982.

Johnson, M. L., Burke, B. S., & Mayer, J. The prevalence and incidence of obesity in a cross-section of elementary and secondary school children. *American Journal of Clinical Nutrition*, 1956, *7*, 231–238.

Kaplan, G. W., & Brock, W. A. Voiding dysfunction in children. *Current Problems in Pediatrics*, 1980, *10*, 4–29.

Kellerman, J. Anorexia nervosa: The efficacy of behavior therapy. *Journal of Behavior Therapy and Experimental Psychiatry*, 1977*a*, *8*, 387–390.

Kellerman, J. Childhood encopresis: A multimodal therapeutic approach. *Psychiatric Opinion*, 1977*b*, May/June, 39–43.

Kingsley, R. G., & Shapiro, J. A comparison of three behavioral programs for the control of obesity in children. *Behavior Therapy*, 1977, *8*, 30–36.

Kimmel, H. D., & Kimmel, E. An instrumental conditioning method for the treatment of enuresis. *Journal of Behavior Therapy and Experimental Psychiatry*, 1970, *1*, 121–123.

Lavigne, J. V., & Daruna, J. H. A comment on Epstein et al.'s "Comparison of family-based behavior modification and nutrition education for childhood obesity." *Journal of Pediatric Psychology*, 1982, *7*, 95–98.

Levine, M. D. Children with encopresis: A descriptive analysis. *Pediatrics*, 1975, *56*, 412–416.

Lifschitz, M., & Chovers, A. Encopresis among Israeli kibbutz children. *Israeli Annals of Psychiatry*, 1972, *10*, 326–340.

Linscheid, T. R. Eating problems in children. In C. E. Walker and M. Roberts, *Handbook of clinical child psychology.* New York: Wiley, 1983.

Linscheid, T. R. Disturbances of eating and feeding. In P. R. Magrab (Ed.), *Psychological management of pediatric problems:* (Vol. 1) *Early life conditions and chronic diseases.* Baltimore: University Park, 1978.

Linscheid, T. R., & Cunningham, C. E. A controlled demonstration of the effectiveness of electric shock in the elimination of chronic infant rumination. *Journal of Applied Behavior Analysis*, 1977, *10*, 500.

Linshaw, M. A., Hipp, T., & Gruskin, A. Infantile psychogenic water drinking. *Journal of Pediatrics*, 1974, *85*, 520–522.

Lovibond, S., & Coote, M. Enuresis. In C. Costello (Ed.), *Symptoms of psychopathology*. New York: Wiley, 1969.

Madden, N., Russo, D. C., & Cataldo, M. F. Environmental influences on mouthing in children with lead intoxication. *Journal of Pediatric Psychology*, 1980, *5*, 207–216.

Marshall, S., Marshall, H. H. A practical approach to nonorganic enuresis. *Medical Times*, 1973, *101*, 58–61.

Mayer, J. Obesity during childhood. In M. Winnick (Ed.), *Childhood obesity*. New York: Wiley, 1975.

McGlynn, F. D. Successful treatment of anorexia nervosa with self-monitoring and praise. *Journal of Behavior Therapy and Experimental Psychiatry*, 1980, *11*, 283–286.

McKendry, J. B., & Steward, D. A. Enuresis. *Pediatric Clinics of North America*, 1974, *21*, 1019–1020.

McLain, L. G. Childhood enuresis. *Current Problems in Pediatrics*, 1979, *9*, 4–36.

McTaggert, A., & Scott, M. A review of twelve cases of encopresis. *Journal of Pediatrics*. 1959, *54*, 762–768.

Mesibov, G. B., Schroeder, C. S., & Wesson, L. Parental concern about their children. *Journal of Pediatric Psychology*, 1977, *2*, 13–17.

Miller, P. M. An experimental analysis of sphincter control training in the treatment of nocturnal enuresis in two institutionalized adolescents. *Behavior Therapy*, 1973, *4*, 288–294.

Minuchin, S., Baker, L., Rosman, B., Liebman, R., Milman, L., & Todd, T. A conceptual model of psychosomatic illness in children. *Archives of General Psychiatry*, 1975, *32*, 1031–1038.

Minuchin, S., Rosman, B., & Baker, L. *Psychosomatic families: Anorexia nervosa in context*. Cambridge: Harvard University, 1978.

Mitchell, D., Winter, W., & Morisaki, C. M. Conditioned taste aversion accompanied by geophagia: Evidence for the occurrence of "psychological" factors in the etiology of pica. *Psychosomatic Medicine*, 1977, *39*, 402–412.

Morgan, R. T. T. Relapse and therapeutic response in the conditioning treatment of enuresis: A review of recent findings of intermittent reinforcement overlearning and stimulus-intensity. *Behavior Research and Therapy*, 1978, *16*, 273–279.

Nelson, W. E., Vaughan, V. C., & McKay, R. J. *Textbook of pediatrics*. Philadelphia: Saunders, 1969.

Nettelbeck, T., & Langeluddecke, P. Dry-bed training without an enuresis machine. *Behaviour Research & Therapy*, 1979, *17*, 403–404.

Novick, J. Symptomatic treatment of acquired and persistent enuresis. *Journal of Abnormal Psychology*, 1966, *71*, 368.

O'Neil, P. M., White, J. L., King, C. R., Jr., & Carek, D. J. Controlling childhood rumination through differential reinforcement of other behavior. *Behavior Modification*, 1979, *3*, 355–372.

Oppel, W. C., Harper, P. A., & Rider, R. V. Social, psychological, and neurological factors associated with nocturnal enuresis. *Pediatrics*, 1968, *42*, 627–641.

Palmer, R. L. The dietary chaos syndrome: A useful new term? *British Journal of Medical Psychology*, 1979, *52*, 187–190.

Palmer, S., Thompson, R. J., Jr., & Linscheid, T. R. Applied behavior analysis in the treatment of childhood feeding problems. *Developmental Medicine and Child Neurology*, 1975, *17*, 333–339.

Palmer, S., & Horn, S. Feeding problems in children. In S. Palmer and S. Ekvall (Eds.), *Pediatric nutrition in developmental disorders*. Springfield, IL: Charles C. Thomas, 1978.

Paschalis, A., Kimmel, H. D., & Kimmel, E. Further study of diurnal instrumental conditioning in the treatment of enuresis nocturna. *Journal of Behavior Therapy and Experimental Psychiatry*, 1972, 3, 253–256.

Perlmutter, A. D. Enuresis. In T. P. Kelalis & L. R. King (Eds.), *Clinical pediatric urology*. Philadelphia: Saunders, 1976.

Pertschuk, M. J., Forster, J., Buzby, G., & Mullen, J. L. The treatment of anorexia nervosa with total parenteral nutrition. *Biological Psychiatry*, 1981, *16*, 539–550.

Pierce, C. M. Enuresis. In A. M. Freedman and H. I. Kaplan (Eds.), *The child: Vol I*. New York: Atheneum, 1972.

Pierce, C. M. Enuresis and encopresis. In A. M. Freedman, H. I. Kaplan & B. J. Sadock (Eds.), *Comprehensive textbook of psychiatry II*. Baltimore: Williams & Wilkins, 1975.

Physician's Desk Reference. Oradell, NJ: Medical Economics Company, 1982.

Pierloot, R. A., & Houben, M. E. Estimation of body dimensions in anorexia nervosa. *Psychological Medicine*, 1978, *8*, 317–324.

Pinkerton, P. Psychogenic megacolon in children: The implications of bowel negativism. *Archives of Diseases in Childhood*, 1958, *33*, 371-380.

Poole, A. D., & Sanson, R. W. A behavioral program for the management of anorexia nervosa. *Australian and New Zealand Journal of Psychiatry*, 1978, *12*, 49–53.

Pyle, R. L., Mitchell, J. E., & Eckert, E. D. Bulimia:

A report of 34 cases. *Journal of Clinical Psychiatry*, 1981, *42*, 60–64.

Ravitch, M. M. Pseudohirschprung's disease. *Annals of Surgery*, 1958, *147*, 781–795.

Resnick, M. E., & Patterson, C. Coma and convulsion due to compulsive water drinking. *Neurology*, 1969, *19*, 1125–1126.

Ringdahl, I. C. Hospital treatment of the encopretic child. *Psychosomatics*, 1980, 21, 65–71.

Rivinus, T. M., Drummond, T., & Combrinck-Graham, L. A group behavior treatment program for overweight children: Results of a pilot study. *Pediatric Adolescent Endocrinology*, 1976, *1*, 55–61.

Rocklin, N., & Tilker, H. Instrumental conditioning of nocturnal enuresis. *Proceeding of the 81st Annual Convention of the American Psychological Association*, 1973, 915–916.

Rosen, L. W. Modification of secretive ritualized eating behavior in anorexia nervosa. *Journal of Behavior Therapy & Experimental Psychiatry*, 1980, 11, 101–104.

Rosen, J. C., & Leitenberg, H. Bulimia nervosa: treatment with exposure and response prevention. *Behavior Therapy*, 1982, *13*, 117–124.

Ross, A. O. *Child behavior therapy: Principles, procedures, and empirical basis*. New York: Wiley, 1981.

Russell, G. Bulimia nervosa: An ominous variant of anorexia nervosa. *Psychological Medicine*, 1979, *9*, 429–448.

Sajwaj, T., Libet, & Agras, S. Lemon juice therapy: The control of life-threatening rumination in a six-month-old infant. *Journal of Applied Behavior Analysis*, 1974, *1*, 557–563.

Salmon, M. A., Taylor, C. D., & Lee, D. On the EEG in enuresis. In I. Kolvin, R. C. MacKeith, & S. R. Meadows (Eds.), *Bladder control and enuresis*. Philadelphia: Lippincott, 1973.

Schachter, S. Some extraordinary facts about obese humans and rats. *American Psychologist*, 1971, *6*, 129–144.

Schmitt, B. D. Nocturnal enuresis: An update on treatment. *Pediatric Clinics of North America*, 1982, 29, 21–36.

Schroeder, C. S. Psychologists in a private pediatric practice. *Journal of Pediatric Psychology*, 1979, *4*, 5–18.

Schultz, R. B., & Parra, A. Relationship between body composition and insulin and growth hormone responses in obese adolescents. *Diabetes*, 1970, *19*, 492.

Schwartz, A. S. Eating problems. *Pediatric Clinics of North America*, 1958, *S*, 595–611.

Schwartz, D. M., & Thompson, M. G. Do anorexics get well? Current research and future needs. *American Journal of Psychiatry*, 1981, *138*, 319–323.

Selvini-Palazzoli, M. *Self-starvation*. New York: Jason Aronson, 1978.

Shane, M. Encopresis in a latency boy: An arrest along a developmental line. *Psychoanalytic Study of the Child*, 1967, *22*, 296–314.

Shaw, W. J. Enuresis; Survey articles. *Journal of Pediatric Psychology*, 1976, *4*, 4–6.

Singh, R., Phillips, D., & Fischer, S. C. The treatment of enuresis by progressively earlier waking. *Journal of Behavior Therapy and Experimental Psychiatry*, 1976, *7*, 277–278.

Sours, J. A. *Starving to death in a sea of objects: The anorexia nervosa syndrome*. New York: Jason Aronson, 1980.

Sours, J. A. The primary anorexia nervosa snydrome. In J. D. Noshpitz (Ed.), *Basic handbook of child psychiatry* (Vol. 2) New York: Basic, 1979.

Sours, J. A. Physical, mental, and therapeutic aspects of anorexia nervosa. *International Journal of Child Psychotherapy*. 1973, 2, 419–439.

Strober, M. A. Comparative analysis of personality organization in juvenile anorexia nervosa. *Journal of Youth and Adolescence*, 1981*a*, *10*, 285–295.

Strober, M. A. The significance of bulimia in juvenile anorexia nervosa: An exploration of possible etiologic factors. *International Journal of Eating Disorders*, 1981*b*, Autumn, 28–43.

Strober, M. A. Personality and symptomalogical features in young, nonchronic anorexia nervosa patients. *Journal of Psychosomatic Research*, 1980, *24*, 353–359.

Strober, M. A., Goldberg, I., Green, J., & Saxon, J. Body image disturbance in anorexia nervosa during the acute and recuperative phase. *Psychological Medicine*, 1979, *9*, 695–701.

Stuart, R. B., & Davis, B. *Slim chance in a fat world: behavioral treatment of obesity*. Champaign, IL.: Research Press, 1972.

Stunkard, A. J., & Mahoney, M. J. Behavioral treatment of eating disorders. In H. Leitenberg (Ed.) *Handbook of behavior modification and behavior therapy*. Englewood Cliffs, NJ: Prentice-Hall, 1976.

Tapia, F., Jekel, K., & Demke, H. R. Enuresis: An emotional symptom. *Journal of Nervous and Mental Diseases*, 1960, 130, 61–66.

Toister, R. P., Condron, C. J., Worley, L., & Arthur, D. Faradic therapy of chronic vomiting in infancy: A case study. *Behavioral Therapy and Experimental Psychiatry*, 1975, *6*, 55–59.

Vaughan, V. C., McKay, R. J., & Nelson, W. E. *Textbook of pediatrics.* Philadelphia: Saunders, 1975.

Walker, C. E. Toilet training, enuresis, and encopresis. In P. R. Magreb (Ed.), *Psychological management of pediatrics problems:* (Vol. I.) Baltimore: University Park, 1978.

Walker, C. E., Hedberg, A., Clement, P. W., & Wright, L. *Clinical procedures in behavior therapy.* Englewood Cliffs, NJ: Prentice-Hall, 1981.

Wells, K. C., & Forehand, R. Childhood behavior problems in the home. In S. M. Turner, K. S. Calhourn, & H. E. Adams (Eds.), *Handbook of clinical behavior therapy.* New York: Wiley, 1981.

Wermuth, B. M., Davis, K. L., Hollister, L. E., & Spinkard, A. J. Phenytoin treatment of the binge-eating syndrome. *American Journal of Psychiatry,* 1977, *134,* 1249–1253.

Werry, J. S. Enuresis: A psychosomatic entity? *Canadian Medical Association Journal,* 1967, *97,* 319–327.

Werry, J. S. Enuresis—On etiologic and therapeutic study. *Journal of Pediatrics,* 1965, 67, 423.

Werry, J. S. Psychosomatic disorders, psychogenic symptoms and hospitalization. In H. C. Quay & J. S. Werry (Eds.), *Psychopathological disorders of childhood.* New York: Wiley, 1979.

Werry, J. S., & Cohrssen, J. Enuresis: An etiological and therapeutic study. *Journal of Pediatrics,* 1965, *67,* 423–431.

White, J. H., & Schnaultz, N. L. Súccessful treatment of anorexia nervosa with imipramine. *Diseases of the nervous system,* 1977, *38,* 567–568.

Wolters, W. G. H. A comparative study of behavioral aspects in encopretic children. *Psychotherapy and Psychosomatics,* 1974, 24, 86–97.

Wolters, W. H. G., & Wauters, E. A. K. A study of somatopsychic vulnerability in encopretic children. *Psychotherapy and Psychosomatics,* 1975, *26,* 27–34.

Wright, L. Handling the encopretic child. *Professional Psychology,* 1973, *4,* 137–144.

Wright, L. Conditioning of consummatory responses in young children. *Journal of Behavior Therapy and Experimental Psychiatry,* 1971, *10,* 363–367.

Wright, L., Schaefer, A. B., & Solomoans, G. *Encyclopedia of pediatric psychology.* Baltimore: University Park, 1979.

Wright, L., & Thalassinos, P. A. Success with electroshock in habitual vomiting. *Clinical Pediatrics,* 1973, *12,* 594–597.

Wright, L., & Walker, C. E. A simple behavioral treatment for psychogenic encopresis. *Behavior Research and Therapy,* 1978, *16,* 209–212.

Wright, L., & Walker, C. E. Treatment of the child with psychogenic encopresis. *Clinical Pediatrics,* 1977, *16,* 1042–1045.

Yates, A. J. *Behavior therapy.* New York: Wiley, 1970.

Young, G. C. A staggered-wakening procedure in the treatment of enuresis. *Medical Officer,* 1964, *111,* 142–143.

Young, G. C., & Morgan, R. T. T. Overlearning in the conditioning treatment of enuresis. *Behavior Research and Therapy,* 1972 (a), *10,* 147–151.

Ziai, M., Janeway, C. A., & Cooke, R. E. *Pediatrics* (2d. Ed.). Boston: Little, Brown, 1975.

CHAPTER 9

Depressive Disorders

John M. Reisman

Depression refers to an emotional state of lowered initiative and responsiveness to stimulation, of gloomy and self-critical thoughts, of sadness and dejection. Almost everyone has experienced such "blue" or "down" periods, with the difference that here the affect is so severe that the person finds it difficult to perform routine tasks or to function in a satisfactory way.

For some time the romantic notion of the carefree, happy innocence of childhood made it difficult, even for professionals in the field of mental health, to seriously think that children might be depressed. Often the subject was ignored, or it was argued that children did not exhibit the symptoms of depression in the same manner as adults, which is to say that childhood unhappiness might be expressed through other symptoms of disturbance, such as delinquency or physical complaints (Hughes, 1984). Accordingly there was much interest in the concept of "masked depressions" or "depressive equivalents," and many of the conduct disturbances and antisocial behaviors of juveniles were seen as reversals of painful, unhappy affect.

At the same time it is difficult to see how depression could not be involved in almost every form of psychopathology. The various theories of personality speculate on the existence of unhappy and depressing feelings and cognitions at the core of human development, with ineffective means of dealing with these concerns expressed by abnormalities. Unacceptable, troublesome impulses and wishes (Freud), feelings of inferiority and inadequacy (Adler), feelings of insecurity and rejection (Horney), worries about being abandoned or not being true to oneself (Rank), self-dissatisfaction (Rogers), and so on certainly imply depressive associations. Thus it becomes reasonable to argue that depression is everywhere in childhood and adulthood and hence we must be careful to specify under what conditions it is to be regarded as pathological.

DSM-III provides one of the first attempts of a psychiatric nomenclature to recognize and identify depressive disorders in infancy and childhood. Five such disorders with special relevance to children are described, though of course as youngsters grow through adolescence, they are more apt to exhibit symptoms characteristic of depressive syndromes in adulthood and would be so diagnosed. First we shall discuss these five disorders, and then we shall discuss suicide, which is a depressive symptom and not a diagnostic category in DSM-III.

Reactive Attachment Disorder of Infancy

Drawing upon reports at the beginning of the twentieth century of high infant mortality rates among institutionalized children, Rene Spitz described a condition which he called *hospitalism* (1945, 1946a). He speculated that infants taken from their mothers and placed in institutional care, though they received adequate nutrition and medical attention, suffered damage to their intellectual and physical development and were prone to contract and suffer the effects of ill health. His speculations were supported by his observations of the superior progress of infants raised by their own mothers in a prison nursery as compared with those youngsters given to the care of a foundling home; the latter were reported to be lethargic, unresponsive to stimulation, and retarded both physically and mentally.

Spitz (1946b) also noted a condition that he termed *anaclitic depression,* in which infants of about six months of age or older who were separated from their mothers reacted with distress. If the relations with the mother were "good" and if the separation continued for three or four months, the infants lost weight, became withdrawn and listless, and evidenced fear when approached by adults. This particular pattern was evidenced by 19 of 123 infants. Fortunately, the disturbance appeared reversible when the infant was reunited with the mother within five months (Spitz, 1965, p.275). The term "anaclitic" was used by Spitz to refer to the dependent relationship of the infant upon the mother for nurturance and emotional support, as contrasted to the more complex types of relationships that subsequently occur based upon love and more advanced psychological development.

In both hospitalism and anaclitic depression the infant seemed to be reacting to a loss. In hospitalism there was supposed to be a chronic loss of mothering, while in anaclitic depression there was a loss of the mothering person. Both conditions seemed instances of response to *maternal deprivation,* and hence the disorders might be countered through the provision of mothering or reunion with a mothering person.

To conscientious staffs of institutions Spitz's work had clear implications: They were to hold and attend to infants and to interact with them so as to convey affection and care. However, among psychologists there were questions about the adequacy of the studies, the specific variables associated with the infants' disorders, and the long-range consequences of deprivation.

Spitz's studies were severely criticized (Pinneau, 1955), and the irrefutable point was made by Yarrow (1961) that it had not been established that the deleterious effects observed were due to maternal deprivation in particular, rather than the more general variable of sensory deprivation. Nevertheless, everyone agreed separation from one's mother was not a salubrious experience, and the chances were it was stressful, if not harmful. It was also agreed relatively simple measures, such as holding infants in one's arms while feeding them instead of leaving them in their cribs with nursing bottles propped against their mouths, could avert the consequences of whatever deprivation was involved and therefore should be implemented.

The point was also made by Prugh and Harlow (1962) that children could be raised within the bosoms of their families and still not have their psychological needs met. These infants would exhibit the condition of hospitalism, despite the facts of their not having been separated from their mothers or placed for prolonged periods in institutions that neglected them. They were presumably the victims of parental neglect or *masked deprivation* and in certain instances might be better served by caring institutions than by indifferent or rejecting mothers and fathers.

Among many practitioners who dealt with infants the terms *hospitalism, anaclitic depression, maternal deprivation,* and *masked deprivation* were supplanted by the more neutral designation *failure to thrive.* This last term highlighted the retardation in growth of affected infants without implicating mothers or caretakers. Still evidence suggested parental disturbances were somehow involved, since affected infants living at home would gain weight if placed in hospitals or institutions that ministered to them. A careful study of these infants by Fischoff (1975) indicated failures on the part of their mothers to feed them. Even when the mothers were supplied with sufficient food, some did not dispense all of it to their children, though they reported they did! In his study Fischoff demonstrated failure to thrive is not necessarily a byproduct of depression or *affect hunger,* but can be a failure to be fully fed. At least in some cases, the syndrome observed by Spitz may have been due to some extent to malnutrition or starvation.

The concept of anaclitic depression was further enlarged and elaborated upon by Bowlby (1973; 1982), who has come to view attachment behavior as an innate response. Children of six months to six years who are separated from their mothers for a prolonged period may be expected to evidence an unlearned three-stage reaction of mourning. First there would be a relatively short stage of *protest.* During this time, which lasts no more than a few days, the child might cry, exhibit temper tantrums, and appear obviously distressed. The second stage, *despair,* is longer than the first and may persist for months or years. Here the child might evidence retardation in development, social withdrawal, reduction in activity, and other signs of mourning or depression. A third state, *resignation,* suggests an eventual lessening in the severity of obvious symptoms as the separation persists, though the child may show a defensive *detachment* in human relationships or attitudes of wariness about becoming involved.

There has been some disagreement among authorities as to the consequences, if any, that occur during the third stage, but there is consensus, particularly in view of the reproducibility of these findings among young monkeys (Suomi &

Harlow, 1977), that stressful or depressive reactions can occur among infants and children following separation from the mother, and these reactions can be terminated or reversed by reunion with the mother or the provision of mothering.

Reactive attachment disorder of infancy is the DSM-III designation for anaclitic depression, hospitalism, failure to thrive, and so on *when the symptoms have their onset before eight months of age.* It is also required that there be some identifiable precipitating factor, such as neglect, deprivation, or separation from the mothering person; that the symptoms not be attributable to some other disorder: and that the symptoms be reversed by the provision of adequate care. For the diagnosis to be made the infant must exhibit at least three of the following: hypomotility; little responsiveness to stimuli; excessive sleep; weak cry; poor muscle tone; weak rooting (a reflex involving head-turning and mouth-opening movements when the cheek is stroked); and grasping in response to feeding. There should also be signs of a lack of appropriate social responsiveness, such as not smiling to faces by an infant older than two months or not playing games with a caretaker by an infant older than five months, and significant failure to be of the expected weight.

Prevalence. Even among the infants observed by Spitz who were separated from their mothers, anaclitic depression or a reactive attachment disorder was evident in only 15 percent. However, it should be noted that an actual separation is not necessary to make the diagnosis and that many of the symptoms could be byproducts of nutritional as well as psychological impoverishment. Thus the disorder could be prevalent among infants where adequate care and nourishment are not readily provided, but exact figures are not known.

Diagnostic Issues. Although DSM-III specifies symptoms, it does not make explicit the criteria that should be employed in assessing them. Thus, for example, it is not made clear how far below in weight an infant should be in order for that weight to be judged of pathological significance. In the study by Fischhoff (1975) this was operationally defined as "weight, below the third percentile on the Stuart growth grids." Hopefully, these operational deficiencies will be remedied in subsequent revisions of the nomenclature. Meanwhile, the reliability of diagnosis may be expected to be attentuated by the subjectivity involved in determining the symptoms.

Etiology. This is one of the few disorders in DSM-III where an etiology is specified. In fact if it is not thought the symptoms are due to some inadequacy in caretaking, such as neglect or social deprivation, the diagnosis should not be made.

Treatment. The provision of adequate care (mothering) and food seem successful in reversing the symptoms. Moreover, if the symptoms are not reversed by the provision of adequate caretaking, the diagnosis of reactive attachment disorder of infancy is suspect. Clearly, this is a disorder where populations at risk can readily be identified and where presumably relatively simple measures can be taken to prevent its occurrence.

Outcome. The consequences of early and prolonged deprivation are somewhat controversial. No one contends deprivation has salubrious effects, but beyond that there is disagreement about whether the effects are truly reversible and whether there are subtle consequences about which there should be concern.

Basically, there have been two major

findings at issue. One is that institutionalized infants—and the earlier and more prolonged the institutionalization the more likely the deleterious effects—suffer intellectual retardation, particularly in verbal skills (Goldfarb, 1955; Provence & Lipton, 1962). The second is that these infants even when given the opportunity to form attachments to parental figures fail to do so; they are reported to be indiscriminately friendly, suggesting a lack of depth and involvement in their relationships (Provence & Lipton, 1962), and prone to delinquent and antisocial behaviors (Tizard & Rees, 1975).

There are several problems in interpreting these results: (1) Children are not randomly assigned to institutions, foster homes, or adoptive parents. It is possible that less responsive and more likely retarded infants are placed in institutions and are less readily accepted for adoption and foster home placement. (2) These infants are more apt to suffer economic (nutritional) deprivations, in addition to parental and stimulus deprivations. (3) These infants are more likely to experience social stigmatization and frequent disruptions in interpersonal relationships, as well as institutionalization and separation from their natural mothers. (4) Institutions and parents vary widely in their quality and care.

In an early review of the studies bearing on these issues Yarrow (1961) concluded: ". . . Severe sensory deprivation before one year of age, if it continues for a sufficiently long period of time, is likely to be associated with severe intellectual damage. Direct observation of children undergoing the experience of maternal separation shows a variety of immediate disturbances in behavior, permitting the simple conclusion that this is a stressful experience for children. There is no clear evidence that multiple mothering (as in Israeli collective settlements), without associated deprivation or stress, results in personality damage. With regard to the long-term effects of early deprivation or stress associated with institutionalization or maternal separation, no simple conclusions can be drawn."

Later reviews have emphasized the corrective effects of later experiences and the complexities of the variables involved. Depending upon the quality of the institution and caretaking, institutionalized children have been found functioning within the normal range of intelligence. Evidently it is not the simple fact of institutionalization or maternal deprivation that brings about retarded performances. Similarly, antisocial behaviors have been found associated with harsh, inconsistent, neglectful parenting; parental discord and disruptions; and the stresses of economic deprivations, whether children do or do not undergo actual separations from their parents (Hetherington & Martin, 1979). Children adopted by four to six years of age seem able to develop deep bonds of affection toward their adoptive parents, so deprivation experiences in infancy need not preclude the acquisition of trusting, intimate relationships. A lack of infant responsiveness has been found to be a temperamental characteristic which can be countered or intensified, depending upon whether the caretakers react with greater efforts at stimulation and involvement or whether they respond with rejection and neglect. Moreover, the fact that many infants do not appear harmed by deprivation would suggest more than one stressor needs to operate, or an interaction of variables needs to be in effect (genetic or temperamental vulnerability, rejecting or neglectful caretakers, and so on), for the infant to be adversely affected (Rutter, 1980). Unfortunately, as Bowlby (1982) noted, the infant who has suffered a loss is very likely to encounter additional stressors.

Chess and Thomas (1982), who have devoted much of their careers to the study of infancy and temperament, concluded: "Just as the child's nutritional requirements can be met successfully with a wide range of individual variation, so can his psychological requirements. Once mothers can appreciate this, that the neonate separated from his mother is not permanently damaged by the experience as such . . . they can perhaps relax and actually become better parents." Although the issue is not settled, the mood among professionals about the long-range consequences of this disorder is less pessimistic than it was. Thomas and Chess (1984) have been, perhaps, most optimistic: "In reviewing the developmental course of our subjects, we have been deeply impressed by the human capacity for flexibility, adaptability, and mastery in the face of all kinds of adverse and stressful life situations."

Adjustment Disorder with Depressed Mood

By definition, DSM-III regards adjustment disorders as reactions to specific and identifiable psychological stressors. The maladjustment, which results in social or school impairment or other symptoms, occurs within three months of the onset of the stressor, and it is assumed that the disturbance is transitory. An improvement should be evident when the stressor ceases or when the person is helped to come to grips with the problem.

Although almost anything can be a stressor (Holmes & Holmes, 1970), the impressions of mental health professionals emphasize the aspect of *loss* as a precipitating factor in depression. In particular, loss of mothering or caretaking has been mentioned in connection with anaclitic depression, or to put it more broadly, a loss of sensory stimulation. Subsequent losses, arranged somewhat in developmental order, are: loss of the mother or mothering person, where the child reacts with distress to the loss of a specific person to whom an attachment has been formed; loss of a body part or function, the response that might be occasioned by an amputation, hearing loss, memory impairment, perceptual handicap, serious accident, or illness; loss of any being for whom fondness was felt, such as a friend or pet; and loss of self-esteem, which is usually regarded as one of the more developmentally advanced reasons for depression since it can be solely a failure to meet one's own standards or values.

Many of the differing theories of depression are variations on the theme of loss. For example, analysts emphasize the self-punishment, self-blame, and self-criticism in depression, which are super-ego functions that can come into play following some loss; Beck's cognitive theory of depression sees early losses predisposing the person to depression, with the depressive thoughts of being helpless and at fault in need of correction (Beck, 1967); Lewinsohn (1974) and Ferster (1973) have emphasized a loss of positive reinforcements; and Seligman (1975), with his learned helplessness model—animals in an unsolvable situation become passive—sees it applicable to humans in terms that affect loss of self-esteem (Abramson, Seligman, & Teasdale, 1978). Where these theories differ is not in the significance they attribute to loss in the generation of depression but where their energies would be directed in effecting treatment: reducing the demands of one's standards, being more reasonable, giving reinforcement or helping the person act so as to obtain rewards, and helping the person cope more effectively. Loss, then, seems to be regarded as the primary class of stressors, if not the only kind, that brings about depression.

An adjustment disorder with depressed mood is diagnosed when the major criteria for an adjustment disorder are satisfied and the predominant symptoms involve depression, such as hopelessness, tearfulness, unhappiness, and so on.

Case Illustration: George was eleven years old when his mother phoned to ask for help. She described her son as a reasonably happy, well-adjusted boy until two months before the phone call. It was then that his father, with whom George had been very close, had left the family to live with another woman. Since then the father had not made any contacts with his children and the mother had been compelled to go to work. According to his mother, George's major problems were his moodiness and irritability. He would tease his nine-year-old sister and hit her without provocation. Also, his grades in school, which had been good, had dropped and were close to failing.

During his first meeting with a psychologist George was quiet and morose. He could not understand why he was having difficulties, but wept softly as he spoke of his love for his father and of his father's love for him. They had been great pals and companions, and this made it all the harder to reconcile how his father could suddenly abandon him. Gradually, he stated an explanation that was an elaborate, convoluted bit of logic: Not loving his daughter and not wanting to take her with him, yet not wanting to hurt her feelings unduly, George's father had been forced to leave him behind. George had been abandoned out of consideration for the feelings of his sister. In school, he could not concentrate on his work because all too often these thoughts and feelings about his father would intrude.

In all, George was seen for twelve sessions of psychotherapy. Immediately after his sessions began he stopped tormenting his sister. Within a month his grades in school improved. What he came to see in therapy was the complexity of his hurt and emotions toward his father: anger and hate and disappointment, as well as love.

Prevalence. No accurate figures for this adjustment disorder are available, but it is probably less prevalent among children than among adults. Children below the age of ten infrequently receive a diagnosis of depression, and less than 5 percent of adolescents do, as compared to 20 percent of adults (Weiner, 1982, pp. 266–267); these figures refer to diagnoses within psychiatric populations, so the percentages within the general population would be much less. The likelihood is that less than 1 percent of the general population of children and youth would be regarded as depressed in the DSM-III sense of the term. However, see below.

Diagnostic Issues. Two important points must be noted in relation to this disorder. First, there must be an identifiable stressor associated with the onset of depressive symptoms. A distinction sometimes made about depressions is that some are *exogenous*—their onset can be attributed to a crisis or stress that ordinarily brings unhappiness—and some are *endogenous*—there is no identifiable stressor and presumably the depression originates from factors within the individual. An adjustment disorder with depressed mood is, by definition, an exogenous depression.

Second, the depressive behaviors have to be more severe and handicapping than what would normally be expected. If George felt sad about his father's abandonment, but this sadness did not interfere with his schoolwork or with his ordinary functioning, it is unlikely that he would receive this diagnosis. This is to say that people can be unhappy about one thing or another, but should not necessarily be regarded as depressed in the psychopathological sense, unless there is an evident decrement in performance.

It is not uncommon for surveys to be conducted of child populations by questionnaires or similar measures (Kazdin, 1981) and to get estimates of the prevalence of "depression" that are quite high. Typically, a list of depressive symptoms is presented to children or to someone who knows the children and the items descriptive of a particular child are checked off. The mean number of symptoms checked on the questionnaire is calculated, a standard deviation is computed, and those who score one standard deviation above the mean are considered "depressed" (Kovacs & Beck, 1977; Lefkowitz & Tesiny, 1980; Rehm, 1981). Thus it is guaranteed by statistics and the method employed that a percentage, usually 16 percent, will be identified as depressed, and although the researchers probably recognize that this percentage does not correspond to the number who would receive a DSM-III diagnosis of depression, the unbridled use of the term depression in relation to the measures employed does not help clarify the issue (Lefkowitz & Burton, 1978).

It is also worth noting that a major attribute of an adjustment disorder is its improvement with treatment and/or time. Now how is one to satisfy this criterion at the outset? Clearly, one cannot, so that the diagnosis of an adjustment disorder becomes suspect when the symptoms persist. That is the reason why adjustment disorders are more frequently diagnosed before treatment and why more serious diagnoses are assigned the patient if the symptoms prove refractory. The change of diagnosis does not necessarily mean the patient has become worse during the course of treatment, as has sometimes been suggested and as might be supposed.

Etiology. An adjustment disorder is attributed to a psychosocial stressor, by definition.

Treatment. Some form of crisis intervention is usually employed. Generally the aims are to: (*a*) indicate to the child that the particular stress is ordinarily upsetting to people and therefore the child's reaction is not that unusual; (*b*) explain that these reactions are usually temporary and that in time improvement is to be expected; and (*c*) help the child deal with the stressor effectively. How much of this would be conveyed to a child explicitly in words depends upon the age of the child—the older the child, the more likely some sort of explanation would be communicated—and the conceptualization the child gives the problem.

Often depressive symptoms are accompanied by, or manifested in, eating problems (eating too much or too little), sleeping problems (sleeping too much or too little), headaches, somatic complaints, abdominal pain, enuresis, and so on (Blumberg, 1978; Hughes, 1984; Leon, Kendall, & Gaber, 1980). Behavioral psychologists and psychiatrists might focus on one or another of these complaints and employ behavioral techniques or medications for their amelioration. Since this discussion is about adjustment disorders, which are presumed to have a favorable prognosis with relatively modest therapeutic effort, perhaps the treatment of choice is psychotherapeutic intervention.

Outcome. By definition, adjustment disorder with depressed mood has a favorable outcome.

Uncomplicated Bereavement

This disorder refers to a normal depressive reaction to the death of a loved one. The symptoms may consist of insomnia, weight loss, unhappiness, poor appetite, and guilt. However, the symptoms are not prolonged or so severe that functioning is seriously impeded. Uncomplicated bereavement is not considered a mental disorder, but an essentially normal response to loss. It is a milder form of adjustment disorder with depressed mood in reaction to a very specific stressor.

Case Illustration: Jim was a six-year-old referred for evaluation following the death of his grandfather. He had told his mother that he thought he saw his grandfather standing in his bedroom at night. She was concerned that he might be hallucinating and this "visitation" was the onset of a serious disorder.

In the evaluation it became clear Jim was not psychotic. He was very close to his grandfather and recognized this death was a loss. Yet he hoped that somehow his grandfather would come back to him. At night he would lie awake, and in the shadows one evening he imagined he saw the form of his grandfather; however, he knew he did not actually see him. Similarly, Jim reported he had dreams in which his grandfather returned and played with him, but these were only dreams.

His mother was reassured about the normality of Jim's reaction, and at a follow-up three months later stated her son was doing fine and presented no problems.

Prevalence. Given the conditions, this is very prevalent among adults and probably less so among children, particularly youngsters who see death as reversible.

Diagnostic Issues. This is a new diagnostic category. For a time psychiatrists toyed with the idea of diagnosing reactions such as this as healthy reactions, but it probably seemed somewhat inconsistent to make such a diagnosis when the person was suffering under stress. It is a very benign straightforward disorder, and thus should be diagnosed with high reliability. Morticians recommend that children below seven to eight years of age not attend funerals since their understanding might lead them to think their loved ones are being buried alive, which could be most distressing.

Etiology. By definition, this is an exogenous depression with the stressor specific to the loss of a loved one.

Treatment. Crisis intervention and/or psychotherapy would seem the treatment of choice, when professional help is indicated. Support from relatives and the community are usually sufficient to help the bereaved through the process of mourning.

Prognosis. By definition, very favorable.

Phase of Life Problem

This is not a mental disorder but a problem associated with some change in life circumstances. The symptoms could be of any sort in connection with the stress and presumably they could also be depressive in nature. A child who feels homesick when separated from parents at summer camp, or who is despondent about going away to school might receive this diagnosis. Similarly, children and adolescents reacting with unhappiness to the divorce of parents or the burdens of making decisions about their occupations might be diagnosed as phase of life problem.

Prevalence. This is a new diagnostic category and no prevalence figures are available, though they would probably bear some correspondence to the prevalence of the stressors.

Diagnostic Issues. Given the existence of adjustment disorder with depressed mood, it is difficult to see why this category would need to be employed when the reaction to the phase of life stress is depressive. Hopefully, it will not be used, since almost any conceivable reaction could be diagnosed here and it could constitute a very prevalent and heterogeneous category of behaviors and symptoms. It is mentioned only in the interests of comprehensiveness and to alert the reader to the possibilities for confusion.

Etiology. By definition, a reaction to a specific, external demand or change.

Treatment. See discussion under adjustment disorder with depressed mood.

Outcome. Presumably very favorable.

Dysthymic Disorder

The rather esoteric term *dysthymia* is used by DSM-III to designate what used to be called a "depressive neurosis." The major point is that this is not as serious a disorder as a major depression, which can involve delusions, hallucinations, mutism, and an almost catatonic immobility; dysthymic disorder has none of those symptoms. It does consist of an unhappy mood that extends far beyond what would be regarded as the normal reaction to stress. For children and adolescents the depressive symptoms must have lasted for at least one year (two years for adults) before the diagnosis can be made; during this interval the child may have experienced periods of remission of relatively brief duration, but the predominant mood was that of sadness and/or loss of interest in school and ordinary activities.

At least three of the following symptoms must have been evidenced: sleeping too much or too little; chronic tiredness or little energy; self-deprecation; lowered performance in school; decreased attention, concentration, or ability to think clearly; social withdrawal; loss of interest in and enjoyment of pleasurable activities; irritability and anger expressed toward parents or caretakers; no pleasurable response to praise or rewards; less active or talkative, or feels slowed down or restless; expressions of pessimism, or feels sorry for self; crying or unhappy facial expression; thoughts of death or suicide.

Prevalence. The criteria indicate that this is a relatively serious disorder in that the symptoms must have been evident and of some concern for a period of at least a year. Epidemiological studies suggest this disorder is probably uncommon among young children (below five years) and that it becomes more prevalent in later childhood and adolescence. In an English study done on the Isle of Wight, only about 3 children out of 2,000 would have been likely to have received this diagnosis, but among older children and adolescents, the prevalence was probably ten times greater (Rutter et al., 1970; 1976)—which figured out to about 1.5 percent. That dysthymic disorder is rare below five years of age and increases in frequency through the years of childhood and adolescence is an oft-reported and yet-to-be adequately-explained finding. It is also widely reported that prevalence figures are inflated as diagnostic criteria become less stringent and percentages are reported from psychiatric or clinic populations, instead of the general population (Carlson & Cantwell, 1980a; Gittelman-Klein, 1977; Graham, 1979, p. 203).

Case Illustration: Jeff was 16 when his parents referred him for evaluation. He was an outstanding student at school and was holding down a part-time job, yet at home he was moody and irritable. He would spend long periods of time in his room sulking, complained bitterly to his parents about his unhappiness, and had threatened to commit suicide. It was that threat that had compelled them to seek help.

When interviewed, Jeff reported he had felt "down" for over a year. There was no particular reason for the onset of his unhappiness, and in fact neither he nor his parents could understand why he was miserable. Superficially he had every reason to be happy: His grades in school were high; he was popular; his family was well-to-do; and he was involved in many activities. Yet he claimed to derive no enjoyment or satisfaction from any of these things. Instead, he felt alienated, despondent, and alone.

In assessing the seriousness of his suicide threat, Jeff minimized its importance. He indicated he had told his parents that he might kill himself so they would appreciate the seriousness of his situation and bring him for help, but if given the opportunity to get professional assistance, he had no intention of carrying out his threat. He readily accepted the possibility of being seen in psychotherapy, which was something he desperately wanted, even though he wasn't sure why.

Diagnostic Issues. For some years a controversy has raged within the literature about whether young children have depressive disorders and whether the symptoms they exhibit when they suffer from depression are identical to those of adults. Hence the concepts of masked depressions and depressive equivalents: the former refers to depressions that are soon revealed; the latter to antisocial behaviors, conduct problems, hyperactivity, and so on which can be symptoms indicative of depressions in childhood, but where depressed behavior may never become evident (Leese, 1983).

Factually, depressive equivalents helped explain the lower prevalence of the symptoms of depression among younger children; while there is no shortage of depression among youngsters, it is expressed differently than it is among adults. Theoretically, the psychoanalytic position on depression emphasized self-blame and self-castigation as super-ego functions; hence a true depression could not occur until the superego was formed, which did not take place until around the time of the Oedipus complex, at four to five years or so. It was also contended children could not long tolerate feelings of depression and would speedily deny them or reverse them, by being very active rather than despondent. On theoretical grounds, then, children below a certain age were not expected to show the usual depressive behaviors.

However, clinicians looking for depressive symptoms in childhood have been able to find them (Bemporad, 1978), and the conviction has grown that the same manifest behaviors of depression exist in childhood and adulthood (Cytryn, Mc-

Knew, & Bunney, 1980). Moreover, the analytic position has somewhat softened. For some time Melanie Klein (1932) and her followers argued that the psychosexual development described by Freud occurred in early infancy and that by nine months of age children might experience a depressive anxiety, a form of guilt brought about by the anger felt toward parents who were rejecting. Buttressed, if not prodded, by the mounting research in infant psychology, analysts are now inclined to recognize autonomous functions of the ego, and though Klein's view remains a minority position, there is some acceptance of forerunners of super-ego development taking place in infancy (Blanck & Blanck, 1979). The result of this empirical and theoretical activity is reflected in DSM-III. For the first time the nomenclature presents depressive syndromes for children with symptoms similar to those for adults, and the notion of depressive equivalents is not officially recognized.

The presence of a stressor is not mentioned in connection with the diagnosis of dysthymic disorder, quite unlike the situations for the previously discussed depressive disorders, where an identifiable stress is required. Thus dysthymic disorder may be an endogenous or an exogenous depression, when the symptoms have persisted for the required length of time—a year. This heterogeneity and lack of distinction within this category could prove to be a source of confusion in evaluating research. Exogenous depressions may come to be diagnosed here for a number of reasons—persistence of the stressors, ineffectiveness of the treatment provided—and contaminate findings. It would seem prudent to separate data in dysthymic disorder between those who have exogenous and those who have endogenous depressions.

It is also disconcerting to find this disorder diagnosed largely on the basis of how long the symptoms have been evident. Nor is it clear why children are privileged to receive this diagnosis after one year of misery while adults are required to suffer two years; perhaps this criterion has something to do with the relative durations of childhood and adulthood. At any rate there is something unsatisfactory about making a diagnosis dependent upon duration of symptoms when so many variables affect the maintenance of behaviors. Here is another possible and probable source of confusion as children enter treatment with a relatively benign disorder, such as uncomplicated bereavement, only to emerge with a more serious disorder when, for whatever reasons, their symptoms prove refractory. Hopefully, consideration will be given these concerns in DSM-IV.

Etiology. Since this is essentially an endogenous disorder, every kind of explanation has its proponents. Existentialists claim people feel depressed when they fail to accept responsibility for their own behaviors and fail to genuinely accept the realities of life. Rank saw depressed feelings arising when children fear they are not being true to themselves and their own inclinations. Psychoanalysts suggest depressive symptoms are self-punishments for unacceptable wishes or impulses (Hall & Lindzey, 1978; Munroe, 1955); Jeff, for example, might have had his repressed sexual longings for his mother intensified during adolescence and thus his symptoms—in which he avoided her, claimed to feel alienated from others, and said he derived pleasure from nothing—acted to protect him from a situation that threatened loss of control.

Behaviorists might argue depressed feelings come about when the individual feels incapable of dealing with specific problems and circumstances or when the environment is deficient in rewards. The latter explanation does not seem to fit Jeff's case, since he was doing very well in school and since according to both him and his parents he was the constant recipient of primary and secondary rewards.

As biological techniques become more sophisticated, there is ever-present speculation about the significance of genetic and physiological variables determining endogenous depressions. To date, the findings remain inconclusive and equivocal (Orvaschel, Weissman, & Kidd, 1980). There is statistically significant evidence that the offspring of manic-depressive parents are more apt to be depressed (Kuyler et al., 1980), but in the study cited this finding was based on interviews with the parents and not on actual contacts with the children.

Puig-Antich and his associates have been investigating psychobiological variables associated with adult major depressive disorder to determine if they are of similar diagnostic significance in childhood. The most powerful psychobiological marker of endogenous depression in adults is hypersecretion of cortisol, which occurs in about *half* such cases. Among prepubertal endogenous depressives a hypersecretion of cortisol was found in "some" (Puig-Antich & Gittelman, 1980). The reliability and validity of this finding are unknown. Other variables under investigation include hyposecretion of growth hormone after injection of insulin and shortened sleep patterns, with thus far inconclusive results.

Treatment. Consistent with what is known about etiology, every form of treatment has its proponents. Jeff was seen in individual psychotherapy. After about two months of sessions he began to feel better and decided to register for an educational program at an Ivy League university to see if he was interested in accelerated studies leading to the doctorate. Upon his return, he continued to make progress and reported an increasing interest in heterosexual activities. A year after his psychotherapy terminated, he asked to see his therapist "just to let you know that everything is going well and I'm feeling fine." Despite the favorable outcome of his treatment, there did not appear to be any significant insight imparted or gained during its course.

Laufer's (1975) report on the early use of medication with children is appropriate here: "When Dr. Bradley was questioned concerning these results [the positive effects of amphetamines in reducing the hyperactivity of children] and why this agent should have such an effect, he communicated the concept that the children came to Bradley [Hospital] because of difficult behavior, which was their way of showing that they were desperately unhappy or unsatisfied in their lives; that amphetamines are euphoriants and that as the children were enabled to feel happier as the result of the medication, there was less need for them to display their deviant behavior, whether withdrawing or aggressing." It is now thought that among children amphetamines do *not* act as euphoriants, but as normalizers of seriously deviant behaviors (Conners & Werry, 1979).

In short, drugs are tried with children in the hope that they might be effective (Freud, 1962), and in many cases, about 75 percent, one or another antidepressant medication seems to be helpful. Among the medications more frequently used is imipramine (Tofranil) (Puig-Antich & Gittelman, 1980).

Behavioral treatments are highly ingenious and diverse in their refinements for the individual case and depend upon the particular conception of what has brought about the depression. One strategy is to train and reward the person for engaging in behaviors that would be expected to be pleasurable, and thus generate a pattern of activities that are intrinsically and extrinsically rewarding. Another strategy is to get the person to think positive self-thoughts. For example, an adolescent was instructed to recite something positive about himself each time before he urinated, the urination serving as a reward for the positive self-statements; within two weeks the depression seemed to lift (Wilcoxon, Schrader, & Nelson, 1976). There is no shortage of inventiveness and daring in behavioral approaches, but the very existence of such a great number of techniques and approaches points again to how much yet remains to be determined.

Outcome. The prognosis for dysthymic disorder among children is not known since this is a new diagnostic category. However, the likelihood is it is favorable, since anxious-withdrawn or neurotic children, a grouping which includes depressive symptoms, has a "good prognosis" with varying percentages of recovery reported that average out to about 67 percent (Kohlberg, Lacrosse, & Ricks, 1972; Robins, 1979).

Major Depression

This category refers to a profound depression, which may be a single episode or recurrent. It may also be the case that the child exhibits a "major-depressive episode" alternating with manic phases, what used to be called a manic-depressive psychosis and is known in DSM-III as a bipolar disorder. All these, including dysthymic disorder, are referred to as affective disorders because the primary symptoms involve disturbances of emotions or mood. There may or may not be "psychotic features" (delusions, hallucinations, mutism, catatonic stupor), and if they are evident, their presence is noted.

The symptoms for major depression and major depressive episode are the same; the distinction between the two is that major depression is not associated with manic episodes. A dysphoric mood, which is prominent and persistent, characterizes the child; this may be inferred in children under six by a persistently sad expression. In addition, at least four of the following symptoms must have been evidenced daily for a period of at least two weeks (in children under six at least three of the first four): (1) insomnia or hypersomnia; (2) hypoactivity or restless agitation (in children under six, only hypoactivity); (3) eating too much or too little with associated significant gains or losses in weight; (4) loss of interest in usual activities (in children under six, signs of apathy); (5) loss of energy; (6) feelings of worthlessness and guilt; (7) difficulties in concentration or thinking; and (8) recurrent thoughts of death or suicide.

Prevalence. Unknown. Until recently the existence of major depressions in adolescents and children was considered exceedingly rare. Such cases were reported anectdotally from time to time, but the disorder was so infrequent as to hardly merit mention in texts of child psychiatry. Converging bits of evidence suggest the disorder may be diagnosed more often. Depressive adults report having had depressive episodes during their adolescence, but claimed their problem was not so diagnosed. Suicide among adolescents is a matter of growing concern. The DSM-III criteria should not be overlooked as a significant factor in the growing clinical recognition that children can have the same depressive symptoms as adults (Carlson & Cantwell, 1980b). Of seventy-six adolescents who had psychiatric hospitalizations, fifteen appeared to have been diagnosable as major depressions (Friedman et al., 1982). There are other reports suggestive of the existence of this disorder among prepubescents (Puig-Antich, 1980, 1982) which, taken all in all, make the disorder worthy of attention. Nevertheless, major depression is still regarded as highly unlikely to be evidenced in children below the age of six and as an uncommon disorder in older children and adolescents.

Case Illustration: Bill was seventeen years old and had just graduated from high school when his parents were alarmed to discover he was spending day after day in bed. He would not eat, talk, or leave his room. There was no explanation they could provide for his behavior. Bill had been moody before, but never to this extent. Hospitalization for Bill was arranged when it was obvious he was seriously depressed: His head was downcast and he would not move, but remained standing wherever he happened to be placed; if told to sit down, he ignored any nearby chair and simply sagged to the floor; his facial expression was troubled and preoccupied; he was mute, though he might mumble something to himself if pressed to respond; due to his lack of eating, there had been a significant drop in his weight, and there was concern that if feeding was not provided, he might starve. The diagnostic impression was of a major depression with mood-congruent psychotic features.

Diagnostic Issues. For the first time diagnostic criteria are specified in DSM-III for the diagnosis of major depression in children, even those youngsters below the age of six. Accordingly, there cannot help but be an increase in the prevalence of this disorder. What is bound to be confusing is that major depression may or may not have psychotic features, which is to say this may or may not be a psychotic disorder. It would also be remarkable if confusion between this disorder and major depressive episode does not occur. As a matter of fact, in a study by Puig-Antich (1982) the term *major depression* is used without specification about psychotic symptoms and included major depression, major depressive episode, and dysthymic disorder without distinctions between them. Add to this Pandora's box the DSM-III category of atypical depression, in which there are depressive symptoms whose duration and onset do not quite meet the criteria for the disorders discussed!

No stressor is mentioned in connection with the onset of major depression, and presumably this is an endogenous depression, though conceivably there could be cases where it could be argued the disorder is exogenous. At any rate, the possibilities for confusion and uncertainties in evaluating research results exist, which could have been prevented and which hopefully will be prevented in DSM-IV. For the time being the DSM-III category of affective disorders looks sadly in need of revision.

What has been clarified is the psychiatric position with regard to depressive disorders in childhood: They do exist, their symptoms are similar to those in adulthood, and the notion of depressive equivalents has been dismissed.

Etiology. What was said in relation to dysthymic disorder can be repeated here, with additional emphasis given to genetic and physiological variables. Since this is a severe, presumably endogenous depression, medical model explanations tend to be favored. This is one of the few disorders where females tend to outnumber males, a difference in prevalence that increases through adolescence and rises to 2:1 in adults (Weiner, 1982, p. 268), and which does not appear to be totally explicable by sociocultural factors. Further, in addition to physiological markers, such as cortisol and dexamethasone suppression (Poznanski et al., 1982), the concordance for depression among identical twins, though not 100 percent, is significantly higher than the concordance for fraternal twins (40 versus 11 percent) (Allen, 1976). The lack of 100 percent concordance for identical twins indicates a genetic etiology is not the sole explanation, if indeed it is any explanation at all because the interpretation of findings is by no means unequivocal (Solnit & Leckman, 1984).

Treatment. Although all the approaches described under dysthymic disorder have been used in the treatment of major depression, the severity of the disorder, particularly when it is accompanied by psychotic symptoms, has favored the use of drug interventions such as imipramine, either exclusively or to prepare the patient for psychotherapy or behavior therapy. Bill was treated with intravenous feedings and electroconvulsive therapy, but shock procedures are used rarely since the advent of drugs, especially not on children. However, the beneficial response to drugs is slow and there may be an immediate favorable response to electroshock, so it is conceivable that where there is a suicidal risk both treatments may be employed by some clinicians (Martin, 1977, p. 427).

Prognosis. Unknown, but presumably less favorable than for exogenous and less severe depressions. Puig-Antich (1982) reported that of sixteen prepubertal boys with major depressions, thirteen agreed to treatment with imipramine; these youngsters also were diagnosed as having conduct disorders. All had their depressive symptoms relieved by the medication, and eleven of the thirteen no longer gave evidence of conduct disorders. Eleven of these thirteen children also received other therapeutic interventions. Nevertheless, six were recommended for residential treatment and seven of the eleven who responded favorably in depression and conduct relapsed and had another depressive episode and conduct disorder pattern shortly after treatment ceased.

Strober and Carlson (1982) conducted a four year follow-up of sixty adolescents who had been hospitalized for major depression. All sixty required some form of medical or psychotherapeutic assistance during the follow-up period: twelve developed mania and thus exhibited a bipolar disorder; eleven had one or more additional episodes of major depression; four had intermittent episodes of depressive symptoms; and thirty-three were relatively asymptomatic.

From these studies it would appear that about half the children with major depression have a relatively long-lasting, favorable response to treatment. When psychotic symptoms accompany the major depression, the prognosis is less favorable.

Suicide

Suicide and the threat of suicide are symptoms associated with depressive disorders and are not listed as specific diagnostic categories in DSM-III. Nevertheless they are subjects of considerable importance and merit some discussion.

It is profitable to make the following distinctions:

1. There are suicides that are *rational,* in which the individual reasonably evaluates a situation and decides death is preferable to life. The suicides of George Eastman, founder of the Eastman-Kodak Company, and Paul Federn, a psychoanalyst, are examples of men well along in years who determined the pain they faced was not worth enduring. In view of their young ages, children and adolescents would rarely be regarded as rational suicides.
2. There are suicides that are *cultural,* in which the society sanctions the taking of one's life. Committing suicide for country in time of war is highly regarded, as is suicide in the Orient as an expression of deep shame and regret for a mistake. As a rule, our culture does not approve of children and adolescents killing themselves; thus our concern is with neither cultural nor rational suicides.
3. There are suicides that are *unintentional,* in which the person attempts suicide for one manipulative reason or another, has no real wish to die, but inadvertently is successful. The suicide of the actress Marilyn Monroe, who seemed to try to get help after she took an overdose of pills, was probably unintended.
4. There are suicides that are *pathological,* in which the person commits suicide from irrational reasons or fears. The situation was not as hopeless and the options were not as meager as the individual believed; the suicide is regarded by the living as a tragedy and a waste.
5. There are suicidal *gestures,* in which the person is unsuccessful in self-destruction and is not too unhappy about it. The attempt on one's life was designed to impress, to communicate, to influence someone else. However, there is a danger that if due recognition is not given the gestures, the attempts will escalate to become unintentional or pathological suicides. Our concern, then, is with this interrelated group of suicidal gestures and unintentional and pathological suicides: The aim is to prevent them and to assist the person to more effective and less dangerous means of expression and coping.

Prevalence. Kanner (1935) reported that in the United States during the 1920s about thirty to fifty-five children between the ages of ten and fourteen committed suicide each year; under the age of ten was rare, but occasionally did occur; many more whites than blacks killed themselves; and boys killed themselves much more often than girls, by a ratio of 2:1. The favored means for suicide were firearms and hanging; leaping from heights, which was frequent in other nations, was rarely employed by children in this country. He supposed that many more children attempted suicide than actually succeeded. When population changes are taken into account, the recent estimates of prevalence are consistent with those of earlier in the century. The race difference noted by Kanner has been explained as an artifact of urban-rural suicide differences (Shaffer & Fisher, 1981).

Suicide in children below the age of ten is still rare, though it does happen; there were two cases in 1978. That year among children ten to fourteen 117 boys and 34 girls in the United States committed suicide (a rate of .8/100,000). Among adolescents of fifteen to nineteen, 1,367 boys and 319 girls committed suicide (a rate of

7.6/100,000); the probability of suicide thus increases dramatically from childhood to adolescence, with boys much more prone to self-destruction than girls, by a ratio of 4:1 (Shaffer & Fisher, 1981). Since girls account for more suicidal attempts than boys (Haider, 1968; Garfinkel, Froese, & Hood, 1982), males appear to be much more intent on killing themselves when they resort to a sucidal act than are females.

It is also estimated that a certain percentage of accidental deaths, which is the leading cause of fatality among adolescents (a rate of 57.4/100,000), may have been suicidal behaviors (*Vital Statistics*, 1979), and that attempts are involved in 10% of adolescent referrals to outpatient psychiatric clinics (Pfeffer, 1981) and .25% of pediatric admissions to emergency rooms (Garfinkel, Froese, & Hood, 1982).

Diagnostic Issues. There is nothing very subtle about the diagnosis of suicidal behaviors. In general, children who are depressed, who talk about committing suicide or death and dying, who attempt suicide, or who engage in dangerous activities or place themselves in dangerous situations are regarded as suicidal risks. According to existentialists, suicide may appear a reasonable alternative to the futility of living; according to psychoanalysts, self-destruction is an unconscious force within each of us. Thus the issue is to determine to what extent the possibility of suicide is flirted with and seriously entertained.

Case Illustration: Al was seventeen years old and had been expelled from school because he was truant and rude to his teachers when in attendance. He had no friends or useful activities. For years he had been a problem, disobeying his parents and authorities and acting angrily and impulsively when any effort was made to discipline him. His mother reported: "Al spends all day racing his car in the empty lot near our house. Back and forth. Back and forth. Around and around . . . just missing running into a tree or the brick wall of the factory near us." Both parents wanted help in getting Al to work or into school again. When told his behavior was seriously suicidal, they received that as a bit of good news, suggesting some relief that their burden might soon be lifted from them.

Etiology. There are many reasons for people trying and committing suicide. Students may kill themselves from shame (loss of self-esteem) when they feel they have not done as well in school as they should; their actions may be precipitated by conflict with or the loss of a loved one; they may be angry with someone ("I'll kill myself and show them. Then they'll be sorry."); a parent or close relative may have been depressed and suicidal—Goethe's novel, *The Sorrows of Young Werther*, in which the hero kills himself when his love is not returned, seemed to prompt a wave of romantic suicides in nineteenth century Europe.

Shaffer and Fisher (1981) note three major etiological models for suicide: as a consequence of illness or depression (medical); as a result of unconscious conflicts, such as wishing to punish or be united with a loved one (psychodynamic); as an understandable outcome of the person's intolerable social circumstances (systems or ecological) i.e., training for an occupation in which the economy offers scant employment and does little to promote happiness. There is some support for all these models.

Case Illustration: Agnes was a seventeen-year-old who attempted suicide by taking an overdose of pills. She explained that the attempt had not been serious. Her steady boyfriend had been killed several months before in an automobile accident. Though she had mourned him for a time, she soon recovered and was looking forward to going on dates and the social activities of her senior year. However her classmates didn't know how to respond to her; the boys felt to ask her out would be disloyal to the memory of their friend. Agnes said she became depressed again and thought suicide might rally her classmates to her assistance; she was pleased to report her plan had worked. While recovering in the hospital she had been visited by several boys who told her they would try to help her overcome her grief by taking her to movies and dances.

Case Illustration: Pete was a lonely, alienated adolescent who had been hospitalized after slashing himself on his forearms. He would go to anyone who would listen, tell of his suicide attempt, and offer to remove his bandages so his audience would know how close he had come to death. After a few days he began to feel people were no longer caring and sympathetic. One morning he used his shirt to hang himself from a tree by the employees' cafeteria, apparently expecting the employees to rescue him. Unfortunately they were delayed at breakfast that day and when Pete was discovered he was dead from strangulation.

Case Illustration: Mike took an overdose of barbiturates and turned himself in to the hospital before the drugs took effect. His stomach was pumped, and he was hospitalized. He stated he was a member of a group of teenagers who were involved with marijuana and narcotics. The police were after him for information, and in order to save himself from prosecution, he helped the authorities to plan a bust. The suicide attempt was a cover to give him an alibi for not being with the group when the police arrived.

Treatment. There is no specific treatment for those who talk of or attempt suicide and all that has been said with regard to the treatment of depression is appropriate here. In each case it is necessary to evaluate the probability that there will be a more or less serious attempt. This probability depends upon the supports available to the child, the attitudes of the child and those involved, and the difficulties of the circumstances. At the very least we can be among those who appreciate the seriousness of the act and be available to provide whatever help we can to the child to deal with the situation more constructively. Depression is likely to be a growing problem among children and adolescents—the peculiarities of DSM-III in diagnosing depressive disorders practically guarantees it.

REFERENCES

Abramson, L. Y., Seligman, M. E. P., & Teasdale, J. D. Learned helplessness in humans: Critique and reformulation. *Journal of Abnormal Psychology*, 1978, *87*, 49–74.

Allen, M. Twin studies of affective illness. *Archives of General Psychiatry*, 1976, *33*, 1476–1478.

Beck, A. T. *Depression: Clinical, experimental and theoretical aspects.* New York: Hoeber, 1967.

Bemporad, J. Manifest symptomatology of depression in children and adolescents. In S. Arieti & J. Bemporad, *Severe and mild depression.* New York: Basic, 1978.

Blanck, G., & Blanck, R. *Ego psychology II.* New York: Columbia University, 1979.

Blumberg, M. L. Depression in children on a general pediatric service. *American Journal of Psychotherapy,* 1978, *32,* 20–32.

Bowlby, J. *Separation: Anxiety and anger.* New York: Basic Books, 1973.

Bowlby, J. Attachment and loss: Retrospect and prospect. *American Journal of Orthopsychiatry,* 1982, *52,* 664–678.

Carlson, G. A., & Cantwell, D. P. A survey of depressive symptoms, syndrome and disorder in a child psychiatric population. *Journal of Child Psychology and Psychiatry,* 1980, *21,* 19–25. (a)

Carlson, G. A., & Cantwell, D. P. Unmasking masked depression in children and adolescents. *American Journal of Psychiatry,* 1980, *137,* 445–449. (b)

Chess, S., & Thomas, A. Infant bonding: Mystique and reality. *American Journal of Orthopsychiatry,* 1982, *52,* 213–218.

Conners, C. K., & Werry, J. S. Pharmacotherapy. In H. C. Quay & J. S. Werry (Eds.), *Psychopathological disorders of childhood.* New York: Wiley, 1979.

Cytryn, L. McKnew, D. H., & Bunney, W. E., Jr. Diagnosis of depression in children: A reassessment. *American Journal of Psychiatry,* 1980, *137,* 22–25.

Ferster, C. B. A functional analysis of depression. *American Psychologist,* 1973, *28,* 857–870.

Fischhoff, J. Failure to thrive and maternal deprivation. In E. J. Anthony (Ed.), *Explorations in child psychiatry.* New York: Plenum, 1975.

Freed, H. *The chemistry and therapy of behavior disorders in children.* Springfield, IL: Charles C. Thomas, 1962.

Friedman, R. C., et al. DSM-III and affective pathology in hospitalized adolescents. *The Journal of Nervous and Mental Disease,* 1982, *170,* 511–521.

Garfinkel, B. D., Froese, A., & Hood, J. Suicide attempts in children and adolescents. *The American Journal of Psychiatry,* 1982, *139,* 1257–1261.

Gittelman-Klein, R. Definitional and methodological issues concerning depressive illness in children. In J. G. Schulterbrandt & A. Raskin (Eds.), *Depression in childhood.* New York: Raven, 1977.

Goldfarb, W. Emotional and intellectual consequences of psychologic deprivation in infancy: A re-evaluation. In P. Hoch & J. Zubin (Eds.), *Psychopathology of childhood.* New York: Grune and Stratton, 1955.

Graham, P. Epidemiological studies. In H. C. Quay & J. S. Werry (Eds.), *Psychopathological disorders of childhood.* New York: Wiley, 1979.

Haider, I. Suicidal attempts in children and adolescents. *British Journal of Psychiatry,* 1968, *114,* 1113–1134.

Hall, C. S., & Lindzey, G. *Theories of personality.* New York: Wiley, 1978.

Hetherington, E. M., & Martin, B. Family interaction. In H. C. Quay & J. S. Werry (Eds.), *Psychopathological disorders of childhood.* New York: Wiley, 1979.

Holmes, T. S. Holmes, T. H. Short-term intrusions into the life-style routine. *Journal of Psychosomatic Research,* 1970, June, *14,* 121–132.

Hughes, M. C. Recurrent abdominal pain and childhood depression. *American Journal of Orthopsychiatry,* 1984, *54,* 146–155.

Kanner, L. *Child psychiatry.* Springfield, IL: Charles C. Thomas, 1935.

Kazdin, A. E. Assessment techniques for childhood depression. *Journal of the American Academy of Child Psychiatry,* 1981, *20,* 358–375.

Klein, M. *The psycho-analysis of children.* New York: Norton, 1932.

Kohlberg, L., Lacrosse, J., & Ricks, D. The predictability of adult mental health from childhood behavior. In B. B. Wolman (Ed.), *Manual of child psychopathology.* New York: McGraw-Hill, 1972.

Kovacs, M., & Beck, A. An empirical clinical approach towards a definition of childhood depression. In J. G. Schulterbrandt & R. Raskin (Eds.), *Depression in childhood: Diagnosis, treatment, and conceptual models.* New York: Raven, 1977.

Kuyler, P. L., Rosenthal, L., Igel, G., Dunner, D. L., & Fieve, R. R. Psychopathology among children of manic-depressive patients. *Biological Psychiatry,* 1980, *15,* 589–597.

Laufer, M. W. In Osler's day it was syphilis. In E. J. Anthony (Ed.), *Explorations in child psychiatry.* New York: Plenum, 1975.

Leese, S. The masked depression syndrome. *American Journal of Psychotherapy,* 1983, *XXXVII,* 456–475.

Lefkowitz, M. M., & Burton, N. Childhood depression: A critique of the concept. *Psychological Bulletin,* 1978, *85,* 716–726.

Lefkowitz, M. M., & Tesiny, E. P. Assessment of childhood depression. *Journal of Consulting and Clinical Psychology,* 1980, *48,* 43–50.

Leon, G. R., Kendall, P. C., & Garber, J. Depression in children. *Journal of Abnormal Child Psychology,* 1980, *8,* 221–235.

Lewinsohn, P. M. A behavioral approach to depression. In R. J. Freidman & M. M. Katz (Eds.), *The psychology of depression.* Washington, DC: Winston, 1974.

Martin, B. *Abnormal psychology.* New York: Holt, 1977.

Munroe, R. L. *Schools of psychoanalytic thought.* New York: Dryden, 1955.

Orvaschel, H., Weissman, M. M., & Kidd, K. K. Children and depression. *Journal of Affective Disorders,* 1980, *2,* 1–16.

Pfeffer, C. R. Suicidal behavior of children: A review with implications for research and practice. *American Journal of Psychiatry,* 1981, *138,* 154–159.

Pinneau, S. R. The infantile disorders of hospitalism and anaclitic depression. *Psychological Bulletin,* 1955, *52,* 429–462.

Poznanski, E. O., Carroll, B. J., Banegas, M. C., Cook, S. C., & Grossman, J. A. The dexamethasone suppression test in prepubertal depressed children. *American Journal of Psychiatry,* 1982, *139,* 321–324.

Provence, S. & Lipton, R. C. *Infants in institutions.* New York: International University, 1962.

Prugh, D., & Harlow, R. G. "Masked deprivation" in infants and young children. In *Deprivation of maternal care: A reassessment of its effects.* World Health Organization, Public Health Papers, No. 14, Geneva: WHO, 1962.

Puig-Antich, J. Affective disorders in childhood. *Psychiatric Clinics of North America,* 1980, *3,* 403–424.

Puig-Antich, J. Major depression and conduct disorder in prepuberty. *Journal of the American Academy of Child Psychiatry,* 1982, *21,* 118–128.

Puig-Antich, J., & Gittelman, R. Depression in childhood and adolescence. In E. S. Paykel (Ed.), *Handbook of affective disorders.* London: Churchill Livingstone, 1980.

Rehm, L. P. *Empirical studies of childhood depression.* Symposium presented at American Psychological Association, Los Angeles, 1981.

Robins, L. N. Follow-up studies. In H. C. Quay & J. S. Werry (Eds.), *Psychopathological disorders of childhood.* New York: Wiley, 1979.

Rutter, M. Maternal deprivation, 1972–1978: New findings, new concepts, new approaches. In S. Chess & A. Thomas (Eds.), *Annual progress in child psychiatry and child development.* New York: Brunner/Mazel, 1980.

Rutter, M., Graham, P., Chadwick, O. F. D., & Yule, W. Adolescent turmoil: Fact or fiction? *Journal of Child Psychology and Psychiatry,* 1976, *17,* 653–686.

Rutter, M., Tizard, J., & Whitmore, K. *Education, health, and behavior.* London: Longman, 1970.

Seligman, M. E. P. *Helplessness: on depression, development, and death.* San Francisco: Freeman, 1975.

Shaffer, D., & Fisher, P. The epidemiology of suicide in children and young adolescents. *Journal of the American Academy of Child Psychiatry,* 1981, *20,* 545–565.

Solnit, A. J., & Leckman, J. F. On the study of children of parents with affective disorders. *American Journal of Psychiatry,* 1984, *141,* 241–242.

Spitz, R. A. Hospitalism: An inquiry into the genesis of psychiatric conditions in early childhood. *The Psychoanalytic Study of the Child,* 1945, *1,* 53–74.

Spitz, R. A. Hospitalism: A follow-up report. *The Psychoanalytic Study of the Child,* 1946, *2,* 113–117. (a)

Spitz, R. A. Anaclitic depression. *The Psychoanalytic Study of the Child,* 1946, *2,* 313–342. (b)

Spitz, R. A. *The first year of life.* New York: International Universities, 1965.

Strober, M., & Carlson, G. Bipolar illness in adolescents with major depression. *Archives of General Psychiatry,* 1982, *39,* 549–555.

Suomi, S. J., & Harlow, H. F. Production and alleviation of depressive behaviors in monkeys. In J. D. Maser & M. E. P. Seligman (Eds.), *Psychopathology: Experimental models.* San Francisco: Freeman, 1977.

Thomas, A., & Chess, S. Genesis and evolution of behavioral disorders from infancy to early adult life. *American Journal of Psychiatry,* 1984, *141,* 1–9.

Tizard, B., & Rees, J. The effect of early institutional rearing on the behavior problems and affectual relations of four-year-old children. *Journal of Child Psychology and Psychiatry,* 1975, *16,* 61–73.

Vital Statistics of the United States, 1975 & 1976. Vol. II. *Mortality* (Parts A & B). Hyattsville, MD: National Center for Health Statistics, 1979.

Weiner, I. B. *Child and adolescent psychopathology.* New York: Wiley, 1982.

Wilcoxon, L. A., Schrader, S. L., & Nelson, R. E. Behavioral formulations of depression. In W. E. Craighead, A. E. Kazdin, & J. J. Maloney (Eds.), *Behavior modification: Principles, issues, and applications.* Boston: Houghton Mifflin, 1976.

Yarrow, L. J. Maternal deprivation: Toward an empirical and conceptual reevaluation. *Psychological Bulletin,* 1961, *58,* 459–491.

CHAPTER 10

Anxiety and Neurotic Disorders

Richard J. Lawlor

Anxiety, what Levitt (1980, p. 2) called "our official emotion," may refer to a mood, a symptom, an emotion, or a state of psychopathology. The focus in this chapter is on anxiety as an abnormal emotion and a symptom of pathology.

Many of the disorders presented here are no longer important because of their prevalence but because of their historical significance. The anxiety disorders stimulated Freud and led to the various theories of psychodynamics. Also the study of fear and phobia led to the early applications of behaviorism and behavior therapy. Anxiety is an important theoretical and motivational construct, but whether it has the pervasive significance given it by clinicians is questionable.

We shall begin by examining those anxiety disorders characteristic of childhood and adolescence, and then move to a discussion of those, such as somatoform disorders, which are not too common among adults and even less frequent among children.

Separation Anxiety Disorder

According to DSM-III (American Psychiatric Association, 1980, pp. 50–57), the essential characteristic of separation anxiety disorder is "excessive anxiety on separation from major attachment figures or from home or other familiar surroundings." The anxiety may reach such profound proportions that the child reacts with panic and manifests some or all of the following: difficulty in breathing (dyspnea), dizziness, sweating, paleness, fainting or feeling faint and weak, trembling, and feelings of unreality. Such a panic attack is, however, a secondary symptom in this disorder and is not essential to the diagnostic picture.

Case Illustration: Robert was a nine-year-old boy who refused to attend school. This school refusal began after Christmas vacation, during which Robert's grandmother had been seriously injured in an accident. Robert was of superior intelligence, in advanced academic programs in all areas, and achieved excellent grades. His peer relationships were good with advanced pupils, but only marginally adequate with other classmates, who teased him because of his lack of physical abilities and for being slightly overweight. On non-school days Robert engaged in a number of activities such as bike riding and playing with his older brother, but on school days he would waken with stomachaches and severe headaches, which at times were so severe they caused him to vomit. Allowed to stay home, he would rest for a few hours and then get up, do some schoolwork, or help his mother around the house. During the course of extensive diagnostic interviewing it became apparent that Robert had many concerns which he rarely talked about, including a fear his mother would somehow be injured.

Robert's symptom picture illustrates a number of features found in separation anxiety disorder. Unrealistic worries about harms which could befall people are associated, as here, with a refusal to attend school, and no specific aspects of the school situation seem to account for the refusal. Physical complaints, especially headaches and abdominal pain or nausea, are common and generally occur only on school days. During these times away from school the child may resolve to return at the next opportunity, seem to look forward to and plan for the return, and then have the same symptoms recur when the return to school approaches. These behaviors often confuse both the child and the parents, and family discord is a frequent consequence if the symptoms persist.

Less frequently seen symptoms, but important indicators nonetheless of separation anxiety disorder, include vague fears of catastrophes which might prevent the child from getting home or back to the parent; difficulty leaving the parents or others in order to go to sleep (though this normally occurs with younger children); nightmares involving loss or separation; temper tantrums when forced to leave home alone or when the parents leave the child with a babysitter (again, normal with youngsters); and, especially after the separation problems have persisted, gradual withdrawal from, lack of enjoyment of, and avoidance of peers.

In early childhood, from one to three years of age, separation anxiety is considered normal. Even when tantrums or crying spells are associated with separation from attachment figures at five or six, the upset is generally not viewed as pathological unless it persists and meets the criteria for a true panic. In pervasive developmental disorders and other disorders, anxiety is secondary to the major symptoms (see Chapter 5). So what we are discussing is serious distress experienced by an older child when faced with separating from parents.

Prevalence, Sex, and Familial Considerations

Exact figures on the prevalence of this disorder are unavailable, but it is considered by clinicians to be a relatively common problem. Gittelman-Klein and Klein (1971) noted that this disorder is one of the few psychiatric emergencies seen in outpatient clinics, and most clinicians believe prompt intervention is essential to prevent further deterioration, entrenchment of the symptoms, and insurmountable academic deficiencies. Adams (1979) suggests that the disorder is found in about 1 percent of children in the general population and that children of all levels of intelligence show the disorder. Waldfogle, Coolidge, and Hahn (1957) found no sex differences in prevalence, and that it occurs most often between grades 1 and 3. Episodes which manifest for the first time in high school are not rare and have a less favorable prognosis than cases which occur earlier. School refusal in adolescence is often unrelated to separation anxiety and may be brought about by any number of problems. It has also been found that the prevalence of the disorder is greater in higher socioeconomic classes and in families seen as striving and upwardly mobile (Coolidge, 1979). Separation anxiety disorder can also be diagnosed in adults if the symptoms appeared prior to age eighteen and the person does not meet the criteria for a diagnosis of agoraphobia, a fear discussed later in this chapter.

Much of the early research pertinent to separation anxiety disorder of childhood is found under what used to be called "school phobia." In DSM-III, however, a true fear of the school situation would be classified as either social phobia, when the basic fear is of humiliation and a desire to avoid scrutiny and embarrassment, or as a simple (specific) phobia, when what the individual desires to avoid is a threatening object or place and avoidance of others is not a major consideration. Doubts that school phobia was a true phobia arose early (Johnson, 1941; Johnson, 1957), and these early researchers suggested that not fear of school but fear of separation was the major difficulty; the validity of this suggestion has been recognized in DSM-III.

A number of studies have yielded different classifications of school phobia "types" (Adams, 1979; Hampe, 1973; Sperling, 1974; Waldron et al., 1975), but there seems to be a great deal of overlap in these categorizations. Fear of separation from parents has consistently been found a significant feature, often associated with family interaction patterns which present the child or adolescent with conflicting messages, usually from the mother, about the degree of independence the parent can tolerate or allow.

A second major factor is an extreme dread of impending destruction or injury at home, often experienced by the child as a vague foreboding about the well-being of the mother.

Sperling (1967) noted that especially with children where the onset of the problem with separation has been relatively sudden and associated with a clear-cut precipitating event, such as illness of a close relative or friend, the basic fear is of separation. Often this fear of separation symbolizes for the child an unconscious or unrecognized fear of death of the mother and of the child's own death. Those children labeled "acute" by Coolidge, Hahn, and Peck (1957), tend to be ones whose basic personality functioning, other than for the disruption in the school area, remains intact. They continue to function with their friends outside school and, where it is necessary to utilize homebound tutoring, continue to develop intellectually and academically.

With older youngsters and adolescents who refuse to attend school, those who show definite characterological (enduring personality traits; see Chapter 13) manifestations and a gradual insidious onset denoted by chronic shyness, avoidance of peers, and embarrassment in social situations, the picture is a graver one and the severity of the disturbance more marked. In these cases the "phobic" picture often resembles more the agoraphobic (agoraphia is a fear of public places) features seen in true phobic disorders, and panic attacks within the school situation are far more likely to occur. In many of these cases with older children, one aspect of the problem seems to be an inability to solve adolescent developmental issues of identity and separation as a result of inadequate development of independence at earlier age levels, often fostered by parents who have highly ambivalent feelings toward their own independence-dependence conflicts as well as toward their children's struggles with dependence and independence. There is some evidence that separation anxiety disorder may even be a precursor in some cases of later "work phobia" in adults (Pittman, Langsley, & DeYoung, 1968), and when close scrutiny of the history of such adults is done, one often finds signs of earlier separation anxiety. Further evidence of the diagnostic importance of this category, particularly the chronic or characterological subtype, is found in the research of Liebowitz and Klein (1974), who found that 20 percent of the outpatients and 50 percent of the inpatients they observed as adults with agoraphobia and panic attacks had histories of separation anxiety in childhood, often with school refusal. Another finding which suggests that separation anxiety disorder may be a variant or precursor of agoraphobia is that treatment of nonpsychotic school phobic children with imipramine (a tricyclic antidepressant medication) resulted in all showing significant improvement in their panic symptoms. (Gittelman-Klein & Klein, 1971; Robinson, et al., 1973). In adults with agoraphobia it has consistently been found that administration of imipramine is an effective treatment in eliminating or greatly reducing panic attacks. The effectiveness of this antidepressant medication is not, as might be expected, correlated with their initial level of depression. (Thoren et al., 1980; Zitrin, Klein, & Woerner, 1980). This finding strongly suggests that imipramine does not act solely as an antidepressant, but also tends to decrease the general anxiety level of the patient (Zitrin, Klein, & Woerner, 1980). Imipramine and other antidepressant medications, however, seem to have no effect on the anticipatory anxiety often associated with separation anxiety disorders, and little improvement in social functioning is noted (Thoren et al., 1980; Zitrin, Klein, & Woerner, 1978) without further psychotherapy or often with antianxiety medication (minor tranquilizers) as an adjunct.

Treatment

Controversy abounds concerning treatment of separation anxiety disorder, and the summary of the issues by Weiner (1970) is still the clearest exposition of the various viewpoints. Essentially, the major treatment decision is whether to defer or compel the child's return to school. Clinicians who recommend a deferred return (Waldfogel, Coolidge, & Hahn, 1957) suggest the major focus has to be on the effort to correct pathological family relationships, particularly the hostile-dependent relationship between mother and child. They argue that early return, while often superficially successful, leads to early termination of therapy and a greater probability of relapse (Hersov, 1960).

Immediate and early return of the child to school as the preferred approach was first suggested by Klein (1945) and elaborated on by many authors and clinicians Eisenberg, 1958; Levanthal et al., 1967). The strategy recommended requires the clinician to assure that the child is unable to manipulate or intimidate any of the adults (parents, school officials, and therapist) with symptoms, often extremely dramatic at this stage. Control and the struggle for power in the family are major issues and the child's efforts to maintain control can be frightening.

Two Case Illustrations: After a complete diagnostic workup and confirmation of the diagnosis of separation anxiety disorder, James, an eleven-year-old who had been absent from school for three months, was told during a disposition conference that his severe headaches, nausea, and diarrhea were not physical problems and that he would have to return to school the following day. James at that point began to perspire profusely, became extremely pale, and doubled over with abdominal pains and a severe headache. He said he was going to vomit, but did not. Both parents became extremely anxious, but listened as the therapist assured them that the symptoms, dramatic and frightening as they were, were not life threatening. It was also predicted that James would have these symptoms the following morning, but that the parents had to promise to take him to school, kicking, screaming, and nauseated if necessary. The appropriate school officials were also notified in James' presence and similarly told what to expect and what to do. Surprisingly, on the following morning James complained of only mild nausea and fear, rode to school with only minor verbal protests, made it successfully through the first day. Within three days he ceased even these verbal complaints. Unfortunately, however, James and his parents withdrew from formal therapy after three sessions and it was not felt that the family problems had been adequately resolved.

In contrast, Billie, an eight-year-old responded calmly to similar recommendations during the disposition conference and promised he would return to school. The following morning, however, he developed severe abdominal pain and locked himself in the bathroom. His parents unlocked the door and with help from two older brothers physically carried Billie to the car. Billie was carried kicking and screaming into the principal's office. There he was given the choice of remaining or proceeding to his class. He chose to stay in the office, but volunteered to return to class after an hour, and had no further difficulties that day. Similar scenes were repeated, with somewhat less intensity for several days, and Billie was eventually able to go to school without further disturbance. During this period he continued to see a therapist, initially twice a week. The focus of treatment was on his areas of success as well as resolution of his underlying concerns over his mother's health and his even more repressed ambivalent feelings toward his relationship with her. Collateral therapy with the parents and family sessions helped to resolve many of these issues.

Some investigators (Coolidge, Brodie, & Feeney, 1964; Liebowitz & Klein, 1979; Rodriguez & Eisenberg, 1959), concerned about the high prevalence of prior separation anxiety disorders in agoraphobic problems, suggest the following hypotheses about prognosis. First, the younger the child and the more sudden the onset, especially in the presence of a clearcut precipitating event and few or no characterological features, the more likely an early return to school and the effectiveness of relatively brief psychotherapy. Second, the older the child and the more gradual the onset of the separation difficulties, especially with several early behavior difficulties in peer relationships or academic functioning, the more likely the child may need long-term treatment, possibly in conjunction with medication to avoid panic attacks (Sperling, 1967).

A large psychoanalytic literature traces the origin of school phobia to underlying sexual, and usually oedipal, fantasies of the child and the displacement of these fantasies onto the social environment, especially the school (Prince, 1968). Consistent with this psychodynamic orientation is a therapeutic approach which requires resolution of the underlying conflicts.

On the other hand, other professionals have suggested that the disorder may have a biological base and that there are significant variations among individuals, based on constitutional or temperamental factors, in their susceptibility to difficulty in this area (Bowlby, 1960; Klein & David, 1969). An inference to be drawn from this constitutional view is that psychotherapy, at best, is helpful but that significant change in the underlying biological base of the anxiety threshold is unlikely. The only thing psychotherapy can accomplish in this view is to help the child or adolescent to learn to cope with anxiety through the development of more effective coping mechanisms.

Gittelman-Klein and Klein (1971), however, suggest that, while there seems to be strong evidence for a "pathologic process intrinsic to the child," they still find parental cooperation essential in overcoming the child's anticipatory anxiety which has become part of the clinical picture; medication is effective only in controlling the panic which ensues with separation, not the anxiety the child has developed over time about separation or returning to school. The child still needs psychotherapy and parental pressures to force the required venturing into feared social situations and away from the major attachment figures.

Behavioral approaches to children and adolescents with this disorder have ranged from systematic desensitization, forced immersion, aversion relief, and modeling. With *systematic desensitization* (Wolpe, 1961) the child is first taught relaxation techniques. Following this a hierarchy of feared objects is developed, and the child is asked to imagine situations involving increasingly intense fears, the idea being that by pairing relaxed states with these feared situations he or she will learn to approach the feared situation while relaxed and comfortable. The child may also be led to experience feared situations hierarchically and actually *(in vivo)*, thus gradually going closer and closer to school.

Forced immersion has two variations, flooding and implosion. When flooding is used, the child is brought into immediate confrontation with the feared situation (the school), whereas with implosion, the child uses imagination to suddenly confront and overwhelm the anxiety defense (Emmelkamp & Wessels, 1975).

Aversion relief (Sheehan, Ballenger, & Jacobson, 1980) involves administering shock, usually to a finger, until the feared object appears or is imagined, and then discontinuing the shock. *Modeling* involves having someone else, often a person who has developed a relationship with the child, approach the feared object (Bandura, 1969) while the child observes this person's nonanxious response. In all behavioral approaches there are reports of success without any discernable negative consequences.

Avoidant Disorder of Childhood or Adolescence

The clinical picture in avoidant disorder is marked by "a persistent and excessive shrinking from contact with strangers" (DSM-III, p. 54), so severe that it interferes with the child's social development. Coupled with this shrinking from contact, however, is a strong desire to be liked, accepted, and to have friends.

Case Illustration: Mary Ann, a seven-year-old, performed adequately in school, but was described by her teacher as a social isolate. She never talked with other children, stood quietly near the teacher at recess, refused overtures from peers to get involved in activities, and talked only to her teacher in frightened one syllable responses. At home, she was a "delightful child" with her parents and younger sister, but would hide behind the couch or leave the room whenever her grandparents, other relatives, or family friends arrived. When seen by the school psychologist, Mary Ann would not look directly at her, kept placing her index finger in her mouth, and stood mute. Whenever she was asked a question, she would sign, tremble slightly, and continue to stare ahead.

The prevalence of this disorder is low and children with anxiety as crippling and disabling as Mary Ann's are seen infrequently. Nevertheless, the severity of social inhibition and sense of insecurity is so striking when the disorder is encountered that the clinician generally has no difficulty distinguishing the anxiety from normal or even moderately severe shyness. Moreover, the anxiety in this disorder is relatively circumscribed, often being focused exclusively on contact with strangers; with close family members the child is often relaxed, friendly, spontaneous, and talkative.

PREVALENCE, SEX, AND FAMILIAL CONSIDERATIONS

No body of research exists which suggests any particular or specific etiological factors in this disorder, and the rarity of its prevalence makes systematic collection of data difficult. The clinical impressions of many therapists suggest that the disorder may be self-limiting, in that there is little documentation, clinical, anecdotal or otherwise to suggest that the disorder becomes chronic.

With young children, a combination of play therapy and gradual desensitization procedures are common therapeutic approaches. For example, Mary Ann was treated with a combination of gradual desensitization to situations in which contact with strangers was fostered, often with successive approximations of communication behaviors. At the start, Mary Ann was essentially mute but gradually she was reinforced successfully for slight head movements, nods of the head, lip movements, whispered responses, louder one word responses, responses with eye contact, and eventually short sentence responses. The prognosis in this disorder, then, based on clinical impression, is that the disorder does not usually persist into adulthood, at least not to the same severe extent, and does yield good results with both psychotherapy and behavioral approaches.

Overanxious Disorder

Overanxious disorder is the child and adolescent version of what is called generalized anxiety disorder in persons over eighteen; the symptoms are similar in both the adult and child disorders. The "predominant disturbance is excessive worrying and fearful behavior that is not focused on a specific situation or object (such as separation from a parent or entering new social interaction) and that is not due to a recent psychosocial stressor" (DSM-III, p. 55).

As Adams (1979) noted, excess anxiety

is one of Freud's original classifications of an "actual neurosis," and the complete emotional and behavioral symptom picture is fear of impending doom; feelings of inferiority; general unease; restlessness; insomnia; constant seeking of reassurance; physical complaints, such as headaches, nausea, diarrhea, dry mouth, palpitations and sweating; and preoccupations with past failure and wrongdoings. The younger the child, the more diffuse and general this anxiety seems to be, and it is often noted that it is only as the child becomes older that the symptoms become more elaborated and specific.

Case Illustration: Jennifer was a bright twelve-year-old who had always achieved good grades in school. She began to have increasing attacks of vomiting and nausea and worried about her ability to keep up her grades and concentrate. When seen for evaluation she was extremely anxious. Her palms were sweaty and she fidgeted nervously in her chair, biting her almost nonexistent nails continuously. She had a few close friends at school, but felt she was unpopular with most children, blaming this on their jealousy over her achievements.

Jennifer's symptoms are relatively common among children and they seem to affect boys more than girls. Unlike avoidant disorder, where there is little evidence of persistence into adulthood, it is felt that this disorder may persist, either as a generalized anxiety disorder or as a social phobia. In milder form, however, where symptoms consist primarily of nailbiting, shrinking from social contact except for a few friends, excessive worrying, etc., it is felt that there is a good prognosis for well-adjusted adult behavior (Robins, 1966). In more severe cases, particularly in cases where the children are seen as "pseudomature" (acting more like adults than is appropriate) and overly compliant, the prognosis for good adjustment without significant anxiety manifestations as an adult are less certain. During childhood it is rare to see this disorder in a form so severe that it becomes incapacitating.

One of the major difficulties in this area stems from the paucity of research on the development of emotions in children, (Lewis, 1979). There is also no research which specifically answers questions about familial patterns in this disorder, in contrast to the documented family pattern seen in separation anxiety disorder.

Treatment

Treatment of overanxious disorder is heavily dependent on the theoretical orientation of the clinician. Dynamic or psychoanalytically oriented clinicians tend to view the disorder as resulting from misdirected somatic or sexual energies, fears resulting from masturbation, or excessive sexual tension when no appropriate discharge is available (Adams, 1979). Essentially, they conceptualize anxiety in children in ways which parallel those of adult neuroses (May, 1979) and most agree that these disorders are seldom seen prior to school age.

Chess (1965) and Thomas, Chess, and Birch (1968) describe "precursors" of anxiety in infants and young children as the "difficult child with irregular rhythms, withdrawal from new stimuli, frequent negative mood, intense reactions, and slow adaptability to change," and note that these may be temperamental features significant in the development of anxiety disorders later in childhood. Therapy done by adherents of a dynamic approach utilize a psychotherapy aimed at uncovering underlying sexual or aggressive conflicts and helping the child develop insight into them. Behavioral approaches, on the other hand, generally utilize a combination of relaxation and desensitization techniques.

Oppositional Disorder

Oppositional disorder has been described as a transitional diagnostic category "between a period of greater plasticity and one of fixity" (LaVietes, 1980). The transition is between normal developmental stages in which negativism, disobedience, and rebelliousness are normal or common and a chronic symptom picture of late adolescence or adulthood called passive-aggressive personality disorder. Oppositional disorder is defined as "a pattern of disobedient, negativistic, and provocative opposition to authority figures"(DSM-III, p. 63). This pattern is focused especially on parents and teachers, and one of its most striking characteristics is its persistence and refractoriness to treatment or intervention even when the behavior is self-defeating.

For example, a child may be failing in school and be told by a teacher that he is to complete a certain amount of work in order to pass a course, but refuse to do the work in spite of the obviously negative consequences. Attempts at reasonable discussion of the problem frequently result in argumentative behaviors and at times even temper tantrums. At other times the child exhibits a facade of conforming behaviors, agreeing verbally and outwardly, but continuing to provoke the adult with continual delays, stubbornness, and other negativistic behaviors which seem to represent an extreme degree of underlying anger and resentment. This continuous opposition characterizes the relationships between these children and authority, and frustration of adults seems to be both the intent of the behavior as well as the actual result.

Case Illustration: Skip was a nine-year-old, third-grade boy who had recently moved to a large city with his parents. Prior to the move, he had been doing well at school, but had never fully achieved his academic potential. He was described by both teachers and parents as having "a strong will," and would often insist on his way of doing things. His mother recalled him as having been "persistent" as a toddler, giving as an example his quickly learning how to circumvent baby gates in the house and climbing up onto high pieces of furniture despite numerous spankings. Following the family's move, which Skip had objected to because he had to leave his friends, he began to "forget" to bring home assignments, did not get his work done at school, refused to hand in completed lessons, and remained unmoved by all attempts to reward, cajole, threaten, or punish him. Referral to a child guidance clinic was made after several months of increasingly disruptive confrontations.

When seen for evaluation, Skip responded only to direct questions, often waiting several minutes to respond. In general, he denied any of the above problems, and when confronted with further questions would blame his teacher for demanding unreasonable standards of work and his mother for being, "too picky; I do it but she always wants everything perfect." His increasing peer problems and rejection by the group at school were minimized as irrelevant because "I've got other friends I like better at home" (which he did not).

Prevalence, Sex, Etiological, and Familial Factors

In evaluating oppositional behavior clinicians must distinguish between normal and pathological negativism. The prevalence of nonpathological school age negativism has ranged from 8.7 percent with girls (Werry & Quay, 1971) to 22 percent for boys and girls (Greene et al., 1973), with the modal occurrence in five-year-olds. Thus negativism is common in the general population. In addition, oppositional behavior is considered normal during the period between eighteen and thirty-six months, with a peak at about twenty-four months, and again during adolescence.

During both these periods, the focus is on expression of the child's growing sense of autonomy and independence. At the earlier stage, the development of a sense of separateness and individuality is achieved by saying "no." LaVietes (1980) suggests that about 10 percent of these younger children have a constitutional predisposition to be strong-willed and express their negativism in a more intense form than usual. She raises the possibility that these children are at risk to develop an oppositional disorder, especially if environmental circumstances, such as an inordinate need for power and control, exist in the parents. In that case, the child intensifies the struggle in order to defend against overcontrol and loss of autonomy.

In adolescence, children begin increasingly to express a need to be independent of parents, and negative behavior becomes to some degree normal. Again, predisposing constitutional factors (temperament) can play a significant role in conjunction with overreactions by parents or teachers to produce an oppositional disorder. The likelihood of such a development in adolescence is enhanced when negativistic behavior is a means for achieving peer recognition and status (Redl, 1976).

Studies of oppositional disorder are rare, but Gilpin and Worland (1976) do provide some data. Boys were found to exhibit problems of this type more frequently than girls, and a trend toward passive-aggressive personality disorder in fathers of these children was noted. Younger children were referred for treatment as a result of acts of physical aggression (kicking, pinching, spitting), whereas older children were most frequently seen for refusals to comply with demands for adequate school performance. There was also a higher than expected prevalence of depression or depressed features in the mothers of these children.

Treatment Considerations

Only Gilpin and Worland's (1976) data are available on treatment outcomes with children exhibiting this disorder. Their findings suggest a guarded outlook when treatment is undertaken with younger children and a dismal prognosis for older youngsters. One complicating factor in their study is the large proportion of parents who refused treatment, which suggests severe family pathology in the homes of these children and perhaps even oppositional behavior in the parents. As LaVietes (1980) points out, the course of treatment with this disorder is likely to require considerable time and expenditure of effort, but when this effort is made, the results, especially with young children, are encouraging.

Intervention: Skip began family therapy with much reluctance and refused to discuss any of the issues of concern to his parents or the school. With the focus upon family dynamics, including his father's indirect expressions of hostility and overcontrol of anger, as well as support for his mother's attempts to set limits on his behaviors at home, a gradual change began to occur. Initially, his behavior at school improved, and later he began to cooperate more at home. Eventually Skip was able to express his feelings of rage about his family's move and his fantasies that he could return to his old school and house if he made his parents and teachers angry and frustrated enough to try to "bribe" him into "being good" by an offer to return. The therapy itself was not steady progress, but significant improvement was seen by Skip, his parents, and the school.

Elective Mutism

Elective mutism is characterized by a refusal to speak in almost all social situations. In some cases communication by means of gestures, shaking of the head, or brief, narrative responses is seen. There is no biological disability, since these children can and do speak at home or in certain other situations. Often associated with the mutism are excessive shyness, temper tantrums, school refusal, crying, negativism, urinary and bowel problems, and use of passive-aggressive behaviors to control or punish others (Browne, Wilson, & Laybourne, 1963). No predisposing or precipitating factors have been consistently related to this disorder. Some factors suggested include early physical trauma, especially of the mouth (Parker, Olsen, & Throckmorton, 1960), maternal and paternal rejection or disinterest (Elson et al., 1965), maternal overprotection and excessive encouragement of dependency (Adams & Glasner, 1954; Pustrom & Speers, 1964), marital conflicts with the child forced to take sides in the conflict (Adams & Glasner, 1954), and modeling by parents or siblings of silence as a weapon to express anger and control of family members (Silver, 1980).

Despite their refusal to speak, most children displaying elective mutism do learn in school, as seen by their performance on both classroom and written standardized tests. Often, however, they are untestable on tasks which require oral responses, such as on individual tests of verbal intelligence. With prolonged maintainance of the mutism, there is usually a gradual deterioration in school performance or in the child's social relationships with peers, since as the child becomes older, verbal interactions are increasingly required, especially in school. When seen for a mental status examination or psychological interview these children are passive and avoid or ignore any overtures designed to get them engaged in conversation; they usually comply with directions or requests for nonverbal performance.

Case Illustration: Priscilla was a five-year-old kindergarten student who seemed shy upon entering school but complied easily with all requests from her teacher. After several weeks the teacher observed that she never spoke to the other children and managed to comply with nods and shakes of the head to most interactions. In a parent-teacher conference Priscilla's mother described her as shy, but said she did talk "some" at home. No other symptoms were noted.

Prevalence, Sex, and Familial Considerations

Elective mutism is rare, being found in significantly less than 1 percent of clinical populations referred for emotional problems. No epidemiological studies have been done on this disorder recently, but in the early 1950s two different studies found its prevalence in clinics to be from

0.2–1 percent (Morris, 1953; Salfield, 1950). A therapist may never see a child with elective mutism, although refusal to speak as an aspect of other disorders is common. The disorder is more frequent in girls than boys, although the small number of cases makes this finding somewhat uncertain. No evidence of a familial pattern has been found, and siblings are almost never affected.

Children who develop elective mutism usually do so prior to age five, although the disorder may be minimized until the child reaches school age. Until then, the parents and relatives may merely ascribe the child's refusal to talk to shyness, especially if the child does talk to one or more individuals within the immediate family. Pediatricians often do not diagnose the disorder when given this history since many children, especially those with older siblings, have delayed or decreased speech as a result of either being overwhelmed in conversation or because their responses are anticipated by older siblings.

Elective mutism is most common in young children, but there are reports of its initial occurrence among adolescents. In adolescence onset the refusal to speak is more extensive (includes both strangers and family members) (Kaplan & Escoll, 1973).

Treatment

While viewed by some clinicians as a neurotic disorder (Silver, 1980), elective mutism has no accepted etiology. Thus, its categorization as a neurosis, especially if strict analytic criteria are accepted (Nagera, 1966), is questionable. Family dynamics have been elucidated in several studies (Adams & Glasner, 1954; Browne, Wilson, & Laybourne, 1963; Pustrom & Speers, 1964), but no pattern of conflict has been statistically established. Marital conflict is a frequent finding in families of such children, and pressures on the child to form alliances with a particular parent are often seen. Other theorists have concluded that conflicts with control or authority are predominant (Loomie, 1961; Browne et al., 1961) or that the basis is unresolved oral dependency conflicts (Parker, Olsen, & Throckmorton, 1960). Other therapists have conceptualized the problem in terms of differential reinforcement patterns within the family or as a product of anxiety avoidance (Reed, 1963; Shaw, 1971). Overall, however, there is no accepted explanation.

Treatment ranges from individual psychodynamically oriented psychotherapy (Chethik, 1973; Silver, 1980) to family therapy (Pustrom & Speers, 1964) to behavior therapy (Shaw, 1971). Only outcomes with individual cases are available, and this evidence suggests that the disorder does seem to respond fairly well to treatment, especially to a combination of behavioral and family therapy approaches (Laybourne, 1979). Behavioral approaches are reported to work quite well with young children, where careful history taking suggests the behavior has been learned and reinforced, e.g., the parents describe thinking the early signs of shyness and mutism were "cute." In the case of inappropriate parental reinforcement, family therapy with the parents and child, with the focus on altering inappropriate reinforcements and changing the contingencies on the child's behavior, seems effective. Where silence serves the child as a fear reduction mechanism, training the child to be assertive in combination with parental counseling seems to produce good results.

Neurotic Disorders

In DSM-III the term *neurosis* is abandoned, although it is retained in parenthetical form following several diagnoses. This partial elimination of neurosis reflects the atheoretical, descriptive nature of DSM-III and suggests that psychodynamic, and especially psychoanalytic, assumptions have come to define the term. Accordingly, it is important to understand what neurosis means within a psychoanalytic framework. As May (1979) noted, the use of the term neurosis with children requires that there be unconscious conflicts resulting from relatively compromised and unsuccessful attempts to handle sexual or aggressive impulses.

It should be recognized that the prevalence of neurotic disorders is very rare, particularly among children, no matter how one thinks of their etiology.

PHOBIC DISORDERS

The essential feature of phobic disorders (agoraphobia, social phobia, and simple phobia) is fear of a dreaded object or situation which results in a persistent desire, always recognized as irrational by the child, to avoid the object or situation. The possible relationship between agoraphobia and separation anxiety in children has already been discussed, but true agoraphobia, with or without panic attacks, does not usually develop until late adolescence. This disorder is the most common and severe of the phobic disorders.

Simple phobias often begin in early childhood and are thought to be common among untreated populations. They are less severe and disabling than agoraphobia, have a circumscribed stimulus, and a somewhat more favorable prognosis.

Agoraphobia. The essential feature of this disorder is:

> Marked fear of being alone, or being in public places from which escape might be difficult or help not available in case of sudden incapacitation. Normal activities are increasingly constricted as the fears or avoidance behavior dominate the individual's life (DSM-III, p. 226).

If the disorder is accompanied by panic attacks of the type described under the separation anxiety disorders, then the diagnosis becomes agoraphobia with panic attacks.

Prevalence, Sex, Age, and Familial Considerations: While it has been estimated that phobias are found in about 1 percent of the population, outpatient clinic figures suggest they account for 5 percent of all neurotic disorders and that agoraphobia accounts for about 60 percent of phobic disorders (Nemiah, 1980). Females are diagnosed as having this disorder more frequently than males but since the disorder is rarely diagnosed until late adolescence, its prevalence in children and adolescents is extremely low. As previously discussed, precursors of the disorder seem to exist in a subpopulation of those with separation anxiety disorder. Strong familial and genetic factors seem present, and the disorder is usually chronic, although there are often periods of remission.

Case Illustration: Frank was a seventeen-year-old who dropped out of school to join the army. Following successful completion of basic training he was given a two-week leave. Returning to his base after the leave Frank suddenly and without warning experienced a panic attack while driving across a long bridge over a lake. He began to sweat, tremble, and experience shortness of breath. His heart pounded and he thought he was going to lose control of the car and crash through the guardrails. Somehow he made it safely to the other side where he was able to calm himself. Following this incident, Frank began to experience panic reactions on other bridges and took to avoiding them. Because he served his military duty in an area with few bridges, he was able to successfully complete his service duty and was honorably discharged. He had begun to realize, however, that even thoughts of bridges made him increasingly uneasy.

Following discharge as a nineteen-year-old, Frank got a job as an office manager, married, and seemed to be doing well. His company, however, transferred him to a new area which necessitated his travel across two bridges to get to work. Initially he was able to cross the bridges by timing his commutes for the end of the rush hour traffic. After several months, however, he began to increasingly fear the trips to work, stopped going in, and when his "sicknesses" were found to be faked, was fired. In the next several years, Frank lost numerous jobs because he was unreliable about going to work. At the same time he began to develop other fears: tall buildings, long corridors, open spaces, crowded buses, particular rooms at home and at work. Finally even thoughts of these places could precipitate panic attacks and Frank was hospitalized.

Treatment: Frank demonstrates the insidious onset, often in late adolescence, of agoraphobia, as well as the crippling effects of the disorder. Until recently, dynamically oriented therapy and behavior therapy oriented toward desensitization of the phobias were the primary treatment approaches. Clinicians often found these patients developing new phobias as fast as, or faster than, the existing ones could be removed, and some investigators referred to the disorder as *panphobia* and postulated an underlying dynamic of overdependence. The focus of treatment then shifted to assertive training approaches.

Imipramine is an effective method of stopping the panic attacks and with traditional psychotherapy or behavioral techniques, often in conjunction with family therapy designed to gain system support for the patient, constitute the treatment of choice. Until recently the outlook in this disorder was grave, but clinical experiences in the past five to ten years suggest that at least some improvement in functioning can be expected with this combination of treatments.

Social Phobia. Social phobia is essentially a fear of, and wish to avoid, situations in which the person may be humiliated or embarrassed.

Prevalence, Sex, Age, and Familial Considerations: This is an extremely rare disorder, being found in significantly less than 0.5 percent of the population. No information is available on the sex ratio or familial considerations, but it is known that it begins frequently by late childhood or early adolescence and has a chronic but fluctuating course. Rarely is the disorder as severe or disabling as agoraphobia, since the child or adolescent can frequently avoid the anxiety provoking situations. Where this is not possible (e.g., a required public speaking course), the situation can usually be avoided more easily later as an adult.

Therapy with children and adults exhibiting social phobias is most often behavioral, with a combination of relaxation, desensitization, and assertive training techniques. These techniques are relatively effective, although many clinicians

depression. It has been estimated that 20 percent of patients with depressive disorders also show obsessive compulsive symptoms (Nemiah, 1980) and there is further evidence of overlap in the two disorders found in neurobiological and psychopharmacological studies which demonstrate that treatment of obsessive compulsive disorders is sometimes facilitated by administration of a tricyclic antidepressant medication (Thoren et al., 1980a, 1980b.) Jane had no signs of schizophrenia other than the obsessions, which are sometimes seen in the early or prodromal stages of that disorder, and thus the possibility of a psychosis, always a consideration when obsessive-compulsive symptoms are seen, is not likely.

Prevalence, Sex, Age, and Familial Considerations: Epidemiological studies are lacking, but it is felt to be rare, probably being found in significantly less than 1 percent of the population. Nemiah (1980) suggests that the first symptoms of the disorder appear in two-thirds of the patients prior to age 15 and sometimes as early as age 10. Rarely does the disorder begin after age 40. The disorder is thought to be a serious one by clinicians, with impairment from it ranging from moderate to severe. Its course, even though studies of it are rare, is thought to be chronic, with periods of remission or decrease in the symptomatology alternating with periods of acute crisis. Both boys and girls seem to be equally affected, but no conclusions are possible about predisposing or genetic factors.

Treatment: As with most neurotic disorders, psychodynamically oriented therapy has been tried with varying results, but in general psychoanalysis is felt to be relatively ineffective (Hicks, Okonet, & Davis, 1980). When traditional psychodynamic therapy is attempted, the therapist generally tries to uncover and resolve the conflicts resulting from the child's fixation at the anal-sadistic stage of psychosexual development, although this stage is often seen as being a regression from a coexisting oedipal conflict. The typical defense mechanisms seen in this disorder are isolation, intellectualization, undoing, and reaction formation, and the underlying conflicts have to do with both aggressive and sexual impulses, Salzman (1968) has shown that treatment with children and adults exhibiting this disorder has its problems, particularly because of the person's need to be in control and to understand everything at an intellectual level only. Emotions are avoided at all cost. Excessive focusing on details, rapid shifts in ideas, doubts, procrastination, regimentation in behaviors, and intellectualizing make therapy difficult.

Some therapists have used behavioral approaches for obsessive-compulsive symptoms. Specific behavioral techniques such as response prevention and thought stopping (Marks, 1975; Stern, 1970) have been demonstrated to be effective, at least temporarily, with single or focal symptoms, but evidence of significant impact on the disorder is lacking. In addition, it has recently been found that use of tricyclic antidepressants can be an effective adjunct to other forms of treatment, (Thoren et al., 1980a). The success of these medications, however, cannot be explained by ascribing either an antianxiety or antidepressant effect to them, and much further research is needed to clarify how they function.

Somatoform Disorders

This group of disorders includes two disorders (conversion disorder and hypochondriasis) which have typically and historically been conceptualized as separate neuroses and two other disorders (somatization disorder and psychogenic pain) which were previously subsumed under hysteria. The common denominator of all four disorders is the presence of physical symptoms for which no organic basis can be demonstrated. The symptoms are not voluntarily produced as they are in the factitious disorders (DSM-III, pp. 285–290), nor are they false and grossly exaggerated, as in cases of malingering (DSM-III, pp. 331–332).

Conversion Disorder. The most common symptoms of conversion disorder are disturbances in movement (seizures, dyscoordinations, paralyses) and sensations (anesthesia, blindness, tunnel vision, paresthesias). Disturbances can also be found in endocrine and autonomic nervous system functioning.

Case Illustration: Alice was admitted to the adolescent unit of a hospital for evaluation of weakness in her legs which prevented her walking. Complete neurological examination showed sensory and motor nerves to be intact and no organic basis for her disorder could be found. Alice exhibited almost classic *la belle indifference* (lack of concern about the symptom). Both her mother and grandmother suffered from numerous undiagnosed physical complaints, and Alice had a history of frequent school absences with stomach and abdominal upsets. Several weeks prior to the onset of her "weakness," Alice's boyfriend had attempted to fondle her breasts. She felt guilty about this and refused to see or talk to him for several days. On the ward Alice rode her wheelchair and interacted with all the other adolescents and was a model patient. In physical therapy she was uncooperative, even though she adamantly claimed she was exercising as best she could. On one occasion, while accompanying the staff psychologist to her office, which usually took twenty to thirty minutes for the short walk, often with clutching of the wall for support, an elevator door started to close on her as she slowly got off. Without apparently noticing the door, Alice quickly moved the two or three steps necessary to avoid being hit by the door, and then resumed her painfully slow walking. Under hypnosis she was able to walk normally.

From an analytic view, neurotic disorders afford two major advantages to these patients: primary and secondary gains. *Primary gains* refer to the benefits the patient derives by keeping an internal need or conflict out of awareness. Conceptualized from a psychoanalytic perspective, the conversion symptoms are a compromise between impulses, almost invariably sexual, seeking discharge and the defense mechanisms, primarily repression, keeping them from being expressed. These repressed impulses are then converted into physical symptoms when the mechanism of repression begins to fail. The particular symptom is thought to symbolically represent the forbidden ideas or impulses. Thus, in this case, the difficulties in walking symbolically represented the conflict and a compromise between repressed impulses to engage in prohibited sexual behavior and the means of avoiding these impulses without becoming aware of them.

Secondary gains refer to the benefits the patient gets from environmental concern and support. The "illness" brings the patient much attention, care, and solicitude, all of which may reinforce the symptoms and make treatment difficult. This is what behaviorists call secondary reinforcement.

Prevalence, Sex, Age, and Familial Considerations: Most clinicians suggest that conversion disorder is rare today, although it is often seen in times of extreme stress, such as natural disasters and warfare. In adolescents, the group in which onset is most common, precipitating stresses frequently involve sexual and interpersonal conflicts typical of the developmental concerns at this age. There is little research information on the typical course of the disorder or on predisposing or familial conditions, but clinicians report cases which range from relatively brief, transitory symptoms to manifestations of symptoms that become stable and are resistant to all forms of treatment. Slater (1961), in the only moderately well documented outcome study of the disorder, found a 50 percent recovery rate within one year, but also found 30 percent of the patients with some symptoms five years later and 20 percent with symptoms lasting beyond fifteen years. Clinicians also report that females are seen with this disorder more frequently than males, but no systematic studies have confirmed these impressions.

According to Adams (1979) children with conversion disorders have five clinical features which are seen with some consistency: an enchanted world view, extreme expressions of emotion, increased suggestability and identification, disturbed sensory-motor functions, and altered consciousness. The enchanted world view is frequently evident in the child's magical, more infantile view of the world as compared with peers. Problems are solved by the child with imaginary, unrealistic solutions bearing no relationship to reality. These children are also highly dramatic, flamboyant in the expression of emotion, and tend to view the world as centering around them. Their increased suggestability is seen in exaggerated conformity to peers' ideas and behaviors and a tendency to imitate, mimic, and develop the illnesses or symptoms of friends and relatives. The disturbance in sensory-motor functioning has already been discussed. Finally, Adams suggests that many of these children and adolescents show a marked indifference to their surroundings and in extreme form sometimes display a loss of reality involvement which approaches that seen in psychosis. One of the most striking examples of these characteristics was shown by a sixteen-year-old male who, when his older sister became pregnant, developed morning sickness and abdominal pains, gained approximately 25 lb, and went into labor when she did, all the while being relatively unconcerned about his symptoms or others' concerns for him. Following the birth of his sister's child, the symptoms abruptly ended and he apparently resumed his normal activities and relationships with peers.

Therapy: Since conversion disorder is rare in children, little has been written about its treatment. Hypnosis and hypnotherapy have been used successfully (Gardner & Olness, 1980). Some therapists have reported successful interventions utilizing psychoanalysis and some a combination of family therapy and hypnotherapy (Sarles, 1975). In general, however, little is known of the natural course of the disorder, although it is often thought to last for only relatively short periods. Little research knowledge is available to safely allow comparisons among various therapeutic techniques.

Somatization and Hypochondriasis Disorder. These two disorders are discussed together because of the apparent similarity of the surface behaviors, though in DSM-III it is assumed that the two are distinct disorders with subtle but significant differences. In somatization disorder there is a far greater variety of physical complaints and, in general, most of the patients who develop the disorder do so in the early to mid-teens and only rarely in the early twenties. Hypochondriasis, while it can develop as early as adolescence, generally has an onset in the thirties or forties and has fewer, although at times more vague and diffuse, symptoms than somatization disorder.

In previous nomenclatures somatization disorder was lumped with other disorders under the term hysteria, but early research by Briquet (1859), Savill (1909), and Purtell, et al. (1951) led to later studies (Perley & Guze, 1962; Guze and Perley, 1963; Guze, 1967, Guze et al., 1971a, 1971b; Woodruff et al., 1974) indicated its distinctiveness. The complaints of patients with somatization disorder are often vague and imprecise, cover a multiplicity of body organs, and are presented in an exaggerated, dramatic, exhibitionistic manner.

Case Illustration: Melissa was a thirteen-year-old admitted to the hospital with complaints of pains in almost all joints, headaches, nausea, vomiting, diarrhea, painful menstruation, and dizziness. Whenever she would discover what another adolescent's symptoms and diagnosis were she would develop those complaints herself. Prior to her hospitalization she had numerous physical workups and examinations, all of which were negative. During examinations she was petulant and demanding, and if she detected doubts about her symptoms in the physicians, she would become openly angry.

As noted in this case, multiple physical complaints are essential, and the criteria for the diagnosis require at least fourteen separate symptoms for females and twelve for males. The child need not actually have experienced the symptoms; complaining of the symptom is sufficient.

With hypochondriasis, on the other hand, the essential feature is:

> a clinical picture in which the predominant disturbance is an unrealistic interpretation of physical signs or sensations as abnormal, leading to a preoccupation with the fear or belief of having a serious disease (DSM-III, p. 249).

Case Illustration: Joan was a nineteen-year-old who was referred because of a fear that she had cancer of the heart and brain. Despite constant reassurances and numerous medical examinations, she continued to be preoccupied with this concern, to the extent that she had become seriously depressed and had failed to graduate from high school. Her insistence on the presence of the disease was based on what she described as "strange" feelings in the chest and head, accompanied by what she was convinced were abnormal heart beats which she could feel. Periodic diarrhea was also interpreted as a sign of the cancer. No evidence of thought disorder in her thinking could be found.

As can be seen from this description, the symptom picture in hypochondriasis is similar to that of somatization disorder and many clinicians are not at all certain that distinction between the two is warranted (Nemiah, 1980).

Prevalence, Sex, Age, and Familial Consideration: The prevalence of both disorders is extremely rare, the suspected prevalence of somatization disorder being less than 1 percent of the female clinic population and even more rare in males (Woodruff, 1974). Hypochondriasis is also rare, accounting for about 1 percent of the psychiatric population of women, and of course much less than that in the general population (Kenyon, 1964). Again females seem to outnumber males with this disorder (Bianchi, 1973; Kenyon, 1966) in spite of the claim in DSM-III of an equal distribution between the sexes. There is evidence that somatization disorder runs in families (Guze et al., 1971b); it appears that about 20 percent of first degree female relatives share these symptoms. Even more interesting is the frequency of confirmed diagnoses of antisocial personality disorder and alcoholism in male relatives of females with the disorder. No information on genetic or familial factors is available for hypochondriasis, although it is felt that either exposure to a real disease or to relatives with diseases may predispose one to the disorder through the mechanisms of identification or modelling.

Treatment: Both disorders are highly resistant to treatment and the course of each is thought to be chronic with some periods of remission. Some writers (Kenyon, 1964) believe that hypochondriasis is always part of some other syndrome, usually one of the affective disorders, and that fewer than 20 percent of these patients improve even after intensive therapy. Roth et al. (1972) found that when depressed patients had significant hypochondriacal symptoms, the generally favorable course for affective disorders was not seen, and a high proportion either failed to improve or became worse.

There is little agreement about etiology, and Nemiah (1980, p. 1541) suggests it would be best: "to view all the theoretical explanations of hypocondriasis with cautious reservation. They have been constructed from observations made on a small number of patients who are generally limited in their ability to reveal the kinds of psychological introspections on which psychodynamic formulations must be based and tested."

Psychogenic Pain. In psychogenic pain the clinical picture is one in which there is complaint of pain which has no apparent physical basis. This disorder was also previously subsumed under the broad category of hysteria, and early research suggested that pain was a prominent symptom in one-half to two-thirds of patients formerly diagnosed hysteric (Purtell, Robins & Cohen, 1951; Stephens & Kamp, 1962). Pinsky (1978) suggested that rather than the traditional neurotic conflict between expression and repression of impulses, the major problem in these patients lies in an inability to experience and express feelings; this leads to the production of somatic pain rather than anxiety under the stress of external events.

Case Illustration: Brian, a ten-year-old, was hospitalized for severe pain on the soles of both feet. He usually rode in a wheelchair but would, with great difficulty, use crutches if his feet were either padded with several pairs of socks or thick bandages. Physical workups, including neurological evaluation, were negative, and the pain distribution was inconsistent with the anatomic distribution of nerves to the foot. Under hypnosis Brian could walk with no discomfort and he was taught self-hypnosis to control pain, as well as given post-hypnotic suggestions for gradual decrease in the pain. The psychosocial stressor involved in his symptoms seemed to be the recent separation of his parents and the necessity of moving in temporarily with relatives he did not like.

Prevalence, Sex, Age, and Familial Considerations: No systematic studies of the prevalence of this disorder exist, but clinical experience, particularly in general hospital and pediatric settings suggests that it is probably common. The pain can develop at any age, and there is some clinical evidence that the disorder is more frequent among females. There is also abundant clinical evidence from family histories that the patient's family members are more prone to illnesses, including those with pain, than are people in general, suggesting a strong modelling effect in the etiology of the disorder. None of these findings are based on well-designed, replicated studies, however.

Treatment: Psychonalytically oriented therapists suggest that the disorder is "notoriously difficult" to treat (Nemiah, 1980), but other clinicians (Gardner & Olness, 1981) have found hypnotherapy and hypnosis to be quite effective, especially with young children. In fact, other than some of the writings by clinicians using hypnotherapy, little else is known about the treatment of psychogenic pain as a specific disorder. Other therapeutic approaches are similar to those used in the treatment of hypochondriasis and somatization disorder.

THE DISSOCIATIVE DISORDERS (HYSTERICAL NEUROSIS, DISSOCIATIVE TYPE)

The four disorders in this group of disorders—psychogenic amnesia, psychogenic fugue, multiple personality, and depersonalization disorder—are extremely rare conditions but are occasionally reported in children and adolescents. The essential feature of *psychogenic amnesia* is an inability to recall important information about one's life and past; this comes on suddenly and unexpectedly, usually in response to some stress. In *psychogenic fugue,* not only is recall of important events lost, but in this condition the patient suddenly travels away from home or work setting and assumes a completely new identity. *Multiple personality* is the most severe form of alteration in the integrative functions of a person, and is a state in which the person has two or more completely distinct personalities, only one of them dominant at a time, but each having its own memories, social relationships, patterns of behavior, and life style. The transition between personalities is sudden, and each one may be unaware of the others. Finally, in *depersonalization disorder* the person experiences the body with a sense of unreality and may even feel that the hands or legs or head have changed in size. The sense of being outside oneself as an observer or of being in a dream state are common.

Case Illustration: Joe was a sixteen-year-old who was in therapy because of poor interpersonal relationships. During treatment he began to have fainting spells and was hospitalized for a complete evaluation, which produced no answers to the fainting spells. Two weeks after his discharge Joe was arrested, naked and riding a horse to the emergency room of the hospital where he had been evaluated. He had traveled 15 miles, but had no memory of getting the horse, the ride, or what he was trying to accomplish. More episodes of fugue behavior followed over the next several months. Under hypnosis, Joe could recall the events of the fugue state, but could not integrate these events when not hypnotized.

Prevalence, Sex, Age, and Familial Considerations. As noted, all these disorders are extremely rare and little of a scientific nature is known about them. No information exists on familial patterns in any of the disorders, although in amnesia and fugue disorders the presence of psychological stressors is a frequent finding. Typically the disorders first appear in adolescence, although some clinicians speculate that at least some of the personalities in the multiple personality are elaborated during childhood. Depersonalization, in a very mild form, is also thought to be common in about 50 percent of the population at some time during life, usually in adolescence (Nemiah, 1980).

Treatment. Little attention has been given to the various dissociative disorders by analytically oriented theorists, but it is thought that the major defense mechanism is repression, as in many other neuroses, though on a broader scale than in the other disorders. Since dissociation is also linked to the traditional analytic discussion of hysteria, the major focus of repression involves oepidal conflicts. Yet psychoanalysis is not highly successful in treating dissociation and in "more than half the cases it tends to be a long-lasting, chronic condition" (Nemiah, 1980).

The writings on multiple personality (Sizemore & Pittillo, 1977; Thigpen & Cleckley, 1957; Schreiber, 1974) suggest that the disorder is an extremely difficult one to treat. Some clinicians even question whether the disorder is not a psychosis. Behavioral approaches to treatment of dissociative disorders are almost nonexistent, but where they are attempted, they focus on one or two isolated symptoms.

Anxiety in General

With the exception of oppositional disorder, in which anxiety plays a minor role, the other disorders in this chapter are thought by most theorists to involve anxiety. Two major theoretical approaches to the understanding of anxiety are the psychoanalytic and the behavioral. In addition, research findings in the neurosciences and psychopharmacology have raised questions about anxiety. A brief description of these three areas follows.

Psychoanalytic Approach

Psychoanalysis assumes that instinctual drives of a sexual or aggressive nature continually seek discharge in thought and behavior, but ordinarily societal pressure, incorporated into the personality during the phallic stage of development as the superego, utilize the ego and its various defense mechanisms to keep these urges from being expressed. As the urges continue to seek discharge, however, and especially when the primary defense of repression is weakened or begins to fail, fear of the consequences of expression of the impulse causes the state of tension called anxiety. This anxiety acts as a signal of danger and brings into play stronger attempts at repression, or if these fail, other defense mechanisms which allow the impulses to be expressed in disguised or compromise form (symptoms). Freud utilized the term *actual (Aktual) neurosis* to describe neurotic conflicts in which the only defense mechanism is repression. The three actual neuroses are the anxiety reactions, hypochondriacal reactions, and reactive or neurotic depression.

The perception of danger is first experienced by the infant at birth, when stimulation seems uncontrolled and overwhelming (primary anxiety). Later, similar types of anxiety arise, resulting from attempts to discharge sexual or aggressive impulses and to seek immediate gratification of needs, such as hunger, thirst, elimination, and so on (secondary anxiety), which also seem overwhelming. Modern analytic writers (Compton, 1980) tend to believe anxiety results when repressed impulses continually seek to attain consciousness or discharge, and an excessive amount of internal drive and/or external (environmental restrictions) exist; thus there is an insufficient discharge of instincts. This situation produces a "dammed-up state" and anxiety is experienced because the tension is not relieved. If this persists, the individual becomes extremely tense, irritable, and restless, that is, anxious.

In anxiety disorder, whether of childhood or in general, there has been a regression to the phallic stage of development and oedipal conflicts are significant. The anxiety associated with partial breakthrough of the impulses either becomes partially conscious (cognitive symptoms) or is expressed through the autonomic nervous system (physiological symptoms).

Panic attacks are a partial failure of the repressive defenses, and this sudden discharge of affect results in a temporary reduction in the tension of the dammed-up state that was being experienced. Repeated and chronic assaults on the defense system of repression, however, may result in a "pyramiding of defenses" (Levitt, 1980). The original defenses are weakened and each new partial breakthrough of impulses creates further anxiety which then requires elaboration of further defenses, often more primitive and less effective ones, such as denial, a distortion of reality in which the child or adolescent insists something does not exist. The result is deterioration of functioning and increasing susceptibility to further breakthrough of impulses, and thus to development of even greater anxiety.

Much of the empirical research of analysts with children's and adolescents' anxiety has involved the question of when the first signs of anxiety in infancy are observable (Benjamin, 1961; Spitz, 1959, 1965). Spitz felt that precursors of anxiety could be detected within the first month of life and consisted of extremely brief, diffuse reactions to various stimuli, but that anxiety itself was undetectable at this point. Between the second and sixth months, however, reactions could be detected when the mother would leave, which Spitz decided were definite fear reactions. Finally, in the second half of the first year, it was felt that the fear of strangers (stranger anxiety) noted in many children were the first unambiguous signs of anxiety itself.

After a series of studies utilizing both animal and human subjects, Thompson and Grusec (1970) proposed a stage which extends approximately from the sixth month through the second year of human life, and includes overt signs of fear such as stranger anxiety, fear of being left by the parent, development of nightmares, and fears of the dark, as well as what Thompson called phobias. Although May (1979) points out that most analytically oriented clinicians and theorists do not report seeing phobias or any full-blown neurotic symptoms of anxiety at least until school age, behavioral indications of anxiety are often seen in children much younger. These findings suggest that anxiety, as analytically understood, normally occurs and may be observed in early childhood.

Behavioral Approaches

One of the persistent problems for behavioral researchers has been the lack of significant correlations between the three major components of anxiety—subjective reports, autonomic arousal of both surface and internal physiological systems, and apparent behaviors. These theorists agree that these three domains constitute the complete response side of anxiety, but the consistent finding has been of low or zero correlations between these measures (Rachman & Hodgson, 1974). People may look calm and feel anxious, and vice versa. It is generally conceded today that individuals are unique in their patterns of reponses across the verbal, physiological, and behavioral dimensions and that their individualized patterns are susceptible to learning (Lacey & Lacey, 1962).

Initially the question of how anxiety is acquired was thought to be sufficiently answered with a Pavlovian classical conditioning paradigm, such as the model Watson and Rayner (1920) developed. Later research cast doubt on this model when it was discovered that not all stimuli were equally likely to become conditioned to an unconditioned stimulus. Seligman (1971) proposed a biological predisposition for becoming conditioned based on the survival value of what it is that may be conditioned. Later researchers (DeSilva, Rachman, & Seligman, 1977) have disputed what has been called the "preparedness model," at least as a generally applicable principle.

Persistence of fear responses has been extensively explored from a behavioral perspective. Mowrer (1947) proposed a *dual-process theory* to explain the persistence of certain anxiety behaviors. The first process consisted of classical conditioning in which a conditioned (conditional) stimulus becomes associated with shock, and presumably fear. Fear then motivates escape and avoidance behavior through an operant paradigm, in which the avoidance or escape responses are reinforced by the reduction in fear which occurs when escape or avoidance is attained (the secondary process). As an explanation for ritualistic behaviors, like compulsions, the paradigm seems to provide a workable model for designing a treatment program. Bandura (1977) has cast doubt on this paradigm by pointing out that the autonomic reactions associated with fear take longer to develop than the overt avoidance response, thus undermining the explanation that an autonomic response (the fear reduction) reinforces the avoidance response. In addition, other researchers found that obliteration by surgery of the feedback mechanisms involved in fear does not prevent acquisition of avoidance responses (Rescorla & Solomon, 1967), and the avoidance responses are maintained even when the fear reduction (the physiological response) cannot occur (Bolles, 1972).

Reconceptualization of the reinforcing nature of the response and the stimulus situation in the operant paradigm so that stimulus properties of the environment become discriminative stimuli for reinforcement (Bootzin & Nicassio, 1978), as well as research into cognitive variables such as the predictability of consequences and controllability of consequences (Weiss, 1977), have shown that people do acquire emotional responses to symbolic cues such as images, languages, observations of models, and the predictability of the likelihood of punishment or reward. This research has reawakened interest in the cognitive processes underlying the learning of anxiety responses.

In summary, several behavioral paradigms now seem necessary to explain the acquisition, maintenance, and removal of anxiety responses, and no one behavioral theory is adequate to explain all the data available on these three areas of anxiety research (Bootzin & Max, 1980). Increasingly, behavioral models are utilizing cognitive theories and developing cognitive approaches to therapy (Meichenbaum, 1977) which help patients identify, focus on, and change anxiety-producing statements.

The Neurosciences Approach

Levitt (1972, 1980) has consistently pointed out that physiological explanations remain inconclusive despite intriguing and often seeming breakthroughs, primarily because of the extreme methodological difficulties in this area of research (Buss, 1961). And yet to be unaware of the major advances of the 1970s in the study of anxiety in the neurosciences is to ignore an area of research which promises to propel psychological theorizing, currently relatively stagnant in both its psychodynamic and behavioral manifestations, into a new era of development.

In neurochemistry the basic paradigm has involved isolating and describing the functions of various central nervous system (CNS) neuroregulators and correlating these neurotransmitters with both normal and abnormal behaviors. The two most extensively studied neurotransmitters in anxiety research have been the catecholamines (Norepinephrine and Dopamine) and the indoleamines (seratonin).

Recent discoveries of control of behavior, particularly pain responses, through endogenous (normally occurring) opiate-like substances in the brain, such as the endorphins and enkephalins, also seem to have potential for further behavior research into anxiety (Goldstein, 1978). Amino acid neurotransmitters, such as clycine and gamma-amino-butyric acid (GABA), are also being investigated (Aprison, 1977), and the interaction between neurotransmitters and the neuroendocrine systems is beginning to yield promising results (Kizer & Youngblood, 1978). In addition to noradrenergic system correlations with anxiety and stress, other researchers have found relationships with lactate (Pitts & McClure, 1967; but cf. Grosz & Framer, 1972) and also with the beta-receptor sites in the peripheral nervous system which mediate the physiological changes—pallor, flushing, heart rate, etc.—correlated with anxiety (Jefferson, 1976; Gottschalk, Stone, & Goldine, 1974). Interactions of the nonadrenergic system and the opiate receptor systems (Extein et al., 1979) have also led to further findings that elucidate the complexity of this area of research and afford greater knowledge of brain sites (locus coerulus) involved in the production and inhibition of anxiety.

One of the enduring controversies has been whether anxiety is primarily a peripheral or central response. In the psychological literature, this controversy is expressed in the James-Lange and Cannon-Bard theories of anxiety. Briefly, James and Lange, independently in 1884 and 1885, proposed that anxiety consists of the individual's perceptions of the physiological changes in the body brought about by an exciting stimulus. In the 1920s, the physiologists Cannon and Bard showed that emotional responses could occur in animals in whom all autonomic reactivity had been surgically removed. They proposed that the physiological reactions and the emotional experience were simultaneously mediated by the thalamus and hypothalamus. Later, Papez and MacLean showed that the limbic system was definitely involved with emotional expression and control. Thus, the question was: Did the feeling of being anxious cause physiological changes or did physiological changes produce the anxiety?

Studies using propanolol, which blocks beta-receptor sites in the peripheral nervous system, have suggested that "basal or resting" anxiety can be reduced peripherally, but that acute anxiety is mediated centrally (Gottschalk, Stone, & Goldine, 1974). These findings suggest a distinction between *trait anxiety*, the propensity to feel anxious, and *state anxiety*, a momentary condition (Spielberger, 1966, 1972) and that there are separate peripheral and central neurochemical mediators for the two different anxieties. Future research may uncover more varieties of anxiety (McNair & Fisher, 1978).

Izard (1972, 1977) recently conceived

of anxiety as a complex of emotions. Anxiety in his scheme always consists of fear plus two or more other states like guilt, disgust, etc. At this point, little research has been produced based on his theory of differential emotions, but it seems that a multidimensional model similar to this one will eventually need to be developed to account for all the complexities of anxiety being discovered through neurobiological research.

REFERENCES

Adams, M., & Glasner, J. Emotional involvements in some forms of mutism. *Journal of Speech and Hearing Disorders*, 1954, *19*, 56–69.

Adams, P. Psychoneurosis. In J. D. Noshpitz (Ed.), *Basic handbook of child psychiatry* (Vol. II). New York: Basic, 1979.

American Psychiatric Association. *Diagnostic and statistical manual* (3d ed.). Washington, DC: American Psychiatric Association, 1980.

Aprison, M. H. Are some amino acid neurotransmitters involved in psychiatric disorders? In E. Usdin, D. A. Hamburg, & J. D. Barclas (Eds.), *Neuroregulators and psychiatric disorders*. New York: Oxford University, 1977.

Bandura, A. Modelling approaches to the modification of phobic disorders. *International Psychiatric Clinics*, 1969, *6*, 201–223.

Bandura, A. Self-efficacy: Toward a unifying theory of behavioral change. *Psychological Review*, 1977, *84*, 191–215.

Benjamin, J. D. Some developmental observations relating to the theory of anxiety. *Journal of the American Psychoanalytic Association*, 1961, 9, 652–668.

Bianchi, G. N. Patterns of hypochondriasis: A principle component analysis. *British Journal of Psychiatry*. 1973, *122*, *(570)*, 541–48.

Bolles, R. C. The avoidance learning problem. In G. Bower (Ed.), *The psychology of learning and emotion* (Vol. 6). New York: Academic, 1972.

Bootzin, R. R., & Max, D. Learning and behavioral theories. In I. L. Kutash & L. B. Schlesinger (Eds.), *Handbook on stress and anxiety*. San Francisco: Jossey-Bass, 1980.

Bootzin, R. R., & Nicassio, P. Behavioral treatments for insomnia. In M. Hersen, R. M. Eisler, & P. M. Miller (Eds.), *Progress in behavior modification*. Vol. 6. New York: Academic, 1978.

Bowlby, J. Separation anxiety: A critical review of the literature. *Journal of Child Psychology and Psychiatry*, 1960, *1*, 251–269.

Briquet, P. *Traité clinique et therapeutique de l'hystérie*. Paris: Baillière et Fils, 1859.

Browne, E., Wilson, V., & Laybourne, P. C. Diagnosis and treatment of elective mutism in children. *Journal of the American Academy of Child Psychiatry*, 1963, *2*, 605–612.

Buss, A. H. *The psychology of aggression*. New York: Wiley, 1961.

Chess, S., *Your child is a person: A psychological approach to parenthood without guilt*. New York: Viking, 1965.

Chethik, M. Amy: The intensive treatment of a elective mute. *Journal of the American Academy of Child Psychiatry*, 1973, *12*, 482–498.

Compton, A. Psychoanalytic theories. In I. L. Kutash & L. B. Schlesinger, (Eds.) *Handbook on stress and anxiety*. San Francisco: Jossey-Bass, 1980.

Coolidge, J. School phobia. In J. Noshpitz (Ed.), *Basic handbook of child psychiatry* (Vol II). New York: Basic, 1979.

Coolidge, J. C., Hahn, P. B., & Peck, A. L. School phobia: Neurotic crisis or way of life. *American Journal of Orthopsychiatry*, 1957, *27*, 296–306.

Coolidge, J. C., Brodie, R. D., & Feeney, B. A ten-year follow-up study of sixty-six school phobic children. *American Journal of Orthopsychiatry*, 1964, *34*, 675–684.

DeSilva, P., Rachman, S., and Seligman, M. E. P. Prepared phobias and obsessions: Therapeutic outcome. *Behavior Research and Therapy*, 1977, *15*, 65–77.

Eisenberg, L. School phobias: A study in the communication of anxiety. *American Journal of Psychiatry*, 1958, *114*, 712–718.

Elson, A., Pearson, C., Jones, D., & Schumacher, E. Follow-up study of childhood elective mutism. *Archives of General Psychiatry*, 1965, *13*, 182–187.

Emmelkamp, P., & Wessels, H. Flooding in imagination vs. flooding in view: A comparison with agoraphobics. *Behavior Research and Therapy*, 1975, *13*, *7–15*.

Extein, I., et al. Behavior and biochemical effects of FK 33-824, a parenterally and orally active enkephalin analogue. In E. Usdin, W. E. Bunney, & N. S. Kline (Eds.), *Endorphins in mental health research*. New York: Macmillan, 1979.

Freud, S. Analysis of a phobia in a five-year-old boy (1909). In *Standard edition of the complete psychological works of Sigmund Freud* (vol. 18). London: Hogarth Press, 1955, 3–149.

Gardner, G. G., & Olness, K. *Hypnosis and hypnotherapy with children.* New York: Grune & Stratton, 1981.

Gilpin, D. C., & Worland, J. Symptomatic oppositionality as seen in the clinic. In E. J. Anthony and D. C. Gilpin (Eds.), *Three clinical faces of childhood.* New York: Spectrum, 1976.

Gittelman-Klein, R., & Klein, D. F. Controlled imipramine treatment of phobic anxiety. *Archives of General Psychiatry,* 1971, *25,* 204–207.

Goldstein, A. Opiate receptors and opioid peptides: A ten-year overview. In M. A. Lipton, A. DiMascio, and K. F. Killam (Eds.), *Psychopharmacology: A generation of progress.* New York: Raven, 1978.

Gotschalk, L. A., Stone, W. N., & Goldine, C. G. Peripheral versus central mechanisms accounting for antianxiety effects of propranolol. *Psychosomatic Medicine,* 974, *36,* 47–55.

Greene, E. L., Langer, T. S., Herson, J. H., Jameson, J. D., Eisenberg, J. G., & McCarthy, E. D. Some methods of evaluating behavioral variations in children 6 to 18. *Journal of the American Academy of Child Psychiatry,* 1973, *12,* 531–553.

Grosz, H., & Farmer, B. B. Pitt's and McClure's lactate-anxiety study revisited. *British Journal of Psychiatry,* 1973, *120,* 415–418.

Guze, S. B. The diagnosis of hysteria: What are we trying to do? *American Journal of Psychiatry,* 1967, *124,* 491–498.

Guze, S. B. The role of follow-up studies: Their contribution to diagnostic classification as applied to hysteria. *Seminars in Psychiatry,* 1970, *2,* 392–402.

Guze, S. B., & Perley, M. M. Observations on the natural history of hysteria. *American Journal of Psychiatry,* 1963, *119,* 960–965.

Guze, S. B., Woodruff, R. A., Jr., & Clayton, P. J. Hysteria and antisocial behavior: Further evidence of an association. *American Journal of Psychiatry,* 1971, *127,* 957–960. (*a*)

Guze, S. B., Woodruff, R. A., Jr., & Clayton, P. J. A study of conversion symptoms in psychiatric outpatients. *American Journal of Psychiatry,* 1971, *128,* 643–648. (*b*)

Hampe, E. Intelligence and school phobia. *Journal of School Psychology,* 1973, *2,* 66–72.

Hersov, L. A. Refusal to go to school. *Journal of Child Psychology and Psychiatry,* 1960, *1,* 137–45.

Hicks, R., Okonek, A., & Davis, J. M. The psychopharmacological approach. In I. L. Kutash and L. B. Schlesinger (Eds.), *Handbook on stress and anxiety.* San Francisco: Jossey-Bass, 1980.

Izard, C. E. *Patterns of emotions: A new analysis of anxiety and depression.* New York: Academic, 1972.

Izard, C. E. *Human emotions.* New York: Plenum, 1977.

Jefferson, J. W. Beta-adrenergic receptor blocking drugs in psychiatry. *Archives of General Psychiatry,* 1976, *33,* 1389–1394.

Johnson, A. M. School phobia. *American Journal of Orthopsychiatry,* 1941, *12,* 702–7111.

Johnson, A. M., School phobia workshop, discussion. *American Journal of Orthopsychiatry,* 1957, *27,* 307–309.

Kaplan, S. I., & Escoll, P. Treatment of two silent adolescent girls. *Journal of the American Academy of Child Psychiatry,* 1973, *12,* 59–71.

Kenyon, F. E. Hypochondriasis: A clinical study. *British Journal of Psychiatry,* 1964, *110,* 478–488.

Kenyon, F. E. Hypochondriasis: A survey of some historical clinical and social aspects. *International Journal of Psychiatry,* 1966, *2,* 308–325.

Kizer, J. S., & Youngblood, W. W. Neurotransmitter systems and central neuroendocrine regulation. In M. A. Lipton, A. DiMascio, & K. F. Killan (Eds.), *Psychopharmacology: A generation of progress.* New York: Raven, 1978.

Klein, D. F., & Davis, J. H. *Diagnosis and drug treatment of psychiatric disorders.* Baltimore: Williams and Wilkins, 1969.

Klein, E. The reluctance to go to school. *Psychoanalytic Study of the Child,* 1945, *1,* 263–279.

Lacey, J., & Lacey, B. The law of initial value in the longitudinal study of autonomic constitution: Reproducibility of autonomic responses and responses patterns over a four-year interval. *New York Academy of Science Annual,* 1962, *98,* 1257–1289.

LaVietes, R. L. Oppositional disorder. In H. I. Kaplan, A. M. Freedman, & B. J. Sadock (Eds.), *Comprehensive textbook of psychiatry* (3d ed.). Baltimore: Williams and Wilkins, 1980.

Laybourne, P. D. Elective mutism. In J. Noshpitz (Ed.), *Basic handbook of child psychiatry* (Vol. 2). New York: Basic, 1979.

Levanthal, T., Weinberger, G., Stander, R. J., & Stearns, R. P. Therapeutic strategies with school phobia. *American Journal of Orthopsychiatry,* 1967, *37,* 64–70.

Levitt, E. E. A brief commentary on the "psychiatric breakthrough" with emphasis on the hematology of anxiety. In C. D. Spellberger (Ed.), *Anxiety: Current trends in theory and research.* Vol. I. New York: Academic, 1972.

Levitt, E. E. *The psychology of anxiety* (2d ed.). Hillsdale, NJ: Lawrence Erlbaum Associates, 1980.

Liebowitz, M. R., & Klein, D. F. Assessment and treatment of phobia anxiety. *Journal of Clinical Psychiatry,* 1974, *40,* 486–492.

Loomie, L. S. some ego considerations in the silent patient. *Journal of the American Psychoanalytic Association,* 1961, *9,* 56–78.

Marks, I. Behavioral treatments of phobia and obsessive-compulsive disorders: A critical appraisal. In M. Hersen, R. M. Eisler, & P. M. Miller (Eds.), *Progress in behavior modification* (Vol. 1). New York: Academic, 1975.

May, J. G. Nosology and diagnosis. In J. D. Noshpitz (Ed.), *Basic handbook of child psychiatry* (Vol. II). New York: Basic, 1979, 111–144.

McNair, D. M., & Fisher, S. Separating anxiety from depression. In M. A. Lipton, A. DiMascio, & K. F. Killam (Eds.), *Psychopharmacology: A generation of progress.* New York: Raven, 1978.

Meichenbaum, D. *Cognitive behavior modification: An integrative approach.* New York: Plenum, 1977.

Morris, J. V. Cases of elective mutism. *American Journal of Mental Deficiency,* 1953, *57,* 661–668.

Mowrer, O. H. On the dual nature of learning: A reinterpretation of "conditioning" and "problem solving." *Harvard Educational Review,* 1947, *17,* 102–148.

Nagera, H. Early childhood disturbances: The infantile neurosis and the adulthood disturbances. *The psychoanalytic study of the child, Monograph, No. 2.* New York: International Universities, 1966.

Nemiah, J. D. Neurotic disorders. In H. I. Kaplan, A. M. Freedman, & B. J. Sadock (Eds.), *Comprehensive textbook of psychiatry* (3d ed.). Baltimore: Williams and Wilkins, 1980.

Parker, E. F., Olsen, T. F., & Throckmorton, D. M. Social casework with elementary school children who do not talk in school. *Social Work,* 1960, *5,* 64–70.

Perley, M. J., & Guze, S. B. Hysteria: The stability and usefulness of clinical criteria. *New England Journal of Medicine,* 1962, *266,* 421–432.

Pinsky, J. D. Chronic, intractable, benign pain: A syndrome and its treatment with intensive short-term group psychotherapy. *Journal of Human Stress,* 1978, *4,* 17–29.

Pittman, F. S., Langsley, D. G., and DeYoung, C. D. Work and school phobias: A family approach to treatment. *American Journal of Psychiatry,* 1968, *124,* 1535–41.

Pitts, F. N., & McClure, J. N. Lactate: Metabolism in anxiety neurosis. *New England Journal of Medicine,* 1967, *227,* 1329–1336.

Prince, G. S. School phobia. In E. Miller (Ed.), *Foundation of child psychiatry.* London: Pergamon, 1968.

Purtell, J. J., Robins, E., & Cohen, M. E. Observations on clinical aspects of hysteria. *Journal of the American Medical Association,* 1951, *146,* 902–909.

Pustrom, E., & Speers, R. W. Elective mutism in children. *Journal of the American Academy of Child Psychiatry,* 1964, *3,* 287–295.

Rachman, S., & Hodgson, R. Synchrony and desynchrony in fear and avoidance. *Behavior Research and Therapy,* 1974, *12,* 311–318.

Redl, R. Oppositional behavior in everyday life. In E. F. Anthony & D. C. Gilpin (Eds.), *Three clinical faces of childhood.* New York: Spectrum, 1976.

Reed, G. F. Elective mutism children: A reappraisal. *Journal of Child Psychology and Psychiatry,* 1963, *4,* 99–107.

Rescorla, R. A., & Solomon, R. L. Two process learning therapy: Relationship between Pavlovian conditioning and instrumental learning. *Psychological Review,* 1967, *74,* 151–182.

Robins, L. *Deviant children grown up.* Baltimore: Williams and Wilkins, 1966.

Robinson, D. S., Nies, A., Ravaris, C. L., et al. The monoamine oxidase inhibitor, phenelzine, in the treatment of depressive-anxiety states. *Archives of General Psychiatry,* 1973, *29,* 407–413.

Salfield, D. J. Observation on elective mutism in children. *Journal of Mental Sciences,* 1950, *96,* 1024–1032.

Salzman, L. *The obsessive personality.* New York: Science House, 1968.

Sarles, R. M. The use of hypnosis with hospitalized children. *Journal of Clinical Child Psychology,* 1975, *4,* 36–38.

Savill, T. D. *Lectures on hysteria and allied vasomotor conditions.* London: Glaisher, 1909.

Schreiber, F. R. *Sybil,* New York: Warner, 1974.

Seligman, M. E. P. Phobias and preparedness. *Behavior Therapy,* 1971, *2,* 307–320.

Shaw, W. H. Aversive control in the treatment of elective mutism. *Journal of the American Academy of Child Psychiatry,* 1971, *10,* 572.

Sheehan, D. V., Ballenger, J., and Jacobsen, G. Treatment of endogensis anxiety with phobic, hysterical, and hypochondriacal symptom. *Archives of General Psychiatry,* 1980, *37,* 51–59.

Silver, L. B. Speech disorders. In H. I. Kaplan, A. M. Freedman, & B. J. Sadock (Eds.), *Comprehensive textbook of psychiatry* (3d ed.). Baltimore: Williams and Wilkins, 1980.

Sizemore, C. C., & Pittillo, E. S. *I'm Eve.* New York: Doubleday, 1977.

Slater, E. Hysteria. *Journal of Mental Sciences*, 1961, *107*, 359–381.

Sperling, M. School phobias: Classification, dynamics and treatment. In R. S. Eissler, et al. (Eds.), *The psychoanalytic study of the child*, Vol. 22. New York: International Universities, 1967, 375–401.

Sperling, M. *The major neuroses and behavior disorders in children*. New York: Jason Aronson, 1974.

Spielberger, C. D. Theory and research on anxiety. In C. D Spielberger (Ed.), *Anxiety and behavior*, New York: Academic, 1966.

Spielberger, C. D. Anxiety as an emotional state. In C. D. Spielberger (Ed.), *Anxiety: Current trends in theory and research*. (Vol. 1). New York: Academic, 1972.

Spitz, R. A. *A genetic field theory of ego formation*. New York: International Universities, 1959.

Spitz, R. A. *The first year of life*. New York: International Universities, 1965.

Stephens, J. H., & Kamp, M. On some aspects of hysteria: A clinical case study. *Journal of Nervous and Mental Disease*, 1962, *134*, 305–15.

Stern, R. Treatment of a case of obsessional neurosis using thought-stopping techniques. *British Journal of Psychiatry*, 1970, *117*, 441–442.

Thigpen, C. H., & Cleckley, H. M. *The three faces of Eve*. New York: McGraw-Hill, 1957.

Thomas, A., Chess, S., & Bireh, H. S. *Temperament and behavior disorders in children*. New York: University Press, 1968.

Thompson, W. R., and Grusec, J. E. Studies of early experience. In P. Mussen (Ed.), *Carmichael's manual of child psychology* (3d ed.). (Vol. 1). New York: Wiley, 1970.

Thoren, P., Asberg, M., Cronholm, B., Lennart, J., & Traskman, L. Clomipramine treatment of obsessive-compulsive disorders: I. A controlled clinical trial. *Archives of General Psychiatry*, 1980, *37*, 1281–1285. (*a*)

Thoren, P., Asberg, M., Bertilsson, L., Mellstron, B., Folke, S., & Traskman, L. Clomipramine treatment of obsessive-compulsive disorders: II Biochemical aspects. *Archives of General Psychiatry*, 1980, *37*, 1289–1294. (*b*)

Waldfogle, S., Coolidge, J. D., & Hahn, P. B. The development, meaning, and management of school phobia. *American Journal of Orthopsychiatry*, 1957, *27*, 754–780.

Waldron, S., Shrier, D. K., Stone, B., & Tobin, F. School phobia and other childhood neuroses: a systematic study of the children and their families. *American Journal of Psychiatry*, 1975, *132*, 802–808.

Watson, J. D., & Rayner, R. Conditioned emotional reactions. *Journal of Experimental Psychology*, 1920, *3*, 1–14.

Weiner, I. B. *Psychological disturbance in adolescence*. New York: Wiley-Interscience, 1970.

Weiss, J. M. Ulcers. In J. D. Maser & M. E. P. Seligman (Eds.), *Psychopathology: Experimental models*. San Francisco: Freeman, 1977.

Werry, J. S., & Quay, H. D. The prevalence of behavior symptoms in younger elementary school children. *American Journal of Orthopsychiatry*, 1971, *41*, 136–143.

Wolpe, J. The systematic desensitization treatment of neuroses. *Journal of Nervous and Mental Diseases*, 1961, *132*, 189–203.

Woodruff, R. A., Jr., Goodwin, D. W., & Guze, S. B. *Psychiatric diagnosis*. New York: Oxford University, 1974.

Zitrin, C. M., Klein, D. F., & Woerner, M. G. Behavior therapy, supportive psychotherapy, imipramine, and phobias. *Archives of General Psychiatry*, 1978, *35*, 307–316.

Zitrin, C. M., Klein, D. F., & Woerner, M. G. Treatment of agoraphobia with group exposure in vivo and imipramine. *Archives of General Psychiatry*, 1980, *37*, 63–72.

CHAPTER 11

Specific Developmental Disorders

David A. Sabatino and Robert A. Sedlak

The purpose of this chapter is to review the diagnostic and treatment considerations associated with six specific developmental disorders and a related disorder, stuttering.

Specific developmental disorders frequently refer to delays or failures in an academic learned performance, i.e., reading, language, and arithmetic. Deficits in these skills are usually assessed by standardized tests. These disorders are rarely isolated, but impact upon other areas of development, particularly those that promote social learning skills, and often occur as secondary or concomitant disabilities to the primary diagnostic categories described on Axis I. Their "treatment" typically requires educational instruction or tutoring in the deficient areas identified.

Diagnostic Classification of Specific DD and Educational Implications

Certainly, one of the most vexing difficulties in working with specific developmental disorder categories is the number of labels used to describe them. For example, a developmental reading disorder may be: dyslexia, academic underachievement, word blindness, word recognition error, sight vocabulary deficit, reading comprehension problem, etc., which is caused by poor teaching, poor parenting, diet, birth order, siblings, brain injury or malfunctioning, cultural linguistic factors, personality factors or emotional blocks, and/or a developmental lag.

Such a plethora of terminology and cause is not immediately helpful in formulating a corrective program for a given child and provides much confusion to students, professionals, and parents. Using the DSM-III system as a referent can help us conceptionally organize this area and suggest a strategy for a treatment plan.

The determination of a specific developmental disorder in the DSM-III system is generally achieved through the use of individually administered, norm referenced tests in reading, arithmetic, language, or articulation. Whether a deficit skill in one of these areas is considered a *specific developmental disorder* is a function of whether or not the degree of the specific deficiency could be explained by the presence of mental retardation, some relatively common sensory impairment in hearing or vision, inadequate schooling, or some blatant interfering disorder. It is when the deficit is greater than would be expected from other known factors that a specific developmental disorder presumably exists.

For example, a child can receive a diagnosis of mental retardation and also evidence deficiencies in reading, arithmetic, and language without being assessed as having a specific developmental disorder. The reason is the level of achievement in these academic and language skills might easily be accounted for by the mental retardation. In a contrasting case, a student could be diagnosed as mentally retarded and also have a deficiency in reading, arithmetic, or language, when the level of performance is significantly less than would be predicted on the basis of the mental retardation alone. A third example could be a seemingly well-adjusted child with normal intellectual ability and a significant deficit in language, reading, or arithmetic development. This child would probably be diagnosed as having a specific developmental disorder with no identified primary causative condition.

In the following sections the terminology, definitions, prevalence, and diagnostically related theory and practices for each of the specific developmental disorders will be discussed; appropriate tests will be mentioned, and where applicable, informal, or clinically sensitive assessment will also be presented.

Developmental Reading Disorder

Definition and Prevalence

Clinical and school psychologists find reading is the most commonly occurring problem associated with academic underachievement. Data on psychological reasons for referral in schools or to child clinics point to "poor reading" as the primary reason (Gillespie & Johnson, 1974), suggesting the potential to learn is normal (normal or above average intelligence) but the actual level of academic achievement is significantly below that potential.

The Department of Education (NCES, 1979) has estimated the prevalance of reading problems at 10–15 percent. That percentage is a bit misleading and controversial for it represents using the first negative standard deviation (−1 S.D. below the mean) on a reading achievement test to define the potential population of poor readers. A more defensible means of classifying reading disorders for prevalence purposes is to differentiate the student's actual academic achievement from the predicted level based upon one or more intelligence tests or subtests. In studies attempting to describe a limited reading population on this basis, two prevalence groups are observed: a seriously impaired group, representing functional nonreaders who are generally classified as learning disabled, representing 1 to 3 percent of the population (Special Study Institute for Specific Learning Disabilities, 1975); and a second group reading one-and-one-half to two-and-one-half years below predicted grade level. That second group reflects an additional and shocking 10–15 percent of the population, except in those studies of inner city black children, where the percentage exceeds 30 percent (Washington, 1973), or in studies of children who are linguistically different, in which case, the prevalence may approximate 50 percent of that school age population (Illinois Commission on Children, 1977)!

Prevalence figures vary depending on the particular definition of reading disorders used. Reading disability formulas represent one attempt to objectify the diagnosis of a reading problem.

Monroe (1932) was one of the first researchers to define reading disability using a formula combining chronological age (CA), mental age (MA), and an arithmetic achievement score. She expressed all three in grade score (grade equivalents) means, and divided them by a common factor of 3 producing an *expectancy reading grade level*, thus deriving an actual *reading quotient.* If the actual reading level was below the predicted reading level by a quotient of .90, a reading disability was established.

Some thirty years later, Bond and Tinker (1967) devised a formula by which *years in school* × IQ + 1 equalled the predicted or expected reading level. Bruninks and Clark (1972), reviewing these two, and other so-called predicted reading formulas, reported that the various formulas produced widely discrepant results for both third and sixth graders; the formulas failed to establish a one- or two-year criterion level deficiency when a reading disability exists.

Additional difficulties in the use of reading formulas were: (1) the low reliability of the reading tests provided unstable achievement test data; (2) the absence of weighting to adjust for increased age with stable reading performance made the formulas totally dependent upon a comparison between mental age and reading level; and (3) numerous socioeconomic, family, and school behavioral responses known to influence the reading process were omitted.

What has resulted from this wealth of ambiguity and urgency is a belief in authority figures in the field, as opposed to empirical, data-based research, directed at attempting to understand the complex social-psychological-biological and educational mosaic which may relate to reading disability. Do all reading disabled children have all symptoms, forming a common syndrome? The answer is no, because in most cases the reading disability itself cannot be viewed as a primary symptom but rather is *an effect* (as opposed to a cause). Is there a single cause for all reading disability, i.e., brain damage, or severe family pathologies, or poor teaching, or intense emotional problems? No. In most cases, reading disability is not even a diagnostic entity. It is a symptom.

Adding to the complexity of the problem, the labeling of the poor school achiever may become the expectancy, setting into motion a self-fulfilling prophecy toward reading, and in turn influencing the learning of reading and related school behaviors. To view reading as a diagnostic entity, isolated from other considerations is an inexcusable diagnostic myopia long associated with remedial instruction.

Rationale of Process Training and Assessment

Cognitive process trait research with reading disabilities is illustrated by studies in which various test authors (e.g., Maslow et al., 1964) have reported high positive correlations between their tests and reading achievement in the early grades. These studies contrast the skills of good readers with poor readers and have identified traits (measured by specific tests such as the Illinois Tests of Psycholinguistic Abilities and the Developmental Test of Visual Perception) associated with subtest deficiencies in poor readers (e.g., visual closure deficits, auditory sequential memory deficits, etc.)

The rationale for remedial training assumes that the subtest deficiency indicates a deficient psychological process blocking a student's progress in learning to read. Remedy of the process should then open the way for the child to learn. However, reading theorists have clearly stated that the reading process is the conversion of visual symbols to language conceptual relationships, each of which have auditory integrative meaning. Thus, every visually perceived letter has a language conceptual meaning, which when sequenced in a particular manner, generates an integrated whole, for which both the letter parts and the word wholes have a corresponding auditory symbolic value, which can be heard or spoken (read).

That definition of reading makes sense logically, but it also suggests the enormity of the task in measuring the assumed cognitive processes of visual and auditory perception, perceptual integration, perceptual and language memory, and receptive and expressive language in the reading process.

The process training issue has been discussed widely in the professional literature (Mann, 1979, 1971; Newcomer, Larsen & Hammill, 1975; Cruickshank & Hallahan, 1975; Hammill & Widerholt, 1973). Sabatino and Miller (1979) have independently contributed to or reviewed the testing procedures and intervention studies of the cognitive process approach versus the traditional academic remedial training approach and concluded that present, inept research using poorly developed training methods offers little definitive support for either training model.

Nevertheless, recent work with known handicapped populations (both EMH and learning disabled children) has demonstrated highly effective results with a social learning-cognitive process approach (Staats, 1968) over traditional academic remediation (Feuerstein, 1979; Sabatino & Striessguth, 1972), and it is that approach we shall next consider.

Cognitive Process and Reading

Verbal intelligence and reading comprehension scores have correlations ranging from the mid-seventies to mid-eighties that are highly predictive. Accordingly there has been a search for consistent relationships between reading deficiencies and intellectual or cognitive skills.

Farr and Anastasiow (1969) and Spache (1976) summarized the research implications of the Wechsler Intelligence Scale for Children (WISC) subtest patterns as follows:

Poor readers perform badly on the information, arithmetic, digit span, and coding subtests.

Poor readers excel in picture completion, block design, picture arrangement, and, in some studies, object assembly subtests.

Witkin et al. (1962) proposed that WISC subtests fall into three major factors that tap relatively independent functions. These factors are: verbal-comprehension (VC), composed of information, vocabulary, and comprehension subtests; analytic-field-approach (AFA), made up of object assembly, block design, and picture completion subtests; and attention-concentration (AC), composed of arithmetic, digit span, and coding subtests. They suggested a factor score approach would offer diagnostic information of importance in understanding learning problems and should replace subtest profiling or verbal-performance scale contrasting.

Similarly, Bannatyne (1971) reclassified WISC profiles into areas of conceptual learning (comprehension, similarities, and vocabulary), spatial learning (picture completion, block design, and object assembly), and sequential learning (arithmetic, coding, digit span). Dyslexic children normally scored highest on spatial abilities, and lowest on sequential abilities. Schwartz (1974) called a pattern of subtests on which learning disabled children scored lowest ACID profiles (an acronym for low scores on arithmetic, coding, information, and digit span).

To make a long story short, early studies to determine a WISC profile characteristic of reading disorders (Burks & Bruce, 1955; Altus, 1956; Pattera, 1963; Robeck, 1964; Birch & Belmont, 1966) showed considerable promise. The results of more recent studies are less encouraging in their efforts to find a single, clear-cut pattern of WISC subtest scores (Anderson, Kaufman, & Kaufman, 1976). Ackerman, Peters, and Dykman (1971) concluded that, "There are not, so far as the authors can determine, any characteristic WISC patterns which single children with learning disabilities out of the school population" (p. 163).

Work with percepto-cognitive traits began as an outgrowth of Gestalt theory. Clinical measurement of visual perceptual development first appeared in 1937 when Paul Schilder and Lauretta Bender attempted to use nine geometric designs as a differential diagnostic procedure to differentiate brain damaged from emotionally disturbed children. That test is the Bender Visual Motor Gestalt Test. It remains one of the most frequently administered tests to ascertain visual-motor perceptual development. Years of research have established that this test is predictive of early failure in learning to read (Koppitz, 1958). However, more recent studies (Koppitz, 1975) have found it to have a negligible relationship to predicted reading achievement among first graders, probably because of its difficulty and low test-retest reliability in the early school years.

The popularity of tests of visual motor perceptual discrimination is related to the continued emphasis on perceptual problems in reading, begun in the 1920s by S. T. Orton. Orton coined the term *strephosymbolia*, or twisted symbol, to denote the reversals and confusion in visual perception of poor readers. Later he advanced his theories of reading retardation to include word-deafness. The search for impairments of the visual perceptual discrimination process as an avenue blockage to reading continues with a proliferation of tests, such as the Bender, the Frostig Developmental Test of Visual Motor Integration, and the Benton Visual Retention Test.

Auditory perceptual diagnosis has always followed that of visual perceptual development, and so has auditory perceptual test development. Wepman (1958) introduced an auditory perceptual test which required children to discriminate between two spoken words, informing the examiner if the two words sounded the same or different. The research on auditory perception generated correlations with reading achievement test performance somewhat higher than visual perception. The relationships found between auditory perceptual tests and reading range from a low of .56 to a high of .83. In fact, Sabatino and Hayden (1970), in a factor analytic study with a group of 472 reading disabled students on twenty-seven test variables discovered that reading comprehension loaded factorially with both visual-motor perception and visual-auditory perceptual integration.

Sabatino and Ysseldyke (1972) reported data resulting from administering visual and auditory perceptual tests under conditions of immediate perceptual discrimination and short-term memory. They found some children with reading problems were unable to discriminate visual perceptual test items, but performed far above normal on auditory perceptual test items. Others were unable to discriminate auditory perceptual items, but performed well on visual perceptual test items. Another group displayed both perceptual discrimination deficits, also having perceptual memory deficits. Their data support the position that reading disabled children have modality preferences (visual or auditory) for receiving instruction. Hence, administration of perceptual tests should assess both visual and auditory perceptual discrimination. In practice, however, that rarely occurs.

In a now classic study, Birch and Belmont (1965) reported the results of a ten-item visual-auditory perceptual integration test with children having known central nervous system pathologies. The data confirmed the reading theorists' belief that reading is a visual-auditory integration task. Although the reliability for the ten-item measure is limited (.62), the integration trait had predictive power for identifying reading (.70) disability populations. Furthermore, it described a population with a plausible visual-auditory integration trait deficit which, upon treatment, would not profit well from reading remediation.

The importance of visual-auditory perceptual integration to reading has been further supported by Senf (1978). Senf recommended calling children with cognitive process deficits *learning disabled*, while referring to those who fail to read at an expected level, but who do not have measurable cognitive process deficits, as *reading disabled*. This recommendation for differentiating between these two populations has more to commend it than most others proposed to date.

In sum, the complexities of reading make it difficult within the current state of knowledge to identify and measure the specific cognitive processes that may detrimentally affect reading, or to know precisely whether treatment of the reading or the cognitive process should follow such a diagnosis. Currently, some tests use the same name for a trait which is measured differently by another instrument, while other tests use different names for the same cluster of test items. The science of the study between cognitive process and reading is still crude and must be refined if it is to yield usable data.

OPERATIONALIZING READING ASSESSMENT

A viable option to the assessment and training of psychological processes is to examine reading as a task that involves different skills. The identification of a child's deficits in one or more of these skills can be parlayed into an individually tailored training program for that child. Some educators and behavioral scientists believe that an applied behavioral analysis, or task analysis, or criterion referenced reading program is all that is required in the diagnosis of a reading disorder for instructional planning. That would be a simplification. In reviewing informal procedures, a complete assessment of any academic disorder includes: a review of educational history; conferences with previous classroom teachers; review of biological data and medical history; review of any previous psychological, clinical, or social agency reports; conferences with parents; further evaluations, using both standardized instruments (Lloyd, 1979; Buros, 1975) and teacher prepared inventories and tests; and classroom observations and conferences with classroom teachers (Reese, 1976, p. 215).

Reese makes the point that rarely is there a problem of having too little diagnostic data. Instead, the problem is to organize and interpret the massive amount of test and observational information. To that end, most academic diagnosticians suggest that reading performance levels be established for symbolic decoding and reading comprehension. Lloyd (1979) organizes informal reading around type of error and description of instructional activity (shown in Table 11-1).

Any reading material, from a silently read passage to graded word lists, can be used in assessment. The principle is to obtain a sample of a student's actual, on-task performance, with instructional materials that increase in graded level of difficulty. Smith (1959) has such a book of passages graded in difficulty. Another aspect of diagnosis may include differentiating silent from oral reading. Zintz (1975) suggests that two graded passages at each level be administered, one for silent and one for oral reading.

If graded passages are unavailable, vocabulary or comprehension materials may be drawn at random from any graded (basic) reading series. The initial presentation should begin well below the word recognition level and continue in sequential steps until the frustration level of the student is reached. Both the examiner and the student should have a corresponding passage so the diagnostician may mark on the one not being read by the student. Most reading task analyses (Bateman, 1967; Englemann & Bruner, 1973) include: (1) *spatial directions*— left to right orientation; (2) *sound-symbol skills*—knowing the sounds associated with printed symbols; (3) *sound blending*—the attending to the sequential arrangements of connected sounds into words, and between words; and (4) *sound matching*—matching sounds to nonalphabetically arranged graphic symbols, and randomly presented graphic symbols to corresponding sounds.

Reese (1976) and Schmidt (1976) examined the reading process and analyzed it into the following logical components:

1. *Letter recognition*—letter-sound (graphic to sound symbol) matching memory for letters
2. *Word recognition*—letters structural analysis
   Sight word vocabulary
   Word meaning vocabulary
3. *Reading comprehension*—recognition of connected words
   Combine words into sentence meaning
   Combine sentences into paragraph meaning

TABLE 11-1

Conventions for Marking Errors in Oral Reading

Type of Error	Description	Marking
Assistance	Examiner had to supply word after 5 seconds	Underline words aided
Hesitations	Learner hesitated at word but examiner did not have to supply assistance	✓Check above hesitated word
Insertions	Learner inserts word not on page	Put in word or word parts with caret (∧)
Mispronunciation	Learner does not accurately pronounce word	Write in learner's "pronoun-shum" (pronounciation) above the missed word.
Omissions	Learner leaves out a word or words and reads on	Circle the omitted word(s) or punctuation
Order reversals	Learner inverts word order	Mark reversals with this symbol: ⊓⊔
Regressions	Learner reads word(s) and then rereads them	Put a wavy line under word(s) repeated
Self-corrections	Learner makes a mistake but corrects it spontaneously	When the learner sc errors *errs* note the mistake and write sc above it
Substitutions	Learner reads one word as another	When the learner substitutes a word underline the omitted word and write in the given one

From a standpoint of assessment time (efficiency) in ascertaining comprehension of main ideas, directions, sequential organization, word and sentence meaning, many of the formal reading tests (Sipay Word-Analysis, Gates-McKillop, Iowa, Wisconsin) are extremely useful. The strategy here is that after the child's particular performance deficits have been determined, appropriate training in deficient reading skills can progress.

Developmental Arithmetic Disorders

Definition and Incidence

There are no published estimates on the number of children or adults who may have a specific arithmetic disorder. However, extrapolating data from Webster (1980) and using a criterion of at least one year below expected grade level in mathematics achievement, almost 11 percent of a learning disabled population in a suburban school system was considered mildly mathematically disabled. Using a prevalence estimate of 10 percent for learning disabilities would mean that approximately 1.1 percent of the school age population have a mathematics disability. Conversations with teachers in the public schools lead the authors to believe that such an estimate might be low.

Bereiter (1963) points out that because of the nature of mathematics, almost all individuals can reach a level of mathematics at which they will fail. Such failures would not be considered specific developmental disorders but would reflect the complexity of mathematics as a science.

Concern for underachievement in mathematics has long been evident in the literature. In 1925 W. J. Osborn published an article entitled *Ten Reasons Why Pupils Fail in Mathematics.* Osborn suggested that the study of individual differences in learners would identify a large number of reasons for failure. Major difficulties for learners were identified as: (1) problems relating to propositions that involve analogies, (2) problems requiring generalization and transfer (3) tasks in which contradictory conditions exists, and (4) problems requiring the student to select and use correct information. More recently the 1977–1978 National Assessment of Educational Progress (NAEP), (Carpenter et al., 1980) drew similar conclusions. The NAEP results indicated that most learners were reasonably proficient at performing single calculations, making measurements, and identifying basic geometric shapes. Greatest difficulties were noted in higher order applications of these skills, including problem solving, estimation, determing the reasonableness of a result, and applying basic skills to everyday situations.

Selected Types of Arithmetical Disorders

Johnson and Myklebust (1967) identified two types of arithmetical inadequacy—those related to other language disorders and those related to disturbances in quantitative thinking (dyscalculia). *Language disorders* interfere with the learning of, or execution of, mathematics because of the difficulty they create in understanding a teacher's oral discussion of the principles, story problems, or spoken instructions. *Dyscalculia* refers to a disturbance in quantitative thinking and calculating not related to the ability to read or write. The condition is characterized by: (1) higher scores on verbal tasks than nonverbal; (2) poor visual-motor integration (apraxia); (3) confusion between left and right; (4) poor body image; (5) deficient visual-spatial organization and nonverbal integration; and (6) low social maturity.

Goodstein, et al. (1971) were the first to identify a problem among mentally retarded students, which they termed a *rote computational habit.* A discrepancy between computational skills and reasoning (solving of word problems) skills of mentally retarded students had been known for some time (Cruickshank, 1948a; 1948b), but the degree of the discrepancy was even greater than that which would be accounted for by the retardation alone or a related reading problem. Goodstein et al. noted that when given word problems in addition which contained extraneous information, retarded learners were unable to screen out nonessential numbers, but rather added all numbers present. This occurred even though the students were able to read all the words in the problems. Sedlak and Schenck (1981), in a study of strategies for correcting this rote computational habit, found that approximately 40 percent of their mentally retarded students exhibited the problem on both addition and subtraction.

Investigators (including Langford, 1974) have found through the use of an oral interview with grade school children that erroneous or incorrect algorithms (mathematical rules) were the major cause of computation inaccuracy. Roberts (1968) studied errors in computation with students whose IQ's ranged from 107 to 140. He classified the errors made into four categories: wrong operation, computational error, defective algorithms, and random response. Even with the most able students (the top quantile), 39 percent of the errors were due to the use of a defective algorithm. Ashlock (1972) pointed out that incomplete formation of the concept may account for the use of defective algorithms. It should be stressed that students were not taught the defective algorithms, but rather developed them on their own, based on their limited understanding of the underlying principles and concepts. Lepore (1974) found that the major underlying difficulty with the use of defective algorithms was place value. An incomplete understanding of concepts or operations would generally be regarded as a teaching related problem. *Improper teaching may be a significant cause of a specific developmental disorder in arithmetic.*

In the early 1960's mathematics instruction changed in focus from pages of rote memorizations and arithmetic calculation to an emphasis on arithmetic reasoning related to the developmental stages of the child (Flavell, 1977). An assumption was made that mentally retarded children could handle stage appropriate mathematical tasks. However, Vitello (1973) noted that a discrepancy existed between MA and the ability to perform class inclusion problems with the mentally retarded. Cherkes (1975) found learning disabled, mentally retarded, and normal MA matched groups performed similarly on concrete mathematical problems, but normals were decidedly accelerated on abstract mathematical concepts.

One of the few longitudinal studies of a handicapped student with arithmetical disabilities was done by Cohn (1971). He described an eight-year-old boy who reversed numerals as "Γ." Yet by age eighteen the boy was able to solve equations such as $3x + 9y = 7$ and $6x + 9y = 8$. From this example then it would appear that an arithmetic disorder may be highly specific to a particular stage in a student's development.

Cherkes (1975); Goodstein, Kahn, and Cawley (1976); and Cawley et al. (1979) have concluded that mathematics is an area quite distinct and distinctive from reading. Indeed, Goodstein, Kahn, and Cawley (1976) have reported that measured intelligence, reading achievement, and arithmetic computation achievement are all stable and independent functions in learning disabled samples, suggesting the necessity for measuring mathematical process and product performance *routinely.*

Mathematical Assessment

There are four differences between reading and mathematics which need to be discussed in order to understand the assessment process. First, reading is a more abstract process than arithmetic. Physical models can be built to illustrate and prove geometric and arithmetical concepts. Arithmetic is basically a concrete and observable discipline. Second, mathematics can be learned through a lifetime and at all levels of educations, even at the Ph.D. level. Reading has a more limited set of skills. After sixth grade much reading instruction focuses only on the acquisition of new words. In mathematics the scope of the curriculum is considerably more extensive (e.g., geometry, algebra, calculus, statistics, etc.). Third, reading cannot be taught in as many ways as arithmetic. In fact, by its very nature, mathematics encourages diverse teaching approaches. Fourth, arithmetic has a structure that is relatively precise. So precise, in fact, that even machines can follow mathematical directions (i.e., computers) without fail, but reading instructions tend to be ambiguous because of the complexities of language (e.g., "they are eating apples"—note: we do not know if the referent for the word "they" is "apples" or a group of people).

The point to remember in examining these differences between reading and arithmetic is that the structures of the two processes are different and, therefore, the approach to assessment needs to be somewhat different.

Determining what to assess and how to measure it are issues facing those who wish to describe mathematical skills. Based upon the information in the preceding segment, mathematics can be separated into two major operations: (1) calculations and (2) reasoning. (Calculations refer to performing arithmetic functions, such as addition, subtraction, multiplication, and division.)

Mathematics assessment is typically ascertained and reported according to the product and process capability of the student. *Product capability* is typically reflected in a grade level equivalency score obtained by correctly completing a certain number of computation problems. *Process assessment* is the difficult task of attempting to detect and describe the mental process where errors are occurring. A number of processes have been isolated, but agreement exists for at least the following:

Basic mathematical functions
Mathematical logic
Familiarity and practice of mathematic rule learning
Related skills (memory, sequency, cognitive capability)

Generally, formal (standardized) norm-referenced tests provide the measures. On the other hand, informal, criterion-referenced observational systems exist in mathematics as they do in reading. Sedlak and Fitzmaurice (1981) make the point that two children could achieve the same test score in grade equivalents, yet miss different problems, and more importantly, obtain incorrect responses for different reasons. These skill deficits must be observed during the working of a problem if assessment is to be descriptive of the process involved in setting a mathematical principal in operation.

STANDARDIZED MATHEMATICS TESTS

The *Key Math Diagnostic Arithmetic Test* (Connally, Nachtman, & Pritchett, 1976) is one of the best known individually administered tests of arithmetic achievement. Criticism of the test (Goodstein, Kahn, & Cawley, 1976; Sedlak & Fitzmaurice, 1981) include: the limited range of items in specific strands, the wide variation in grade level placement for the items, the lack of independence across subtests, and the limited diagnostic nature of the assessment. Although flawed, there does not appear to be another standardized individual test that is any better.

A widely used standardized diagnostic arithmetic test which is group administered is the *Stanford Diagnostic Mathematics Test* (Beatty et al., 1976). Like the Key Math, the Stanford deals solely with the area of mathematics and is not part of a total achievement battery. The major limitation of a test such as the Stanford is the emphasis placed on reading in its administration.

Informal Assessment Systems

Most math diagnostic systems have the following characteristics:

1. Emphasis is on error analysis.
2. It is more important to understand how students solve problems than whether their answers were right or wrong.
3. In the construction of problems, we need to be aware of the problem dimensions and to control for these dimensions when constructing the problems.
4. The patterns of errors displayed by learners are not due to carelessness or to insufficient drill, but rather are conceptual in nature.
5. The absence of a corrective instructional sequence is ineffective and quite possibly harmful (Sedlak & Fitzmaurice, 1981, p. 480).

Ashlock's Diagnostic Model. One method for diagnosing mathematics deficits is to study error patterns made during calculation. Ashlock (1972) claimed that "patterns of error" are a result of not completely understanding the mathematical concept and then applying false generalization principles. He described thirty-three common error patterns covering whole number usage, fractions, decimals, and measurement conversions operations. Two rules in using his system are (1) the complete collection of data before teaching and (2) determining how deficits do occur as patterns. Remediation emphasizes the learning of correct rules and applications. The following points are observed during assessment:

1. Does the child know the purposes of what (s)he is doing—the possible outcomes?
2. Does the child understand the concept being practiced?
3. Are the steps appropriately sequenced?
4. If the concepts are correct, are the procedures also correct?
5. Does the child organize what has been learned into a meaningful frame of reference for future application?
6. Does the child have the capability to estimate plausible answers?

Cawley's Diagnostic Model. Cawley (1975) advocates a two-step informal assessment process with remedial practice constituting the third step.

Step 1–Administration of the Mathematics Concept Inventory: a domain referenced inventory of mathematical skills and concepts. It contains problems in each mathematic domain, with strength and weakness appraisal made for each. The results place a student into a specific lesson at an appropriate entry level.

Step 2–Administration of the Clinical Mathematics Interview, which requires:

1. Completion of a computational task
2. Verbalization by the person of the procedures used to solve the problem
3. Direct observation of the student solving a problem using sixteen different input and response options and studying the similarities and differences in the student's responses
4. Entry into a remedial module compatible with skill and performance levels

5. Re-administration of the Clinical Mathematics Interview

Assessing Severely Retarded. Math skills have a logically fixed order. Severely retarded students learn math skills *in the same order* as nonhandicapped learners, but learn a more limited set of skills. The skills taught should be those that are deemed to be most functional for the environments in which they will live and work. Functional activities related to math concepts are illustrated by the following:

One-to-one correspondence can be assessed by requesting that a student set the table with plates and silverware for four people.
Sets can be assessed through a prevocational task such as sorting bolts, nuts, and washers.
Event-time relationships can be assessed by asking the student, "Is it time for ______?" (lunch, school, recess, etc.)
Numeral-number correspondence can be observed by playing bingo.

The goal of instruction in mathematics for the severely retarded is the functional use of quantitative skills in problem situations. Most recently, educators have been teaching severely retarded learners to use prostheses, such as calculators, to circumvent some of the memory and skill problems associated with mathematical operations in a problem solving setting.

To this end, then, an assessment system of mathematical skills for severely retarded learners should address four areas of concern:

1. Cover the scope of "functional" mathematical skills required in the learner's environment.
2. Assess the skill in the context of its functional use.
3. Demonstrate one skill across materials, tasks, cues, persons, and settings.
4. Vary the response requirements.

Table 11-2 summarizes a listing of suggested functional math-skills. The person doing the assessment should determine if the student has been taught to use a prosthesis (calculator) in the solution of arithmetic problems and assess competence only under those circumstances. For further information on the assessment of

TABLE 11-2

Functional Areas of Math Assessment

1. Sets
2. One-to-one correspondence
3. One-to-many correspondence
4. Equivalence
5. More and less/some and different
6. Conservation of number
7. Numbers
   a. rote
   b. rational counting to 10
   c. numeral recognition
   d. numeral-number correspondence
   e. ordering numerals
   f. writing numerals
8. Operations*
   a. addition
   b. subtraction
9. Time
   a. event time relationships
   b. telling time
10. Measurement
    a. nonstandard
    b. standard
11. Money
    a. coin recognition
    b. coin values
    c. coin equivalencies
    d. counting change
    e. coin usage

*May use a prosthesis such as a calculator.

mathematics skills of the severely retarded, see DeSpain, Williams, and York (1975) or Williams et al. (1978).

Developmental Language Disorder

DEFINITION AND PREVALENCE

Understanding words and speaking them comprise the most common language practice and the one of central focus for any review of language disorders. Marge (1965) defined language as a purposeful act of using sounds, forms, and meanings, together to allow for the human communications of ideas, thoughts, and feelings.

Language disturbances are classified by Wepman (1968) as: (1) *global*, when little or no speech is available; (2) *jargon*, when speech is unintelligible; (3) *pragmatic*, when speech is useful but no context can be detected; (4) *semantic*, when single words, not connected speech units, are used to express substantive language; (5) *syntactic*, when the syntax or grammar is not used correctly to express feelings or the rhythm native to units of organized thought is impaired.

Simplistically, language disorders include the relative inability to express oneself or to understand the expressed thoughts of others. Within the scope of defining language disorders, Irwin (1972), has attacked the traditional schemes of classifying communicative disorders as an unfortunate development. These schemes, he feels, are not consistent with the manner in which they describe a disorder, either in terms of functional (usage) output, or in terms of condition. *Aphasia* is certainly an example. It literally means without speech, and is used to refer to disturbed speech due to brain lesions. However, there is usually *no* evidence of brain pathology, and the term is often used to describe any serious impairment of central language development or any receptive or expressive language disability.

To offset the historic dependence on a primary single descriptor, Marge (1965) proposed classifying language disabilities according to: (1) the failure to acquire any usable language, (2) delayed language acquisition, and (3) acquired (since birth) language disabilities. Hull and Timmons (1966) report prevalence using the above three-part definition in a more refined Type I, II, III classification structure.

Type I— (0.6% prevalence to age four; 0.08% prevalence from age four to twelve) a language disability of children who fail to show any signs of acquiring the language of their speech community at age four, when some language usage is normally achieved;

Type II—(10.8% prevalence) children have developed some language functions but are delayed in their acquisition when compared with peers. This classification includes the hearing handicapped, mild to moderately mentally retarded, a small percentage of children with emotional disturbances, and a majority of children labeled learning disabled.

Type III— (0.25% prevalence) children who have acquired normal language functions, but who then suffer a reduction in the use of their language. Generally, this category refers to children who suffer personality disturbance or a neurological insult. The age of the onset of the language disability and the severity of the disability are the two most significant factors.

In the section to follow we offer a brief discussion of language, proceeding then to review specific language disorders.

What is Language?

Language is a set of systems that have social, neurophysiological, psychological, and temporal requisites which relate auditory sound to symbolic meaning. It is a means of organizing human communication. In language, the users have a set of symbols to represent the things they desire to communicate, and a method (rules) for combining these symbols into coherent statements expressing what they have in mind.

Miller (1981) has listed seven components of the language system which he feels should be studied diagnostically. They are:

1. *Phonology*—assessed articulation proficiency
2. *Syntax*—assessed as sentence form and ordered sequence of language units
3. *Semantic*—assessed as: (a) sentence meaning, (b) case relationship, and (c) conceptual measuring
4. *Language comprehension*—assessed as the ability to comprehend linguistic units receptively
5. *Motor speech production*—assessed as the capability to correctly produce linguistic units
6. *Pragmatics*—assessed as conversational competency in interpersonal communications
7. *Cognitive development*—assessed as the use of communication skills in displaying intelligent behavior

Thus, language can be viewed as a function which involves a grammatical rule learning, intelligence, and the presence of language models. It is impossible to ascertain language development without attempting to determine the richness of the child's immediate language environment and the opportunities for the youngster to give expression through language.

Language development in preschool children clearly illustrates at least nine distinct linguistic states: *babbling,* occurs from 8–12 months; *single words,* at 10–18 months; *chained single words,* at 18–20 months; *two word utterances,* at 19–22 months; *simple sentences,* at 36 months; and *agreement between subject and verb,* at 41–46 months. Language then is a developmentally sensitive means of communicating, using motor speech and other less efficient communication formats to serve in the exchange of thought and feelings. Simplistically, a language disorder may be described developmentally as a breakdown in a specific language learning level. Functionally, the common practice is to report that aspect, either expressive use or receptive use, which is more impaired, though most children with central language disorders have both expressive and receptive language impairments.

Our dependence upon receptive and expressive language requires at least a working definition of these overworked terms. McLean and Snyder-McLean (1978) clarify:

Receptive Language—deriving a speaker's meaning by decoding a heard linguistic stimulus. Comprehension of heard language requires sensory hearing to perceive meaningful units of sound, and also the ability to integrate and associate word meaning with incoming auditory and visual stimuli.

Expressive Language—the ability to encode linguistic stimuli; the actual production of language; what is said by the speaker.

Problems in Assessing Language

The complexity of language has raised more questions than science has yet answered. Schiefelbusch (1972) has listed eight problems in language which merit consideration:

1. Because of the elusive nature of language, deviant language behavior may be recognized implicitly but be difficult to describe explicitly.
2. Theories and models of language frequently ignore developmental issues, as well as the nature of deviant language behavior and development.
3. Theories and models that are explicitly developmental, often do not relate to broader theories in child development and developmental psychology.
4. Theories and models of language behavior and development vary considerably in their descriptions of language learning, their assumptions about the language acquisition process, the extent of linguistic knowledge attributed to the child through the developmental period, and their completeness of explanation.
5. Developmental data are incomplete, fragmented, and often inconsistent, although in a state of rapid change and expansion.
6. Specific tests and procedures assume different theories or models of language behavior and development.
7. Assessment methodology is incomplete and cannot be employed with all children.
8. Approaches to the assessment of language are often not practical in clinical settings because: (a.) they are often time-consuming and cannot be employed with large numbers of children; and (b.) they fail to provide information relevant to programming, i.e., they may provide scores rather than descriptions of behaviors.

It is ironic that the one behavior which is most easily identified as human is one of the most difficult to classify and diagnose. Language includes vocal motor speech, depends upon sensory intake to a large degree for stimulation, and is more than merely hearing and saying words. The child clinical diagnostician has often considered Wechsler verbal and performance scale subtests as if they were descriptive of the totality of the language process. Vocabulary and comprehension subtests have frequently been referred to as measures of language, the implication being they are global descriptors of the encoding (expressive) and decoding (receptive) language processes, assuming the conceptual association referred to as central language.

Intelligence tests examine the construct of academic relationship, operationally assumed to be the capability to learn. One of the most significant behaviors to be learned, and the one which has a 100-year history of maintaining the highest relationship to academic performance, is verbal intelligence. Verbal intelligence as a motor speech process requires language to make it possible. The absence of measurable verbal intelligence in hearing-impaired, autistic, mentally retarded, or brain-damaged children does not indicate that language as a central thought process is also absent.

At present, there are only a few formal tests which describe language production and concept formation developmentally. There is no standardized test to measure the functional performance of language. Currently, language function is studied clinically by sampling speech and analyzing that sample. Siegel (1975) notes,

"Language tests are available as aids to the clinician. They cannot, however, substitute for informal clinical judgment."

Observing Language Behaviors

Clinically, a developmental history which attempts to establish language performance milestones and any unusual changes or influences in language behavior should be done first. School-age children who have completed many of the critical language developmental stages can then be contrasted in language usage to peers and then reviewed for (1) type and amount of verbalization, (2) intelligibility, (3) comprehension of language, (4) relevant and contextual usage, (5) form, and (6) content.

Form includes: types of words used, length of utterances, completeness of sentences, variety of sentences, appropriateness of morphological endings, and other forms of communication (gestures and manual signs). *Content includes:* capability of describing objects, capability of describing events, capability of stating feelings, and capability of describing relationships between objects, events and people.

Histories taken on chronologically and developmentally young, nonlinguistical children include: descriptions of social interactions, descriptions of preferred activities, medical histories, motor skill development, attention to verbal and nonverbal sounds, and span of attention to preferred and nonpreferred activities.

Actual language samples are usually tape recorded, but some direct observational recording charts are also available. Typically, the procedure for obtaining a spontaneous language sample has been to present the individual with some visual material with which to stimulate discussion of a spontaneous variety. Practically all language sampling procedures attempt to obtain a free sample of speech or speech related behaviors. A minimum of sixty words is necessary for many language sampling procedures. The materials used for eliciting language should be age appropriate. An interview/conversation situation may be used with older, bright children.

Practically all language sampling procedures analyze for: vocabulary usage appropriate for age; syntactic structure, reflecting use of phonological and morphological rules; transformational operations or utterance complexity; semantic functions appropriate to the communicative context; communicative intent; and efficiency of language usage in the communicative process. John Muma (1978) described five steps for a basic linguistic analysis:

Step 1: Analyze each utterance in a large language sample (over several circumstances), usually 200–300 utterances. Make notes about the basic sentence types, transformational operations, alternatives or equivalencies within systems, and restricted structures (linguistic systems that evidence child stages).

Step 2: Map out the various functions or purposes the individual attempts to encode or decode. Describe nominal, verbal, adverbial, and adjectival functions, and utterance modes, such as questions, imperatives, declaratives, and negatives. Record the subfunctions within each of these areas (agent, action, object, states, time, place, manner, cause, duration and so on.)

Step 3: Describe the sentence types, transformation operations, and specific constituents.

Step 4: Record any phonemes the individual has difficulty with. Map out coarticulatory influences.

Step 5: Shift communication system commands to infer alternate coding device adeptness.

A linguistic analysis is obviously complex and requires specialized training; once accomplished, a speech therapist would institute appropriate treatment.

Developmental Articulation Disorder

DEFINITION AND PREVALENCE

Diagnostically, the presence of speech sound additions, substitutions, distortions, or omissions in consonant sound production constitutes an articulation disorder *when* it interferes with communication or draws excessive attention to the speaker.

Articulation of speech sounds is a human process associated with the formation and production of words used in communication. Generally, articulation disorders result from neuromuscular incoordination of the speech production mechanism. An explanation of that process would begin with the diaphragm, as it forces air through the vocal folds which then generate either voiced or unvoiced sounds. For example, /S/ is unvoiced while /Z/ is the voiced counterpart of /S/. The principle organs used to shape sound production are midline structures, such as the tongue, palate, upper and lower jaw (teeth), lips, and the vocal folds themselves. As such, the question of which hemisphere provides the neural innervation has been a serious one. Theoretically, either cerebral hemisphere, or both hemispheres, in a struggle for control, could plausibly drive the speech production mechanisms. Hence the theory of laterality, which offers speculation that in some articulation problems, such as stuttering, the two cerebral hemispheres fight for control over the midline speech production structures.

Like language, it is possible to examine speech production both developmentally and functionally. Developmentally, the motor speech production of sounds can be examined against normative data. Functionally, the articulation of speech sounds can be examined in terms of the site of speech production error. Table 11-3 provides the ages at which certain sounds are produced and the functional articulation needed to produce them.

As one might speculate, the presence and severity of articulation disorders are associated with reading, manual motor, visual motor, auditory perceptual, and language development deficits. Therefore, a child with an articulation disorder may have a speech production problem only, reflecting nothing more than a developmental learning phenomenon, or the speech production error may reflect cultural or linguistic factors. Frequently, articulation disorders occur with reading, and other school related social and academic behaviors as a secondary developmental response to a more primary diagnostic entity, i.e., brain damage, mental retardation, mild to moderate hearing problems, and even emotional maladjustment.

Speech disorders represent the highest prevalence rate of any disability in handicapped children, occurring in about 60 percent of known handicapped children. Generally, the prevalence for speech disorders is about 10 percent of the total school age population.

TABLE 11-3

Sound Development

Phoneme	Age of Development[1]	Place of Articulation[2]	Manner of Articulation[3]	Voicing
m	3 yrs.	Bilabial	Sonarant	Voiced
n	3 yrs.	Alveolar	Sonarant	Voiced
ng	3 yrs.	Velar	Sonarant	Voiced
p	3 yrs.	Bilabia!	Stop	Unvoiced
f	3 yrs.	Labiodental	Fricative	Unvoiced
h	3 yrs.	Velar	Fricative	Unvoiced
w	3 yrs.	Bilabial	Sonarant	Voiced
y	3.5 yrs.	Palatal	Sonarant	Voiced
k	4 yrs.	Velar	Stop	Unvoiced
b	4 yrs.	Bilabial	Stop	Voiced
d	4 yrs.	Alveolar	Stop	Voiced
g	4 yrs.	Velar	Stop	Voiced
r	4 yrs.	Alveolar	Sonarant	Voiced
s	4.5 yrs.	Alveolar	Fricative	Unvoiced
sh	4.5 yrs.	Palatal	Fricative	Unvoiced
ch	4.5 yrs.	Palatal	Stop	Unvoiced
t	6 yrs.	Alveolar	Stop	Unvoiced
th	6 yrs.	Linguadental	Fricative	Unvoiced
v	6 yrs.	Labiodental	Fricative	Voiced
l	6 yrs.	Alveolar	Sonarant	Voiced
th	7 yrs.	Linguadental	Fricative	Voiced
z	7 yrs.	Alveolar	Fricative	Voiced
zh	7 yrs.	Palatal	Fricative	Voiced
j	7 yrs.	Palatal	Stop	Voiced

1. Age norms taken from Templin, 1957. Age when 75% of subjects correctly produced specific consonant sounds.

2 & 3. Place and manner of articulation taken from Singh & Singh, 1976.

Developmental Growth of Sound Production

Diagnostically, it is important to recognize that speech sound production occurs in a developmental hierarchy. Beginning with the front of the mouth, bilabial sounds, which occur first and with greater probability of being accurately produced, are followed by labiodental, and finally alveolar and palatal glottal stops. Males and females develop articulation skills at different rates, with boys taking a year longer to develop the full range of skills. In short, speech production errors in a five-year-old male child may not be clinically significant, as the developmental process is yet being learned. Different cultures also have varying requirements for speech sound production, evidenced in the need for particular sounds to produce words basic to a given language. Most readers of this text would have cultural sensitive speech production errors if asked to roll their /r/'s as required for Spanish words. Manyuk (1972) has reported that by the age of three, children have learned which sound combinations are typical of their language.

Functionally, speech clinicians analyze the formation of speech sounds for therapeutic intervention by noting the place and type of articulation error. There is a vast amount of evidence to support the speculation that speech development is dependent upon anatomical development. The relationship between speech production errors where anatomical differences exist also has ramifications for suggesting that academic and other behaviorally related problems may be present. A glaring example is the presence of a sublingual cleft palate, which is difficult to detect upon physical examination. The palate may look fully developed, but its function is restricted and /n/ and /m/ nasal *(hypernasality)* produced sounds carry over into all phoneme production, excerbating the number and severity of articulation errors. Children so affected may have poor reading, spelling, and school adjustment behaviors.

Motor coordination of the articulators is necessary if the speech mechanism is to produce distinctive speech sounds. Also, it is important to have intact auditory receptive functions which provide the corrective feedback needed to monitor speech sound production. It appears that both apraxia, or disturbance of the speech mechanisms, and *agnosia,* or the inability to distinguish the distinctive features of sounds through auditory perceptual process, may be highly related to articulation disorders. Both apraxia and agnosia occur as a result of brain damage.

Articulation and Concomitant Disorders

Cerebral palsy is a classic example of a condition resulting from damage to the central nervous system where numerous other behaviors may also be atypical. In a longitudinal study of cerebral palsy children (Irwin, Moore, & Rampp, 1972), there was evidence of a 90 percent articulation error prevalence rate, with 75 percent of the population evidencing intelligence below the dull normal level and equally high perceptual and other language related disorders.

The relationship between articulation and reading disorders has been well researched (Wiig & Semel, 1976; Staats, 1968). The overlap between the two conditions is evident by the observation that 50 percent of children with articulation disorders also have reading disorders (Marge, 1965).

The common antecedents, along with

brain damage, are mental retardation (also frequently due to cerebral insult), specific visual and auditory perceptual impairment, central language (aphasia) disability, and cultural-environmental and social-emotional factors. Not all articulation (nor all reading) disabilities are related to a biological-physiological causation. Speech disorders may be learned through inappropriate models, or there may be infantile regression, paralleling childhood-parental overdependancy, or even childhood psychosis.

Children with mild hearing losses frequently fill their speech with nonsyllabic fricative, plosive, and affricate sounds, The fricative sounds are the most vulnerable, but the listener may hear any number of distortions or inaccurate approximations of sibilants, or a generalized imprecision in articulation. Deafness inhibits the development of standard speech sounds. Deaf infants frequently stop babbling because of the absence of auditory feedback. The result is that the untrained utterances of the deaf are undifferentiated vowel-like sounds. The consonant sounds are generally lip and front-tongue adjusted in their production. Sounds such as /k/, /g/, and /th/ are very difficult for deaf students. The fricative and affricates will be greatly distorted. Voicing or sonarancy errors, when voicing occurs for voiceless sounds, is extremely common.

The articulation development of children with auditory perceptual problems may mirror that of the hearing handicapped. Children with severe receptive language disability may function in their speech production similarly to the deaf.

Types of Articulation Disorders

Infantile speech—pedologic or infantile preservations (baby talk)—is the most prevalent articulation disorder among elementary school age children. Generally, the cause is developmental delay in the child's acquisition of phonetic skills, which results in speech production known as developmental delay. The persistence of infantile speech after the age of eight years, particularly when there is evidence that phonemes can be produced normally, may suggest that socio-personal factors need to be examined. One diagnostic identifying and organizing factor useful in differentiating structural (organic) articulation errors from functional ones is the consistency with which the former are produced. Structural and organic problems frequently appear with the more difficult to produce speech sounds, such as /r/, /sh/, /th /, /f/, /z/, /l/, and /ch/. Generally, an easier produced sound is substituted for one of the last to be learned phonemes. An example is the nonsyllabic /r/, yielding "wabbit," for "rabbit."

Lisp—any misarticulation of one or more of the English sibilants (/s/, /z/, /ʃ/, /z/) is considered a form of lisping. Some of the more common varieties of lisping are:

1. *Frontal lips.*—Substitution /θ/ for /s/ ("thee" for "see") and /θ/ for /z/ ("thoo" for "zoo") (also called protrusion or substitutional lisp). The tongue tip protrudes between the teeth and air escapes out the front of the mouth.
2. *Lateral lisp.*—Substitution of a nonstandard sibilant-like sound made with lateral rather than frontal emission of the breath stream, resembles a fricative made with the tongue placement in the approximate position for /L/, then emitting a voiceless breath stream. The resulting distorted sound in place of the /S/ is acoustically unpleasant, accompanied by the rattle of saliva in the mouth, and it is often

seen in children known as "tongue thrusters." Although most common on the /s/, the deficit is also sometimes heard on /z/, /θ/ and on affricates /tθ/ as well. Some speakers may lateralize all of these sounds.
3. *Palatal lisp.*—The tongue placement is too far back and the resulting sound is /θ/ "sh" for /s/ or /z/.
4. *Occluded or occlusion lisp.*—The least common, this lisp approximates the substitution of /t/ for /s/ and /d/ for /z/ and less often /t/ for /θ/ and /d/ for /z/ e.g., "tee" for "see" or "titter" for "sister."

It should be noted that lisping is prevalent among children who have either sensory hearing disabilities or auditory perceptual disorders. It also occurs with increased frequency among children with infantile speech, the major cause seems to be faulty auditory discrimination.

Diagnosing Articulation Disorders

There are several formal tests used to measure articulation disorders. Generally, they are divided by the speech clinician into screening and clinically deep assesssment. To the psychologist, the assessment of articulation disorders may simply be the observation that they exist. In recognition of their existence, a clinically significant question must be asked, similar to the very problem raised in describing a reading disorder.

The presence of a speech problem may suggest that it is a response to, or symptom related to, a more encompassing syndrome, i.e., brain damage, developmental lag, emotional pathologies, hearing loss, unusual cultural-linguistic-familial factors, to name a few. In turn, then, the speech problem may be related to a whole host of secondary factors, ranging from failure to want to talk, to reading problems.

The role of the school psychologist is often to differentially diagnose interrelated causative and secondary response factors. Unless the school psychologist has undergone clinical certification in speech pathology, the skill required to recognize the organic or anatomical structural variation in forming sounds (phonetic elements), given age, sex, and developmental related factors (auditory perception and intelligence), may simply not exist (Bernthal & Bankson, 1981).

Stuttering: Prevalence and Characteristics

Stuttering is not an articulation disorder. It is a disorder of rhythm, affecting some one half of 1 percent of the school-age population. In DSM-III stuttering is not considered a specific developmental disorder, but is placed in a grabbag category of other disorders with physical manifestations. While it cannot be classified as a major disabling condition, it has long been a topic of major popular interest, if not romantic preoccupation.

Explanations for the popular interest in stuttering are not so easily explained. But mention the word and it is amazing that almost everyone has an opinion on the cause and treatment of stuttering. There are several generalities which fascinate both professional and lay persons alike concerning this handicapping condition. Practically all those who stutter can sing without stuttering. Most can whisper without stuttering. But very few, if any, can say their own names without stuttering.

The demographic data on stutterers reveal an interesting profile. First, the majority of those who stutter are average or above intellectually, and rarely does the disability have concomitant or secondary physical or mental handicaps. There does appear to be a familial basis, with more males affected than females, by a ratio of 8:1. There are more stutterers from higher socioeconomic circumstances; and although controversial, more stutterers do appear to be first born.

Definition. Stuttering is by definition a nonfluency in speech production which of course interferes with communication. About 95 percent of all stuttering occurs on the initial syllable of the word and is called a block (stuttering block). That block then, is the act of stuttering and is described as being either tonic or clonic in nature. A *tonic stuttering block* is one of a highly repetitive nature. A *clonic block* is a widely spaced or elongated attempt to produce a sound. Speech and language therapists describe stuttering in terms of the duration and frequency of the block. There is a qualitative clinical aspect to the diagnosis for therapy, which depends on the theoretical point of view of the therapist. There are no formal or informal tests of stuttering and the obviousness of the problem requires two aspects of differential diagnosis. First, some speakers learn to speak rapidly, running words together until intelligibility is hampered, sometimes quite seriously. If these stuttering sounding individuals are asked to speak slowly, they do so poorly, but do it nonetheless. The result is a speech pattern which is uncomfortable for the speaker but improves intelligibility for the listener. This stuttering-like behavior is termed *cluttering.*

The second aspect of stuttering, which moves the problem into the direct domain of the psychologist, is the impact stuttering has on the speaker's attitude toward self and, in particular, the task of speaking. The one point of agreement in practically all stuttering theories is the importance of maintaining speech production for the stutterer, many of whom are reluctant to talk. Then there is also the transference of the stutterer's anxiety, from the task of stuttering to other human performance areas. Most stuttering therapy initiates work on the attitude of the stutterer with the goal being the interruption of the various approach-avoidance conflicts. It is usually true that initial avoidance-reduction therapy will reveal deeper levels of conflict, which have prompted the stutterers to cling defensively to the speech problem.

There is not a "stuttering personality" as such. Stutterers do respond to their disability as one might expect. They feel toward it as they sense others regard them. And that may be dichotomized first into people who don't stutter and those who do. Secondly, they may project the realistic expectancies that they have for their speech. Most stutterers tend to believe that stuttering is an acute problem which will soon right itself or could be corrected by a person who understands. In a stuttering therapy group for college students, the question was asked, "Does the problem of stuttering cause you to feel that you are less a person than you wish to be?" The response was, "No, but other people may think we are less intelligent than we are." Stutterers are often bright, sensitive people, who want to communicate yet fear that they are perceived as being different, even ghastly and grotesque. Therein lie the ingredients for the approach-avoidance conflict.

Current Theories and Therapies. Stuttering theory and stuttering therapy places its current focus on: (1) assisting the stutterer to speak more fluently by eliminating the avoidances and postpone-ments and (2) by drawing out the inhibitors, through advocating acceptance of self and through an avoidance-reduction mechanism that begins with the acceptance of stuttering behavior. Theories by Sheehan (1968) and Van Riper (1978) seem to set the pace for the other more popular therapies of the day. Others, such as Bloodstein (1979), ask the stutterer to forget about quick cures and focus on becoming a more fluent stutterer. Goldiamond (1968) introduced a prolonged speech pattern or pull-out practice, using self-study, data-collecting devices. The stutterers plot their own progress in the reduction of the duration of serious blocks. Webster (1972) introduced precision fluency shaping, which bases its therapy on the observation that stutterers produce most speech sounds incorrectly. Wingate (1966) has developed a vocal modulation process to reduce the production of stressed syllables, increasing the forward flow of the speech pattern. This technique introduces the melody of speech into phonation. Schwartz (1974) has hypothesized that stuttering is a result of a reduction of the normal airflow. He believes the child anticipates the stuttering block and alters the air pressure becoming temporarily speechless. He teaches the stutterer to use the airstream to obtain fluency.

In most cases, the stuttering theory accepted by the clinician provides for the type of diagnosis and the resulting therapy. In short, stuttering is a highly clinician centered practice, Ryan, Bruce, and Vankirk (1974) provides two operant-type data collection forms which may be used in describing stuttering.

The prevalent practice is to teach the stutterer to stutter with techniques that improve fluency. The speech clinician, or more appropriately the stuttering therapist, isolates the type of block and begins an active program of intervention. Simultaneously, most stuttering therapists request that stutterers acknowledge that they display stuttering and respond by accepting themselves as persons with a speech production problem. Restructuring the view of self and the perceived responses of others are currently predominant themes in stuttering therapy, diagnosis, and treatment.

Mixed Specific Developmental Disorder

Definition and Prevalence

DSM-III defines a mixed specific developmental disorder as a multiple handicapping condition where no distinct disability is predominant. The term should be used when the functional performance of the child or youth is fairly equally disabling in several human skill areas. Therefore, this description focuses more on behavioral responses than inherent (to the person) disabilities.

The term *mixed specific disability*, could well be used to describe any number of multiple-handicapping conditions which result from a nondescript etiology of pathology. There is no definitive data on the increase of multiple handicapping conditions in the United States because of the absence of any baseline data. Most child counts, including frequency tabulations of handicapped pre- and school-age students, as required by law (PL 94-142), define students according to one of the twelve classical handicapping conditions defined in the introduction to the chapters. In 1967, the state of Illinois (Graham, 1967) reported statewide survey data which placed the prevalence of multiple handicapping conditions at 1 percent of the total school-age population. Few states have reported data since, because there is no such diagnostic category as multiply handicapped.

The prevalence of multiple handicaps is probably rising because of the increasing capability of modern medical procedures to save the lives of children who, only a few years ago, might have succumbed. The result is an ever-increasing number of children with serious and multiple disability.

Educators concerned with developing programs for developmentally disabled children have been forced to consider degree of severity an issue. Generally speaking, the more severe a disability, the greater the concomitant number of associated handicaps. State agencies, presently those providing services for mental health and developmentally disabled populations, do so under PL 95-602 of the Rehabilitation and Comprehensive Service Act, which includes a Developmental Disabilities Admendment (1978). Developmental disabilities, used in this sense, is a severe, chronic disability present before the age of twenty-two. It is commonly used to describe severely and profoundly mentally retarded children, or those mentally retarded students with IQ's of 35 and below, who have difficulty developing expressive language skills, are frequently nonambulatory, and whose independent living skills and opportunity for competitive employment is sufficiently limited. Therefore, due to the number of disabilities present, they are required to seek continued external maintenance in routine activities of daily living (ADL skills), such as eating, dressing, toileting, and basic mobility.

When DSM-III added the Specific Developmental Disorders Section, it was done in recognition of the wide array of existing learning disabilities which are confusing to classify. The problems in diagnostic clarity become even more pronounced by the fact that educators and psychologists tend to view different aspects of the same issues from a disparate vantage point. Clinicians examine for etiology and pathology. Educators, including school psychologists, try to describe and evaluate those behaviors which have a special bearing on performance in the instructional environment.

In the clinical setting, a psychologist may observe the hyperactivity, short attention span, and distractibility of a "driven" child, low on impulse control, whose symptoms would result in the diagnosis of attention deficit disorder with hyperactivity. However, that same child may display several additional, educationally relevant behaviors. Academic achievement deficits may be present to varying degrees, in several of the reading response areas, specifically in word recognition, or reading comprehension, or reading vocabulary, and in the major areas of mathematics, i.e., arithmetic reasoning or arithmetic calculations. Several other academic task areas, i.e., handwriting and spelling, may also present specific areas of academic disorders. In addition, the child may have visual or auditory perceptual memory deficits. Similarly, he or she may have receptive-expressive or central language disabilities manifested by an inability to retain memory for phonemics, morphemes, or word units. The hyperactivity may be the symptom of the primary diagnosis but may not be the target behavior area critical to classroom performance.

In summary, the complexity of behavioral sequelae in number and type which affect, and are affected by, academic learning is usually quite extensive. This lengthy explanation should make more clear why teachers so frequently complain, "The psychologist didn't tell me anything I didn't already know." And they add, "I still have the responsibility for educating the child."

In an educational setting, a diagnostic scheme which makes considerable sense is to utilize DSM-III to establish its appropriate diagnosis, while also describing the child's behaviors in terms of the *learner characteristics* that affect academic performance.

Atypical Specific Developmental Disorders

This diagnostic category is reserved for those specific developmental disorders not covered by the other categories. Thus, it is a nondescript category and must be used with care lest it become a wastebasket for sloppy assessment practices. There are a number of specific developmental disorders which occur quite rarely and have significant diagnostic characteristics. For example, in *Wartenberg's disease,* the primary diagnosis would probably be mental retardation. However, the clinician seeing the young Wartenberg's child might not recognize the regressive factor, because the mental retardation may not yet be in place and the diagnostic significance of the observable features, i.e., white fetlock of hair, or achromatic features of the eyes (eyes of different color), goes unrecognized (Friel, 1974). Significant to, and paralleling, the mental retardation is a regressive hearing loss. Although the child has a wide nasal root and rolled intercanthic folds, most of these children are referred because they display developmental motor speech problems.

Marfan's disease is another rare, but unique, problem, where examiners from various disciplines may classify the child's disorder as a motor problem with regressive hearing loss (Pyeritz & McKusick, 1979), only to learn that the gross and fine motor movement affecting both gait and balance are deteriorating due to skeletal musculature atrophy.

TABLE 11-4

Descriptor System for Classifying Learner Characteristics

Motor
- Gross
  - Coordination-Balance
  - Strength-Endurance
- Perceptual-Motor
  - Eye-Hand Coordination
  - Directionality
- Body Awareness

Perception
- Visual
  - Discrimination
  - Memory
  - Integration/primary visual input
- Auditory
  - Discrimination
  - Memory
  - Integration/primary auditory input
- Tactile

Language
- Conceptual
  - Concrete
  - Functional
  - Abstract
- Expressive
  - Vocabulary
  - Syntax
- Receptives

Academics
- Reading
  - Letter Recognition
  - Word Attack
    - Phonics
    - Structural Analysis
  - Word Recognition
  - Vocabulary
  - Comprehension
- Spelling
- Writing
  - Manuscript
  - Cursive
- Arithmetic
  - Numeration
  - Computation
  - Measurement

If the diagnosis of specific developmental disorders becomes the search for what is interfering with growth or development and inhibiting academic learning, then physical, mental, and environmental factors are suspect. The enormity of the diagnostic task in the case of observing and reporting developmental disorders is *not* in finding and describing what is wrong, but rather in organizing learner characteristics descriptive of human function and development so that the interrelationship and importance to the learning task can be approximated.

Do remember that not all disabling conditions result in handicap. A handicap is present when a characteristic or behavior of the learner interferes with a developmentally age appropriate performance of an academic task, social interaction, or human function. To assist the diagnostician, Sabatino (1979) has organized a few of the more common motoric, sensory, perceptual, language, and motor learner characteristics associated with developmental disabilities into a descriptive hierarchy, as shown in Table 11-4. The use of these descriptors requires the diagnostician to systematically convey how a student is performing in response to each one. The result is direct attention to critical developmental behaviors and to assess whether they are age appropriate or in need of further evaluation or treatment.

REFERENCES

Ackerman, P. T., Peters, J. E., & Dykman, R. A. Children with specific learning disabilities, WISC profiles. *Journal of Learning Disabilities*, 1971, *4*, 150–166.

Altus, G. T. A WISC profile for retarded readers. *Journal of Consulting Psychology*, 1956, *20*, 155–156.

Anderson, M., Kaufman, A. S., & Kaufman, N. L. Use of the WISC-R with learning disabled populations: Some diagnostic implications. *Psychology in the Schools*, 1976, *13*, 381–386.

Ashlock, R. B. *Error patterns in computation: A semi-programmed approach.* Columbus, OH: Merrill, 1972.

Bannatyne, A. *Language, reading, and learning disability: psychology, neuropsychology, diagnosis and remediation.* Springfield, IL.: Charles C. Thomas, 1971.

Bateman, B. Three approaches to diagnosis and educational planning for children with learning disabilities. *Academic Therapy Quarterly*, 1967, *3*, 11–16.

Beatty, L. S., Madden, R., Gardner, E. F., & Karlsen, R. *Stanford diagnostic arithmetic test.* New York: Harcourt Brace, 1976.

Bereiter, C. *Arithmetic and mathematics.* San Raez, CA: Dimensions Publishing, 1963.

Bernthal, J. E., & Bankson, N. W. *Articulation disorders.* Englewood Cliffs, NJ: Prentice-Hall, 1981.

Birch, A., & Belmont, S., Auditory, visual integration, intelligence and reading ability in school children. *Perceptual and motor skills*, 1965, *20*, 295–305.

Bloodstein, O. *Speech pathology: An introduction.* Boston: Houghton Mifflin, 1979.

Bond, G., & Tinker, M. A. *Reading difficulties, their diagnosis and correction.* New York: Appleton-Century-Crofts, 1967.

Bruninks, R., & Clark, C. R. Auditory and visual paired-associate learning in retarded and non-retarded children. *American Journal of Mental Deficiency*, 1972, *76*, (5), 561–567.

Burks, H., & Bruce, P. The characteristics of poor and good readers as disclosed by the WISC. *Journal of Educational Psychology*, 1955, *46*, 488–493.

Buros, O. *Reading tests and reviews.* Highland Park, NJ: Gryphon Press, 1975.

Carpenter, T. P., Corbitt, M. K., Kepner, H. S., Lindquist, M. M., & Reys, R. E. National assessment: A perspective of students' mastery of basic mathematic skills, In M. M. Lindquist (Ed.), *Selected issues in mathematics education.* Berkeley, CA: McCutchen, 1980.

Cawley, J. F. An instructional design in mathematics. In L. Mann, L. Goodman, & J. L. Wiederholt (Eds.), *Teaching the learning disabled adolescent.* Boston: Houghton Mifflin, 1975.

Cawley, J. F., Goodstein, H. A., Fitzmaurice, A. M., Lepore, A., Sedlak, R. A., & Althaus, V. *Project Math: Mathematics activities for teaching the handicapped, level I and II.* Tulsa, OK: Educational Process, 1976.

Cherkes, M. G. Effect of chronological age and mental age on understanding of rules of logic. *American Journal of Mental Deficiency*, 1975, *80*, 208–216.

Cohn, R. Arithmetic in learning disabilities. In H. Myklebust (Ed.), *Progress in learning disabilities* (Vol. II). New York: Grune & Stratton, 1971.

Connally, A. J., Nachtman, B., & Pritchett, M. *Key Math Diagnostic Arithmetic Test.* Circle Pines, MN: American Guidance Service, 1976.

Cruickshank, W. Arithmetic ability of mentally retarded children: I, Ability to differentiate extraneous materials from needed arithmetic facts. *Journal of Educational Research,* 1948, *42,* 167–170. *(a)*

Cruickshank, W. Arithmetic ability of mentally retarded children: II, understanding arithmetical processes. *Journal of Educational Research,* 1948, *42,* 279–288. *(b)*

Cruickshank, W., & Hallahan, D. *Perceptual and learning disabilities in children* (Vol. 1). Syracuse, NY: Syracuse University, 1975.

DeSpain, C., Williams, W., & York, R. Evaluation of the severely retarded and multiply-handicapped: An alternative. In L. Brown, T. Crowner, W. Williams, & R. York (Eds.), *Madison's alternative for zero exclusion: A book of readings* (Vol. 5). Madison, WI: Madison Public Schools, 1975.

Engelmann, S., & Bruner, E. *DISTAR reading I and II.* Chicago: Science Research Associates, 1973.

Farr, R., & Anastasiow, N. *Test of reading and achievement: A review and evaluation.* Newark DE: International Reading Association, 1969.

Feuerstein, R. *Instrumental enrichment: Redevelopment of cognitive functions of retarded performers.* Baltimore: University Park, 1979.

Flavell, J. H. *Cognitive development.* Englewood Cliffs, NJ: Prentice-Hall, 1977.

Friel, J. P. Dorland's illustrated medical dictionary, Philadelphia: Saunders, 1974.

Gillespie, P. H., & Johnson, L. *Teaching reading to the mildly retarded child.* Columbus, OH: Charles E. Merrill, 1974.

Goldiamond, I. Stuttering and fluency as manipulative operant response classes. In H. Sloan & B. MacAulay (Eds.), *Operant procedures in remedial speech and language training.* Boston: Houghton Mifflin, 1968, 348–407.

Goodstein, H. A., Cawley, J. F., Gordon, S., & Helfgott, J. Verbal problem solving among educable mentally retarded children. *American Journal of Mental Deficiency,* 1971, *70,* 238–241.

Goodstein, H. A., Kahn, H., & Cawley, J. F. The achievement of educable mentally retarded children on the Key Math Diagnostic Arithmetic Test. *Journal of Special Education,* 1976, *10,* 61–70.

Graham, R., The Illinois plan for special education of exceptional children. I. F. Boyles (Comp.), Illinois Dept. of Public Instruction Circular Series, A. No. 12, Springfield, IL: 1967.

Hammill, D., & Wiederholt, J. S. Review of the Frostig Visual Perception test and the related training program. In L. Mann & D. A. Sabatino (Eds.), *The first review of special education.* Philadelphia, PA: JSE Press, 1973.

Hull, F., & Timmons, R. A national speech and hearing survey. *Journal of Speech and Hearing Disorders, 1966,* **31,** *359–361.*

Illinois Commission on Children. *News and Views,* May 1977, *14,* 1–4.

Irwin, J. V., Moore, J. M., & Rampp, D. L. Nonmedical diagnosis and evaluation. In J. V. Irwin & M. Marge (Eds.), *Principles of childhood language disabilities.* Englewood Cliffs, NJ: Prentice-Hall, 1972.

Johnson, D., & Myklebust, H. R. *Learning disabilities: Educational principles and practices.* New York: Grune & Stratton, 1967.

Koppitz, E. M. The Bender Gestalt Test and learning disturbances in young children. *Journal of Clinical Psychology,* 1958, *14,* 292–295.

Koppitz, E. M. *The Bender-Gestalt Test for young children: Volume II: research and application, 1963–1973.* New York: Grune and Stratton, 1975.

Langford, F. S. What can a teacher learn about student's thinking through oral interviews. *The Arithmetic Teacher,* 1974, *21,* 26–32.

Lepore, A. *A comparison of computational errors between educable mentally handicapped and learning disability children.* Unpublished manuscript, University of Connecticut, 1974.

Lloyd, J. Ascertaining the reading skills of atypical learner. In D. A. Sabatino & T. L. Miller (Eds.), *Describing learner characteristics of handicapped children and youth.* New York: Grune & Stratton, 1979.

Mann, L. Psychometric phrenology and the new faculty psychology: The case against ability assessment and training. *Journal of Special Education,* 1971, 3–14.

Mann, L. *On the trail of process.* New York: Grune & Stratton, 1979.

Marge, M. The influence of selected home background variables on the development of oral communication skill in children. *Journal of Speech and Hearing Research,* 1965, *8,* 291–312.

Maslow, P., Frostig, M., Lefever, D., & Whittlesey, J. The Marianne Frostig Test of Visual Perception: 1963 standardization. *Perceptual and Motor Skills,* 1964, *19,* 463–499.

McLean, J. F., & Synder-McLean, L. K. *A transactional approach to early language training.* Columbus, OH: Merrill, 1978.

Menyuk, P. *The development of speech in children.* Indianapolis, IN: Bobbs-Merrill, 1972.

Miller, J. F. *Assessing language production in children: Experimental procedures.*Baltimore: University Park, 1981.

Monroe, M. *Diagnostic reading examination.* Chicago: Stoelting, 1932.

Muma, J. R. *Language handbook: Concepts, assessment and intervention.* Englewood Cliffs, NJ: Prentice-Hall, 1978.

National Center for Educational Statistics (NCES). *Digest of education statistics.* Washington, DC: U.S. Government Printing Office, 1979.

Newcomer, P., Larsen, S., & Hammill, D. A response. *Exceptional Children,* 1975, *42,* 144–148.

Orton, S. T. *Reading, writing, and speech problems in children,* New York: Norton, 1937.

Orton, S. T. Word blindness in school children. *Archives of Neurology and Psychiatry,* 1925, *14,* 58–65.

Osborn, W. J. Ten reasons why pupils fail in mathematics. *The Mathematics Teacher,* 1925, *18,* 234–238.

Pattera, M. E. A study of thirty-three WISC scattergrams of retarded workers. *Elementary English,* 1963, *40,* 394–405.

Pyeritz, R. E., & McKusick, V. A. Current concepts: The marfan syndrome: Diagnosis and management. *New England Journal of Medicine,* 1979, *300,* 772.

Reese, J. An instructional system for teachers of learning disabled children. In D. Sabatino (Ed.), *Learning disabilities handbook: A technical Guide to Program development.* Dekalb, IL: Northern Illinois University, 1976.

Robeck, M. S. Intellectual strengths and weaknesses shown by reading clinic subjects on the WISC. *Journal of Developmental Reading,* 1964, *7,* 120–129.

Roberts, G. H. The failure strategies of third-grade arithmetic pupils. *The Arithmetic Teacher,* 1968, *15,* 422–446.

Ryan, R., Bruce, P., & Vankirk, B. Establishment, transfer, and maintenance of fluent speech. *Journal of Speech and Hearing Disorders,* 1974, *39,* 370.

Sabatino, D. A. Classification for handicapped children and youth. In D. A. Sabatino & T. L. Miller (Eds.), *Describing learner characteristics of handicapped children and youth.* New York: Grune & Stratton, 1979.

Sabatino, D. A., & Hayden, D. Psychoeducational study of selected behavioral variables with children failing in the elementary grades (part I). *Journal of Experimental Education,* 1970, *38,* 49–57.

Sabatino, D. A., & Miller, T. L. (Eds.). *Describing learner characteristics of handicapped children and youth.* New York: Grune & Stratton, 1979.

Sabatino, D. A., & Streissguth, W. O. Word form configuration training of visual perceptual strengths with learning disabled children. *Journal of Learning Disabilities,* 1972, *5,* 435–441.

Sabatino, D. A., & Ysseldyke, J. E. Identification of statistically significant differences between subtest scaled scores and psycholinguistic ages on the ITPA. *Psychology in the Schools,* 1972, *9,* 309–313.

Schiefelbusch, R. L. (Ed.). *Language of the mentally retarded.* Baltimore: University Park, 1972.

Schmidt, C., In D. Sabatino (Ed.), *Learning disabilities handbook: A technical guide to program development.* DeKalb, IL: Northern Illinois University Press, 1976.

Schwartz, G. *The language-learning system.* New York: Simon & Schuster, 1974.

Sedlak, R. A., & Fitzmaurice, A. Teaching arithmetic. In J. M. Kauffman & D. P. Hallahan (Eds.), *Handbook of special education.* Englewood Cliffs, NJ: Prentice-Hall, 1981.

Sedlak, R. A., & Schenck, W. E. Strategies for facilitating verbal problem solving of EMH learners: A comparative study. *Carolina Journal of Educational Research,* 1981, *1,* 30–42.

Senf, G. A perspective on the definition of LD. *Journal of Learning Disabilities,* 1978, *10* (8), 537–539.

Sheehan, J. G. Stuttering and its disappearance. *Journal of Speech and Hearing Research,* 1970, 13, 279–289.

Siegel, G. The high cost of accountability. *ASHA,* 1975, *17,* 796–797.

Singh, S., & Singh, K. S. *Phonetics: Principles and practices.* Baltimore: University Park, 1976.

Smith, N. B. *Graded selections for informal reading diagnosis.* New York: New York University, 1959.

Spache, E. *Reading activities for child involvement* (2d ed.). Boston: Allyn & Bacon, 1976.

Special Study Institute for Specific Learning Disabilities: Proceedings. Tallahassee, FL: State of Florida Department of Education, 1975.

Staats, A. W. *Learning, language, and cognition.* New York: Holt, 1968.

Templin, M. C. *Certain language skills in children.* Minneapolis: University of Minnesota, 1957.

Van Riper, C. *Speech correction: Principles and methods* (6th ed.). Englewood Cliffs, NJ: Prentice-Hall, 1978.

Vitello, S. Facilitation of class inclusion among mentally retarded children. *American Journal of Mental Deficiency,* 1973, 158–162.

Washington, R. A survey-analysis of problems faced by inner-city high school students who have been classified as truants. *High School Journal,* 1973, *56,* 248–257.

Webster, R. E. Short-term memory in mathematics-proficient and mathematics-disabled students as a function of input-modality/output-modality pairings. *Journal of Special Education,* 1980, *14,* 67–78.

Webster, R. L. *An operant response shaping program for the establishment of fluency in stutterers.* Final Report. Hollins College, VA: 1972.

Wepman, J. *Auditory discrimination test.* Chicago: Language Research Associates. 1958.

Wepman, J. M. Aphasia: Diagnostic description and therapy. *Hearing and Speech News,* 1968, *36* (1), 3–5.

Wiig, E. H., & Semel, E. M. *Language disabilities in children and adolescents.* Columbus, OH: Merrill, 1976.

Williams, W., Coyne, P., De Spain, C., Johnson, F., Scheuerman, N., Stengert, J., Swetlik, B., & York, R. Teaching math skills using longitudinal sequences. In M. E. Snell (Ed.), *Systematic instruction of the moderately and severely handicapped.* Columbus, OH: Merrill, 1978.

Wingate, M. Prosody in stuttering adaptation. *Journal of Speech and Hearing Research,* 1966, 9, 550, 556.

Witkin, H. A., Dyk, R., Faterson, H., Goodenough, D. R., & Kays, S. *Psychological differentiation.* New York: Wiley, 1962.

Zintz, M. W. *The reading process, the teacher and the learner* (2d ed.). Dubuque, IA: William C. Brown, 1975.

CHAPTER 12

Psychosexual Disorders

Loretta Haroian

DMS-III divides psychosexual disorders into four groups: *gender identity disorders,* characterized by feelings of discomfort with one's anatomic sex and by persistent behaviors generally associated with the other sex; *paraphilias,* characterized by sexual arousal and gratification in response to nonhuman objects or parts of the body ordinarily nonsexual (fetishes) and which gratifications interfere with affectionate human sexual activity; *psychosexual dysfunction,* characterized by inhibitions in sexual desire or in the psychophysiological changes that characterize the sexual response cycle; and *other psychosexual disorders,* a residual group which includes ego-dystonic homosexuality.

We are going to consider briefly each of these groups and how these disorders are defined by DSM-III. Obviously many of these disorders cannot occur in children and would not be diagnosed until some time in adolescence. Yet there are psychosexual disorders or problems which children may have about which we should be aware. Much of our discussion will focus upon those issues, that DSM-III leaves vague and unspecified, for these constitute a much larger area of concern than the few diagnostic categories appropriate to children.

Gender Identity Disorder of Childhood

This is the only diagnostic group of psychosexual disorders that is specifically related to children. In general, this disorder must originate before puberty. The diagnostic criteria for girls are:

A. Strongly and persistently stated desire to be a boy, or insistence that she is a boy (not merely a desire for any perceived cultural advantages from being a boy);

B. Persistent repudiation of female anatomic structures are manifested by at least one of the following repeated assertions:
   1. That she will grow up to become a man (not merely in role)
   2. That she is biologically unable to become pregnant
   3. That she will not develop breasts
   4. That she has no vagina
   5. That she has or will grow a penis

The diagnostic criteria for boys:

A. Strongly and persistently stated desire to be a girl, or insistence that he is a girl.

B. Either one or two:
   1. Persistent repudiation of male anatomic structures as manifested by at least one of the following repeated assertions:
      a. That he will grow up to be a woman (not merely a role)
      b That his penis or testes are disgusting or will disappear
      c. That it would be better not to have a penis or testes
   2. Preoccupation with female sterotypical activities as manifested by a preference for either cross-dressing or simulating female attire or by a compelling desire to participate in the games and pastimes of girls.

This is not a common disorder and is assumed to lead to transsexualism in adolescence and adulthood (Green, 1974).

Paraphilias

The essential feature of disorders in this subclass is that unusual or bizarre imagery or acts are necessary for sexual excitement. Such imagery or acts tend to be insistently and involuntarily repetitive and generally involve either (1) preference for use of a nonhuman object for sexual arousal; (2) repetitive sexual activity with humans involving real or simulated suffering or humiliation; or (3) repetitive sexual activity with nonconsenting partners. Since paraphilic imagery is necessary for erotic arousal, it must be included in masturbatory or coital fantasies if not actually acted out. In the absence of paraphilic imagery, there is no relief from erotic tension and sexual excitement and/or orgasm is not attained. The imagery in a paraphilic fantasty (rape, sadomasochism, bestiality, etc.) or the object of sexual excitement in a paraphilia is frequently the stimulus for sexual excitement in individuals without a pyschosexual disorder.

Paraphilic imagery or the use of objects would be considered normative in childhood masturbation sexual patterns because of children's limited sexual knowledge and options. In that regard, fetish behavior is not included as a diagnosis in childhood. Before the onset of postpubescent partner sex the criteria of "repeatedly preferred" (to partner sex) is not accessible and when masturbation is the only sanctioned or available sexual option, the use of inanimate objects to enhance the experience is common. When other options (partners) are sanctioned and available the "exclusive or consistently preferred" use of inanimate objects is considered a fetish.

Although the age of onset for fetishes is in childhood or adolescence, paraphilic attachments of childhood and adolescence may recede in their importance or degree of dependency when other sexual options become available. For example, the panty fetish (one of the most common) may begin in childhood as a young boy stimulates himself with thought of, procurement of, and masturbation with or into female panties. However, the adult obsession with collecting panties for sexual use, accompanied by diminished erotic response to partner sex, is not necessarily the eventual result of this early childhood fixation. The adult transition to gratifying partner sex may be smooth and uncomplicated, with childhood sexual patterns giving way to appropriate adult patterns as increasingly varied sexual options and opportunities become available. The adult male's interest in panties as a sexual stimulant may remain but may take a less important role in the overall adult sex pattern. Fantasies about panties as a part of sexual foreplay, etc., may not be considered a fetish because it is not the consistently preferred, necessary, or exclusive sexual pattern.

Sometimes a young boy's erotization of panties leads him to public behavior that is socially unacceptable. Stealing panties from family members or off clotheslines and peeping, especially in the windows of neighbors, may bring a child to the attention of the police or mental health professionals and treatment is required. Such behavior is asocial and may be obsessive but the diagnosis of fetishism is still premature. This and other asocial behaviors, such as public exposing of genitalia, may or may not be accompanied by mental disorder and a differential diagnosis is imperative. Given the contradictory and confusing way Western culture handles sexual development, it is erroneous to assume that asocial sexual acts of children are characterological pathology.

Psychosexual Dysfunctions

Pyschosexual dysfunctions, characterized by inhibitions in sexual desire or the physiological changes that characterize the sexual response cycle, are undiagnosable in children, although there is reason to assume that they may be manifest. There is no help for children who have developmental sexual problems (i.e., arousal, orgasm, pain, guilt, low sensation, etc.). Lack of knowledge and misunderstanding is a major problem and most children and adolescents worry about being normal (Langfeldt, 1981).

What is still lacking in any shape or form in childhood is an open discussion about sexual anxieties, sexual expectations, different sexual acts, and feelings about sex. Many girls (fourteen to eighteen) are not sure if they have had an orgasm because they have no idea what it was supposed to feel like. Most postpubescent adolescents masturbate, but the majority feel guilty, ashamed, dirty, stupid, embarrassed, or abnormal after the act (Hass, 1979).

Although there are no studies on sexual dysfunction in childhood, retrospective sex histories of adults and case histories of children in psychotherapy suggest that all is not well. We have underestimated the significance of sexual interactions and fantasies in childhood. Until we better understand the development of the erotic response through childhood and adolescence, and until normative behavior gradiants are established, children's sexual needs will not be properly addressed by the mental health community.

Ego-Dystonic Homosexuality

Undesired homosexuality is undiagnosable in childhood. Although many adult homosexuals retrospectively identify indications of their adult orientation in childhood events, same sex experimentation in childhood is a common experience in the sex histories of heterosexual adults. It is well to remember that homosexuality is a behavior which is dependent on the preference of same sex partners. Adolescents discover and define the elements of sexual attraction, unique and individual to themselves as an ongoing process of differentiation. Homosexuals discover that they are sexually excited by same sex stimuli in the same way that heterosexuals discover that they are excited by opposite sex stimuli. And, within these categories they both discover even more specific attractants (i.e., body types, body parts, sex acts, positions, odors, words, etc.).

While it is possible for a homophobic adolescent to be disgusted with his or her feelings of attraction to same sex peers and fear the consequences of a gay life, ego-dystonic homosexuality would rarely be diagnosed before early adulthood. We have come to understand that even the most serious love affair with a same sex partner may not be generalized to an ongoing same-sex attraction. Thus adolescence is too early to make a definitive diagnosis.

The lack of child sex syndromes described in DSM-III does not mean that children and adolescents are free from sexual problems or that clinicians are not consulted about the sexual behaviors of children and adolescents. Sexual problems of children, as seen on an out-patient basis by mental or physical health care professionals, are usually public or semipublic behaviors that cause adults (usually the parent) embarrassment and concern because they are a departure from society's expectations. There are many sexual events and/or behaviors that cause children to be referred for psychological evaluation. The parent's decision to seek professional consultation is the solution to their feelings of worry that the child is not normal, fear that if they don't intervene the child will grow up to be a sexually deviant adult, doubt that they have the knowledge or skill to change the behavior pattern, and guilt that they have caused or contributed to the undesirable behavior.

Gender Behavior Disorder

Gender behavior disorder (GBD) in children (mostly males) is characterized by cross-gender or androgynous behavior that is learned and reinforced by the environment, rather than being linked to a persistent belief that they are in fact the other sex. The adult manifestation of GBD is transvestism and effeminate behavior. It is important to differentiate gender identity disorder (GID) from GBD. The GID child believes his/her sex is wrongly assigned and suffers from chronic and severe cognitive dissonance; the GBD child knows his/her anatomical gender, but enjoys androgynous behavior and will suffer only if the environment is punitive and nonsupportive. Rekers (1974, 1978) has argued for the teaching of gender appropriate behaviors to boys who may be suffering peer rejection for their effeminacy. Yet our culture's acceptance of "tom-boyism" raises question as to where corrective efforts should be directed.

Excessive or Compulsive Masturbation

Masturbation frequency is highly variable in an individual child, as well as between children. Although normative frequency data for specific ages is not available, children are often referred to clinicians for excessive or compulsive masturbation. This is a subjective quantification taken to mean that the child is preoccupied with masturbatory activity to the exclusion of other age-appropriate pursuits and/or that the scope of the masturbation activity is resulting in stigmatizing censure from others that may create secondary adjustment problems for the child.

Sexologists believe that masturbation is a viable sexual activity throughout the life span and that it need not be considered a poor postpubescent substitute for sex with a partner (Haroian, 1982). Research in female sexuality (Hite, 1976) and the treatment of anorgasmia in adult women (Barbach, 1975; Chapman, 1977; Dodson, 1974) suggest that masturbation to orgasm is an important developmental step and possibly a prerequisite to becoming reliably orgasmic in adult partner sex. It is often a treatment of choice for adult male and female sexual dysfunction (Kaplan, 1979) and is reported as a childhood activity of some importance by most adults (Kinsey et al., 1948; Hite, 1976, 1981; Hass, 1979).

Sexologists suggest that young boys be encouraged to prolong the arousal stage of their masturbations so as not to condition a rapid stimulus response bond between erection and ejaculation. Young girls are encouraged to look at, and identify, their external genitalia and to connect their erotic feelings and sexual response cycle to appropriate genital body parts. Parents need to understand that childhood masturbation is a normal and beneficial behavior that only needs to be managed to coincide with social etiquette.

Precocious Sexual Interest and Behavior

Clinicians are often consulted by parents who are anxious about their child's interest in sexual topics, masturbation, or sex play with siblings and peers. If the child's basic interest in sex is complemented by unsupervised opportunity to engage in trial and error learning with a partner, sexual rehearsal play is predictable. Some sexologists suggest that not only is sexual rehearsal play quite predictable in children, but that it is advisable and should be encouraged in order to forestall adult sexual problems (Money & Ehrhardt, 1973; Yates, 1979).

Intense and continued or intermittent sexual interest in children should be accommodated as any other interest would be. Age-appropriate books and conversations with parents endorse the child's curiosity about this important part of life and encourage an open and unashamed quest for sexual knowledge.

However, a child who shows little interest or curiosity about sex should not be overwhelmed with sex information by over-zealous parents. Some children personalize their sexuality very early and are uncomfortable with candid sex conversations. They appreciate appropriate sex materials to be used in private and occasional one-on-one talks with a parent to clear up any troublesome sexual ideas or feelings. A few parents may worry about a child with low sex interest, but lack of sex interest is more often considered normal in children.

Of greater concern is the child who is very public with sex talk and sex play, masturbatory or with peers. Parents worry that their children are abnormal genetically or hormonally, that they will be censured by other adults and children, that their sexual behavior will reflect badly on siblings and family, that they will be a target for sexual abuse or exploitation by adults, or will grow up to be promiscuous or perverted.

Case Illustration: Three-year-old Dan was a highly sexed boy who had been involved in sex play with age mates and an older child. He asked his therapist if she wanted to put her mouth on his "dinky." When she replied in the negative, he pleaded "You'll like it," "I'll pay you money," "I'll be your best friend." When asked if he liked to "play dinky," Dan frowned menacingly, clenched his fists, and aggressively replied, "Yes, I like it and I'm not going to stop!"

The child who is pseudomature in any sense is a special child with special needs. They demand more from parents and may be considered a blessing or a curse, depending on the parental value system and resources. Intellectual genius, superior athletic potential, and exceptional musical talent are all considered valuable gifts that should not be wasted. The child who is sexually precocious in development or interest is often shunned and pitied. The parents of these children need help, not only in the management of the child's behavior, but also in considering that precocity in this area need not be thought of as an affliction.

Children Who Report Sexual Contact With an Adult That Cannot Be Substantiated

Psychological literature and the popular press report and often sensationalize the plight of the traumatized child whose story of sexual activity with an adult is not believed and, conversely, of the victimized adult who steadfastly denies the sexual accusations of a child. The most commonly reported pedophilic situation is that of the adult male and the prepubescent female. This is not to say that sex between an adult female and a prepubescent male does not occur, but it would probably not be reported and if it were, it would probably not be considered a traumatic experience for the child.

In Western culture there is a time-honored tradition of young boys being sexually initiated by an experienced older woman. Girls, in contrast, are considered permanently damaged by early sexual initiation by an adult male. The attitude that the child has been damaged by a sexual experience is extended to boys only if the sexual encounter is homosexual or if residual physical damage is sustained. Sexual behavior between an adult female and a female child is the least reported pedophilic possibility and is of least interest to law enforcement and the community.

It is difficult to generalize about adult/child sex because of the variability of age and sex in any individual case. If a sexual encounter did occur and if it was traumatic for the child, the diagnostic process with a clinical child sexologist can be therapeutic. Psychotherapy consists of talking about the traumatic situation in order to bring the experience into cognitive awareness and to work through the feelings engendered by the event. A client is ill-served by a therapist who feels that the child has been permanently damaged by the experience and relates to him/her as a victim.

Many adult women have reported satisfying, nontraumatic, prepubescent, incestuous relationships from which they graduated to postpubescent sex with peers without undue incident. Other patients in psychotherapy report unresolved conflicts in association with childhood sexual experiences, and there is some evidence to suggest that the greater the age differential between participants, the greater the potential for trauma. It is important to note that most reported pedophilic sex is incestuous and that incest is a family rather than an individual pathology.

Postpubescent Sex With a Partner; Heterosexual

Sexologists have attempted to deal with the question of sexual readiness in terms of chronological age. There is a reasonable consensus that around the age of sixteen adolescents are physiologically and psychologically ready. The older adolescent is interested in forming primary relationships outside the nuclear family, and sexual sharing is an integral part of these relationships.

Sexuality is a major concern of adolescence and adolescents are poorly served by the professional community, the family, the school, and the culture (Hass, 1979). The professional mental health worker sees a small fraction of adolescents and may or may not address sexual issues. Family members have little credibility in sexuality if the foundation was not built in childhood. The school is still concentrating on reproductive biology and venereal disease while the adolescent needs help with sociosexual issues, and the culture ambivalently stimulates and misinforms, encourages and prohibits, and punishes and rewards the adolescent for sexual interest and behavior.

The revered notion—that sex is natural, and happens with style, sensitivity, and spirituality when two people love each other—is a myth that departs significantly from most reported first encounters. It does, however, perpetuate a rationale for those who oppose real sex education and dooms the teenager, misinformed by the exploitive messages of the marketplace, to a facade of informed bravado.

Postpubescent Sex With a Partner; Homosexual

Increasingly counselors and therapists are consulted when parents suspect or know that their adolescent is in love with a person of the same sex. Even though societal attitudes are relaxing and homosexuality is no longer a disorder in DSM-III, for the individual family it can be traumatic.

Professional consultation is sought by the parent with the initial purpose of curing the errant child, but the family system is the actual patient or client. Both parents and child need to know that a same-sex love affair does not automatically mean that either participant has a homosexual orientation or that another sex love affair guarantees a heterosexual orientation.

It may be that the love object happens to be of the same sex but the love feelings are unique to that individual and may not be generalized to others of the same sex.

It may be that a bisexual resolution will occur, with either or both sexes being available as primary partners throughout a specific life phase or across the life span. It also may be that the first same-sex love may be the expression of an exclusively homosexual life pattern to come.

It is well to keep in mind that the child is doing what comes naturally. Children experience their erotic and love feelings in association with certain people and events not in association with other people and events.

Less often, but occasionally, an adolescent will seek consultation about homosexual feelings or experiences without parental knowledge. A few adolescents are totally unaccepting of homosexuality and are repulsed by any same-sex attractions they might feel. They are traumatized by a same-sex approach or experience, even though they may have been a willing participant. They seek professional help to get rid of whatever is causing their attraction to and by members of the same sex.

Most parents fervently hope that their child's same-sex preference is a phase they will pass through and are unwilling to disown a homosexual child. However, some families or individual family members may be unwilling or incapable of accepting homosexuality, thus precipitating the gay adolescent's premature emancipation from home.

Sexual Concerns of the Physically and Mentally Handicapped

The myth of the sexual innocence of childhood is most secure in the homes of the handicapped child. Close parental supervision, limited autonomy with peers, identity as a physically handicapped child or child with special needs, and rejection by peers as a potential sex partner all contribute to the negation of sexuality of the physically or mentally handicapped child. Handicapped children have sexual curiosity and sexual feelings. Despite the conspiracy of silence, they need to know both basic sexual knowledge and how they can be sexual given their specific limitations. As adolescents they need opportunities to experience their sexual response cycle, to learn what their individual sexual limitations and abilities are, and, perhaps more importantly, how to negotiate for sex with a partner. The orthopedically handicapped are especially assumed to be incapable of sex by most able-bodied people.

Mentally retarded, physically healthy children pose another type of problem. They may be quite normal in physical and sexual development and as adolescents may be attractive enough to be selected as a potential sex partner by a peer or an adult. Impaired mental function may disallow, however, good judgment in sexual situations. Their own sexual desire, coupled with this lack of discrimination, makes them an easy target for sexual exploitation. Mentally retarded children need explicit sex education; reinforced, plainly stated rules about sociosexual conduct; adequate supervision; and effective birth control for girls at the appropriate age.

Families of handicapped adolescents who live at home and caretakers of institutionalized teens need to facilitate the sexual opportunities of their charges. Even if they can acquire potential partners, the handicapped adolescent needs a safe place, privacy, and perhaps some physical assistance to have a successful sex experience. The issues of birth control and paid partners are complicated for adolescents or young adults in institutions or on public assistance, as charges for these services are not reimbursable by third party payers. As a society we have by default decided that the handicapped shall not have sex lives. The advocacy groups for special syndromes have not provided or demanded sexual equality and sexual rights, which for many handicapped people are as important as access to public buildings or the Special Olympics.

Sexual Guilt as a Factor in the Treatment of the Hospitalized Child

Psychological services for the child hospitalized on the medical or surgical ward have become standard practice in many hospitals. In both routine ward service and psychological referrals, the alleviation of sex (masturbation) guilt is often a significant factor in the understanding and treatment of the physical illness. From the concrete thinking of the young child to the maturing moralism of the teenager, the cause and effect rationale is predominant. The simplistic link from bad thoughts to bad deeds usually includes forbidden sexual behaviors. A frank discussion about masturbation, what it is and what it isn't, allows the therapist to assuage the child's masturbation guilt, to demythologize and disconnect sexual behavior as the cause of injury or illness, to impart accurate information, and to give permission for continued masturbatory behavior in the hospital. It also facilitates trust in the therapist about other personal concerns (e.g., recovery, abandonment, death, etc.).

Most adults are ambivalent about children's masturbation. Medical and hospital personnel may need some help in understanding the purpose of dealing with masturbation when health concerns are primary. Masturbation is an effective tension and anxiety reducer in children and adults and it is self-affirming. It is an activity that reclaims the body and offsets intrusive hospital procedures. Deliberate interference with a regular masturbation pattern constitutes an unnecessary deprivation and added stress to an already stressful situation.

Child Prostitution and Kiddie Porn

The exploitation of children is an anathema in our humanitarian society. We have laws to protect children from unscrupulous adults. However, there is a societal reluctance to intrude on the nuclear family. The campaign for the recognition of the battered child as a syndrome of ongoing abuse was hard fought in the 1960's. No one wanted to believe or admit that it was a widespread phenomenon that had crossed all educational, socioeconomic, racial, ethnic, and religious lines.

Child prostitution and kiddie porn are similarly societal problems that adults are trying hard not to address. Runaways who become street children with no job skills (many are too young to work legally), no money, no shelter, etc., quickly learn that they have only one negotiable commodity, their sexuality. Male or female, they can sell their bodies to adult men. The ranks of street children relegated to prostitution and other forms of sexual exploitation grows consistently.

Some children are encouraged by a parent into prostitution to augment the family income and upgrade the standard of living. These children are usually female, living with a mother as a single parent. The girl in this situation is more apt to come to the attention of authorities and be referred for evaluation and therapy than street children who are rarely seen professionally. Any individual can be psychologically evaluated and can benefit from the self-knowledge gained in psychotherapy. However, child prostitution and kiddie porn are broad-spectrum, societal problems that will not be alleviated by individual psychotherapy.

Other Symptoms of Sexual Significance

Peeping tomism, underwear stealing, and sex with animals are asocial and illegal activities which may be transient attempts to satisfy child or adolescent sexual curiosity, or they may be the development of aberrant patterns of voyeurism, fetishism, and bestiality. The behavior may be in response to a lack of knowledge or an expression of underlying psychopathology. It is helpful to the child if the differential diagnosis is made by a therapist who won't overreact to the symptoms. Society's messages about sex can be contradictory and confusing to children and adolescents. Whether the resultant dissonance is expressed as private worry, fear, and doubt, or erupts into public behavior, children are well served by accurate information, endorsement of the normalcy of sexual feelings and desires, knowledge of their right to be sexual, and an opportunity to learn culturally acceptable sociosexual behavior and skills.

Sexual Health

Sexual health is more than the absence of sexual pathology. The anatomy, gender and function of the human body is the foundation of identity. The awareness of the sexual self as an integrated aspect of identity begins in infancy with the attitudes about the physical body communicated by the caretakers.

The sexual response cycle as described by Masters and Johnson (1966) is present at birth, and there is evidence that the neurological maturation necessary to produce penile erections occurs in utero. The development and expression of the erotic response throughout the human lifespan is not a well-studied phenomenon and normative data have not been compiled for sexual behaviors of childhood and adolescence.

As we know it, the erotic response consists of a complex interplay of physiological and psychological factors that are highly susceptible to familial, religious, and cultural folkways, and mores and attitudes. The styles of acceptable sexual attitude and expression fluctuate historically and culturally between generally positive and generally negative polarities. Our own culture is still preoccupied with imposing sexual constraints rather than promoting sexual competencies as a basic value system. We are certainly less zealous in this pursuit than the repressive Victorians, but fears of sexual excess and pleasure leading to a fall from grace are deeply embedded in the Judeo-Christian ethic. The impact of this often unconscious attitude on child rearing is to overtly and/or covertly discourage sexual interest, curiosity, expression, and behavior of children in the presence of adults and to obscure continually the scientific answer to the question, "What is normal?"

Sexually *permissive* cultures not only allow a less fettered expression of adult sexuality, but may give little attention to the sexual behaviors of children as long as they are not blatantly displayed. Sexually *supportive* cultures, believing that sex is indispensable to human happiness, encourage early sexual expression as means of developing adult sexual competency and positive sexual attitudes. The children in sexually permissive and sexually supportive societies display a similar developmental pattern that is not apparent in sexually *restrictive* and sexually *repressive* societies.

In infancy there is usually manual and oral-genital stimulation of children of both sexes by parents as a means of comforting and pacifying them (most frequently between mothers and sons). In early childhood masturbation alone and in groups leads to exploration and experimentation among children of same and opposite gender. Late childhood (prepubescence) is characterized by heterosexual role modeling and attempted intercourse (girls may begin having regular coitus with older boys). In pubescence girls accelerate rapidly into a phase of intense sexual experience culminating in the acquisition of basic sexual techniques at the adult level of skill mastery. Boys follow a similar pattern, but their learning process is not as rapid nor as complete because they are usually experimenting with younger girls. Heterosexual patterns replace masturbation and homosexual activities for the majority of both boys and girls. In adolescence there is increased sexual activity with peers and adults for both boys and girls, and it is believed that birth control is facilitated by the practice of multiple partners. Marriage is common for late adolescent girls, but boys may delay marriage for economic considerations and continue their adolescent sex patterns for longer periods (Ford & Beach, 1951).

History of Human Sexual Expression

It would appear that human sexual expression follows a logical, orderly, and self-regulating developmental pattern in much the same way as other aspects of human behavior. Psychosexual disorders may be the result of the interruptions of that sequential growth process.

It is well to remember that prior to the Victorian idealization of childhood innocence, children were commonly used and abused physically and psychologically. Eighteenth century aristocratic tradition imposed a barrier between parent and child. It was the height of bad taste to love one's spouse and children, as parenthood was thought to render both men and women less fit for amorous adventure. Infants were removed from their parents, suckled by wet nurses, and mortality was high, even for children who were well cared for. Infanticide was the major method of population control and infants were abandoned, neglected, and intentionally killed by drowning, burning, scalding, potting, and overlaying. Those that survived were often maimed or crippled to make them more poignant beggars and were at the mercy of unscrupulous and exploitive adults. Sexual exploitation of children was freely indulged in until the latter half of the eighteenth century at which time it was fully repudiated. This was a decisive turning point in parent-child relationships in that parents began to punish children for their sexual curiosity and activity (DeMause, 1974).

The Victorian era was a period of sexual schizophrenia for children. The cultural dictum that childhood was free of, and was to remain free from, sexual knowledge, interest, and behavior was contradicted by a constant and continual adult preoccupation with, and surveillance of, children's sexual potential. Freud's attempt to bring some sanity into this schizophenogenic bind was helpful theoretically; however, the sadistic trend in antimasturbatory activity intensified when people became aware of infant sexuality (Spitz, 1952).

The wholesale repression of sexuality made any expectation of sexual health improbable, if not impossible, to achieve. It produced a prevasive negative preoccupation with the sexuality of others and a category of emotional disorders labled psychosexual. In keeping with the contradictions of the time, the sexual referent to all nonsexual symptomatology was diligently searched for or speculated about and direct treatment of sexual symptoms was bypassed in favor of analyzing the "psychosexual" stages of childhood development.

Sexology

The mental health community continues to have a poorly defined concept of sexual health, and is in fact only called upon to attend those who have experienced sexual trauma dysfunction and /or sexual pathology. Although sexuality (i.e., sexual interest, sex drive) is considered by many to be the life force, sexology (sexual science) is less than a hundred years old. *Clinical sexology*, the diagnosis and treatment of sexual concerns and dysfunction, as a specialty is newer still. Sex therapy has been a viable and identifiable health specialty since the 1960s and the clinical sexologist is a phenomenon of the late 1970s. However, the clinical child sexologist is a professional category of the future. Even so, pediatric professionals, in both medicine and mental health, are consulted by parents, caretakers, authorities, and occasionally youngsters themselves about sexual matters. It is no longer conscionable to consider sexual health as the absence of sexual pathology, because sexual pathology is often a religious-cultural definition which fails to consider the broad range of human sexual activity, its developmental aspects, measurable frequencies, and impact on the quality of human life.

Sexual Rights of Children

In Western culture there is great controversy about what adult (parent and professional) attitudes concerning children's sexual expression should be. Many child-rights advocates believe that children are a disenfranchised minority in the age/class system and state that the privilege and responsibility of sexual behavior is one of the many human rights denied them. They suggest that the proper adult stance is one of permissiveness to encouragement (Farson, 1974; Yates, 1979). This argument is more than vaguely akin to the rhetoric of the pedophile groups who have a vested interest in the relaxation or abolishment of child protective (albeit restrictive) laws. Many child experts more conversant with the vulnerabilities of children in a complex pluralistic society opt for laws and social custom that, although somewhat limiting, provide protection from unscrupulous adults. A child, by definition, is not a consenting adult in sexual matters and may need protection from the liability of sexual contracts in the same manner that they are not held accountable for business or labor contracts.

This position does not suggest that there is inherent harm in sexual expression in childhood and we have considerable evidence to the contrary. Sexologically, it is based on the knowledge that the benefits of free sexual expression of children can only occur in a sexually supportive society: where all people have sex for sexual reasons; where sexual knowledge, skill, and pleasure are valued for both males and females; which encourages sexual competency rather than constraint and in which every man, woman, and child can say "yes" or "no" to sex without prejudice or coercion. To encourage children to be sexual in a sexually repressive or permissive (ambivalent) culture is to exploit their healthy sexual interest, as they will be left alone to deal with a double-standard and the sex-negative, self-serving attitudes of peers and adults.

Development of the Erotic Response

In the absence of normative data on the behavioral manifestations of the development of the erotic response from birth through adolescence, we must, for the moment at least, hypothesize a normal distribution. We assume, then, that there will be some highly sexed children to whom sexual concerns and sexual expression will be a dominant theme (positively or negatively expressed) in their lives as a whole, with some fluctuations in the various stages of development and in response to certain circumstances. There will be a like number of children to whom sexual concerns and expressions are a consistently low priority in their organization of life as a whole, with some fluctuations in the various stages of development and in response to certain life events. The middle 68 percent is hypothesized to fall equally distributed between these two extremes and to have a moderate focus on the sexual aspects of human existence with the aformentioned fluctuations. This group would be more responsive to the external cultural attitudes about sexuality and would be more easily influenced by external events (i.e., they would be more liberal in sexually permissive times or cultures and more conservative in sexually restrictive times or cultures, etc.)

With the normal distribution of the population as a theoretical baseline, a wholesale advocacy of more sexual expression in childhood would be as oppressive to the children at one end of the distribution as a societal expectation of no sexual expression in childhood would be to the children at the other end of the continuum. It is a romantic notion that the encouragement of sexual freedom in childhood would produce a society of adults who rise to unparalleled heights of sexual intimacy and ecstasy and who are devoid of sexual dysfunction. If we can hypothesize the normal distribution of sexual interest and drive, can we also project the fluctuations that are subject to age, stage, and life events? A close look at the developmental and sociological literature allows for some cautious extrapolation. Keeping in mind that developmental criteria for normative age and stage behavior is, to a degree, culture bound, we can project some reasonable parameters of expected sexual behavior.

Overview

There are four stages of childhood and adolescence in which the focus of the body shifts between a primary and a secondary concern. The *first stage* is from birth to about 6 years of age. The physical body is primary and sexual interests, curiosity, arousal, and behavior are spontaneously expressed, unless or until the child is taught to repress or inhibit their pleasure orientation.

The *second stage* is from approximately six to pubescence (approximately twelve). The primary attention of the child shifts to the mental realm. The desire for sexual pleasure continues, but most children are thoughtful and discriminating about their sexual behavior and expressions. Their need for privacy and autonomy characterize this stage.

The *third stage* is pubescence to early adolescence (approximately thirteen to fifteen). As sex hormones come into play, the body is once again primary, with rapid growth spurts, development of secondary sex characteristics, sensations of increased intensity, and new awareness of the physical self and its impact on others. Sexual behaviors respond to a stronger biological mandate, becoming a preoccupation which may be characterized by poor social judgment, high-risk behavior, and lack of discrimination.

The *fourth stage* is mid to late adolescence (approximately from sixteen on). The body growth rate slows, hormonal balance is achieved, secondary sex changes are incorporated into the body image, sexual response cycle is accommodated through masturbation or partner sex, and sexual gratification is integrated into the context of a relationship (Haroian, 1976).

The sexual maturation of a child reflects the overall pattern of development, from absorption in and dependency on the family of origin through the gradual acquisition of a sense of the autonomous self to the confidence and desire to establish an intimate bond and form the family of choice. The erotic response of infancy is global, undifferentiated, and polymorph perverse. In childhood it moves toward a genital focus (more surely for boys than for girls) and is expressed through purposefully directed masturbatory activity and perhaps some negotiated social interaction (often with same-sex partners). At pubescence, the genital focus intensifies, the acquisition of opposite sex partners gains importance for heterosexual youth, and sexual experience per se is the paramount goal. In adolescence, this motivation of curiosity and self-gratification emerges into one of sexual reciprocity and mutual sharing. Partnerships are increasingly stable, interdependent, and emotionally intimate (Haroian, 1980).

It is well to note that this developmental scheme appears to be stable in all cultures whether they be sexually repressive, restrictive, permissive, or supportive. It is enhanced by, but not dependent on, the child's ability to engage in sexual behavior and is seen as a mental construct in the absence of sexual experimentation. There is considerable evidence that adult sexual health and pleasure is positively correlated with age-appropriate childhood sexual behavior. The interplay between the individual sex drive (importance of sex to the child) and the sexual values of the culture (sex-negative or sex-positive messages) determines sexual behavior in childhood and adolescence. The strongly sexed child may struggle through what constitutes a repressive childhood in a sexually negative culture, but emerge as a sexually healthy adult because she or he took every possible opportunity to be sexual and maintained a sexual focus despite censure and sanction (typically a male pattern). More at risk in our culture is the moderately sexed child or low sexed child who accepts the culturally negative values and is sexually inactive and unaware during childhood and finds him or herself out of phase with the sexual expectations of adulthood (typically female pattern) (Haroian, 1980).

Although it is popular to attribute all sex specific differences to cultural factors, it may well be that there are inherent sexual pattern differences between girls and boys and men and women. The cultural factors in our sexually restrictive society are so discriminatory against girls and women that they obscure any inherent difference and constitute a major child-rearing concern. A close look at American child-rearing practice suggests that in terms of adult attitudes, boys exist in a sexually permissive culture. "Boys will be boys," which includes sexual experimentation and behavior, and as long as they do not blatantly flaunt their sexual interest and activities in front of adults, they receive little censure.

Girls, on the other hand, are reared in what is essentially a sexually restrictive society in that their sexual interest, and certainly sexual behavior, is not sanctioned and may even be ignored by adults. Girls are expected to be nonsexual in childhood and adolescence. Sexual interest, curiosity, and especially, sexual experience cause girls to be devalued by family and peer group alike. Sexual innocence, inexperience, and ignorance are cultural values for girls. They are permitted to express curiosity and receive information about their future reproductive function as their gender role is programmed. Sexual intercourse is presented as the gift they are to give the man they love, a marital duty, necessary for impregnation, which they might on occasion enjoy. The pleasure aspect is reportedly dependent on love and is not considered sufficient reason for their engaging in sex. (Men have sex because they love sex; women have sex because they love a man). Girls are taught to withhold sex as a means of controlling or punishing men, and without conscious awareness begin to use their sexuality as a negotiable commodity. Concurrently, they are taught to devalue women who sell their sexuality—the prostitute being held out as the greatest threat to the sanctity of female virtue and family values. Girls are expected to be the guardians of cultural mores by restricting or diverting the male sex drive.

Boys are taught that it is their nature and their right to pursue sexual gratification but that girls who, like themselves, seek sexual experience and pleasure are less valued in society than girls who deny them sexual favors. Boys may be more egalitarian in their attitudes about their "sexual partner," expecting her to be uninhibited, willing, and responsive. Although they appreciate and enjoy sex with a responsive partner, they expect her not to engage in sex with others, even though they may give themselves permission to do so. Often without conscious awareness they devalue the sexually responsive girl that they enjoy and dedicate themselves to a relationship of sexual frustration with a girl who uses her sexuality for secondary gain.

The girl who, true to the double standard, has sex to please (and control) the boy, rather then to please herself, offers a sense of security to an unsure male. If she does not enjoy sex or pretends that she is uninterested except to accommodate her partner, he need not worry that she will actively seek nor willingly respond to sex with others. He may seek sex for pleasure outside his primary relationship and value, in a social sense, his nonsexual mate. If her prudishness is a sham, she may also seek outside sexual gratification and be seductive, responsive, assertive, and/or experimental with another partner.

These adult patterns have antecedents in childhood and can be easily traced through the ages and stages of development.

Early Childhood

By three years of age many children can affirm their own sex, "I am a boy," and often in the negative, "I am not a girl." They verbalize sex differences; girls often try to urinate standing up; and there is a desire to touch mother's breasts. They have a great interest in marriage to the other parent and want the family to have a baby. While there may be some basic questioning as to where a baby comes from, there is an intense desire or need to relive his/her own infancy. Parents are urged to repeat the stories over and over. The child may act out being a baby, want to have a bottle or nurse at the breast and be carried in competition with a new sibling, even if the family does not have a baby.

In the latter half of the third year many children begin to feel great tension and express it through many compulsive patterns, such at stuttering, eye blinking, nail biting, thumb sucking, nose picking, masturbation, spitting, and/or chewing on hair or clothing. An intense need for attention, preoccupation with bodily functions, interest and curiosity about reproduction, and increased ability to communicate verbally with adults can culminate in a pseudomature seductive posture, especially in female three-year-olds who have been socialized to be more tractable. It is quite common at a party of adults to see the three-year-old daughter of the host comfortably curled up in the lap or laps of a succession of male guests capturing their attention. She may even request that her "new friend" put her to bed and may hold thoughts of him and make reference to him for days or weeks after the party. This behavioral pattern is not exclusive to girls, but is somewhat more pronounced and is better tolerated in terms of gender role stereotypes by the involved adults than when it occurs in boys.

The potential for sexual stimulation in this situation is obvious and available data confirms the incidence of pedophillic genital fondling at this age (Kempe & Kempe, 1978; Williams & Money, 1980). The accessibility and vulnerability of the child may be beyond the limits of an adult male with poor impulse control. The sexualization of the adult-child relationship is not sin qua non a psychological trauma. The histories of many adult men and women include childhood sexual experiences that were not traumatic or that caused little concern until the sexual activity escalated beyond looking and fondling or until the situation was discovered and responded to negatively by other adults.

Four is an excellent age to test the reproductive interest of the child with accurate and somewhat detailed explanations about procreation. If the environment includes pregnant women or newborns, children's curiosity will be stimulated and they are quite capable of hearing accurate details. If they persist in believing that babies get out through the navel or that they are purchased at the hospital, it is not necessary to make an issue out of their misinformation. At an appropriate time they may again be told the story of reproduction and eventually the information will be assimilated and reported correctly. Many children are quick to grasp the concept of intercourse and may make delightful, albeit inconvenient, reference to their new knowledge. Four-year-old Arnie, in a conversation with his mother, said, "I'm a boy and I have a penis, you're a girl and you have a vagina. We could put ours together. Do you want to, Mom?" Mother answered appropriately that boys and mothers don't put theirs together, just mommies and daddies: "When you're a Daddy, you will put it together with your wife."

Early School Age

Five-year-old boys may still occasionally say, "When I grow up to be a mommy," but respond upon questioning that they are destined to become fathers if they choose to parent. Fives talk of marriage, but expect to marry a family member and live at home with their baby. They may be upset and feel abandoned if the parent insists that they will marry a stranger and leave home.

Although the belly button may be omitted from human figure drawings, genitals are often added, much to the consternation of the kindergarten teacher collecting displays for public school open house. Sex talk is often embarrassing to parents even though it is honest and forthright on the part of the child. Five-year-old Betty said, "Sometimes I see one fly sitting on top of another fly." Her mother replied, "Flies are like that." She continued, "I've thought and thought and I've finally figured it out. That must be her big brother giving her a piggy-back ride."

A five-year-old will often report sexual overtures or sexual behavior, especially from peers, to mother in a matter of fact way. Quite often they have turned down the invitation. Five-year-old Kevin reported to his mother that a twelve-year-old neighbor girl wanted to see his penis and offered to show him her genitals in return. He had social consciousness and explained, "You know, Mom, she doesn't have a brother to look at, but I told her if she wanted to see a penis to ask her dad because he has one."

Although there is little reason to assume peer sex play is a negative experience for five-year-olds, parents may be uncomfortable and concerned about dire consequences at a later date. In point of fact, every child is initially subject to the value system of his or her parents and the arbitrary rules of the household. It is best to investigate and be clear about what the family rules are without burdening the children with fear, doubt, and guilt.

Youngsters show a marked interest in anatomical differences and playing "show" and "doctor" help satisfy that curiosity, especially for children who haven't had opposite gender siblings or playmates. Six-year-old Cathy was crying because her fourteen-year-old brother had locked her out of the bathroom. Her mother explained that he wanted his privacy because his penis was beginning to grow. Cathy continued to cry and bang on the door as she replied, "But he's my brother and I want to see his penis grow."

Penetration, either in masturbation or mutual sex play, may occur and may be vaginal or anal (simulating the taking of body temperature anally, which is in their experiential background). Sex play with older children is also common and a six-year-old's interest and curiosity about sex may be easily exploited by older siblings or extended family members and caretakers. Young children are much more apt to report to mother sexual contacts with older children or adults than peer sex play, which most often goes unreported.

There is still much confusion over sexual facts during these years and many children are not knowledgeable enough or comfortable enough to ask parents the appropriate questions. Parents may be willing to answer if asked and assume that if the question is not forthcoming that it is too early to offer information. Both boys and girls are curious about the total process of reproduction and few can piece together accurately the information received thus far.

Case Illustration: Eight-year-old Chris desperately wanted her mother to have a baby. Her mother said she and her new husband were trying to have a baby, but with little success. When Chris found out that her mother was taking birth-control pills to prevent conception, she angrily refused to communicate with her mother or her stepfather and vowed to have her own children when she grew up. One day she queried her therapist, "If you want to have babies when you grow up, do you have to practice when you're young?" After assurance that most women do not have difficulty getting pregnant and that prepubescent practice was unnecessary, Chris revealed that her friend Peter, aged 12, was suggesting that if she didn't practice now, she might not be able to have a child when she grew up. He was also kind enough to volunteer his services in this regard.

Books of their own, lovingly inscribed by their parents, endorse a child's interest and curiosity about sex and provide a reference that can be returned to and shared with friends. Graphic depiction, photos, or sketches are also important learning aids as our culture becomes increasingly visual. Books and pictures about the body and sex help children understand that human sexuality is a legitimate academic subject that can be explored objectively as well as subjectively. They learn to satisfy a good deal of their sexual curiosity vicariously and become less dependent on trail and error learning.

PREADOLESCENCE

By ten years of age gender differences are pronounced, with girls manifesting social behavior which is considered more mature. Boys' activities tend to focus around gross motor games and sports and their spontaneous play is action oriented, with one challenging the other to informal bouts of wrestling, racing, climbing, etc. Many boys are involved in organized team sports at ten that focus the family on their performance. Girls' physical contacts tend to be affectionate rather than aggressive. They hold hands or walk with their arms around each other and they are more interested in relationships. They gossip, write notes, keep diaries, and play dolls to act out their interest in romance, weddings, marriage, and children. Girls operate in smaller, more personal groups and they are more aware of their appearance and their expectations of others. Girls have more interest in love and romance and peer boys are consistent disappointments in this regard. Girls at this age are often in love with a considerably older boy or adult male.

Girls and boys at ten are about equal in size; however, many girls will experience nipple enlargement and the beginnings of pubic hair in their tenth year. Girls have an increasingly practical interest in menstruation, some looking forward to it as a symbol of maturity and others resisting and denying that it will happen to them. Girls are less likely to tell sexual jokes, but are interested in the parental sexual relationship and may ask personal questions about it. If parents are divorced and dating, daughters may probe for the intimate details of the new relationships.

Boys are less likely to question parents about sexual matters, more apt to repeat sexual and elimination jokes and rhymes and to use sexual words as perjoratives. Most are aware of the male's role in reproduction, understand the fundamentals of intercourse and have had some sexual experience. Few have noticeable physical changes, but may require bathroom and dressing privacy from mother and sisters. These same boys may peek at sister and friends whenever possible. Boys begin to differentiate sex jokes that can be shared appropriately with mother or girls and a few ten-year-old boys develop a strong attraction for a specific girl. Boys and girls consider their mother a friend, confide in her, request private time with her, and think up nice things to do for her (i.e., gifts, surprises, breakfast in bed, etc.). Fathers are often idolized and companionship with father is sought by both boys and girls.

Friends are paramount at this age and everpresent if allowed. Sleeping over is a favorite activity and sex talk and experimentation is common. Few children are encouraged or allowed to entertain opposite sex friends overnight so there is a tacit parental endorsement of same-sex acts. Most children feel that same-sex experimentation is normal and age appropriate, but that heterosexual coupling should be reserved for adulthood and reproduction. That is not to say that heterosexual play does not occur at ten, because it does for some. However, it is wise to consider that the age specific division of the sexes, the earlier focus on reproductive information, and the parental unconcern over the sexual potential of same-sex friends all combine to produce in the mind of a ten-year-old a tacit adult approval of homosexual experimentation, all the while producing quite a different mind set about heterosexual experimentation.

Many girls at eleven are still in an antiboy stage and have a consuming interest in horses. As girls begin to develop secondary sex characteristics, they gain status among girls and popularity with boys. The more mature boys court and tease the developing girls, wanting to know bra size, trying to see up skirts, etc. Recreation centers are the meeting place for physical activity and group discussion. Preoccupation with the physical female form is well-serviced in the athletic arena. Not only is sports attire revealing, the periodic water balloon fights, if well directed, produce a spontaneous wet T-shirt contest.

Girls at twelve experience their most rapid growth in both height and weight, achieving 95 percent of their mature height. Breasts fill out and nipples darken, auxiliary hair sprouts, and menarche occurs near the end of the twelfth year. Body odors change and intensify and hygiene needs increase. Self-consciousness about breast development may be expressed in some girls by attempts to minimize their changing form, while others augment nature and flaunt their new proportions. Girls need acknowledgment and endorsement of their emerging sexuality from family members if they are to integrate their sexual self into their total self-concept. It is important that parents neither overvalue or undervalue (ignore) the physical changes of pubescence, but rather that they celebrate reproductive potential as the passage from childhood to adulthood that it truly signifies. It is an artifact of complex civilization, not biology, that girls will probably delay childbearing for close to another decade even though the physical and psychological readiness to reproduce is a phenomenon of adolescence.

Many girls look forward to the menarche, but even so, may be ambivalent when it occurs. Twelve-year-old Anne, eagerly anticipating menarche, began her first period on a Friday and that evening asked to spend the night with her grandma. Her mother asked if she had included sanitary napkins in her overnight bag. She had not, and asked if it was necessary. Mother explained that Grandma would not have any at her house and that she should take at least two. As Anne went off to get them, she muttered, "This having your period isn't as wonderful as I thought it was going to be."

As girls adjust to the rituals of menstruation and their periods become more uniform in nature and regular in occurrence, they become more positive about growing up and more knowing about sexual matters in general. Because the early periods are not usually accompanied by premenstrual signals, most girls experience the embarrassment of spotting and/or they may be excused from P.E. or showering, which serves notice to peers that they have reached the milestone of menstruation. Girls who mature more slowly may be pleased that they do not have to experience the inconvenience of menstruation and/or are concerned that they are not one of the group. Girls talk in the abstract about sexual matters and may need to clarify previously held misconceptions with peers, parents, and/or other adults. Sometimes a specific teacher develops a reputation as a reliable source of sex information and is queried regularly to clarify the myths and misconceptions that reliably surface during these junior high years. It is remarkable that sex jokes and stories, despite their inaccuracies, are perennial, resurfacing at the same age, generation after generation.

Boys are more interested in hearing and repeating sexual jokes and in acquiring sexually graphic material. By twelve they have a good sense of humor and wit and love the double entendre. They can be embarrassed by sexual situations or jokes, especially if the joke is on them, i.e., sexual naivete or ignorance in the midst of others knowing. The sexual components or meanings of heretofore nonsexual words and actual sexual vocabulary is a major task of the pubescent child. It is a rite of passage that separates childhood and adolescence. Boys are usually more conversant with sex words and meanings than girls, but they too must learn. Social customs dictate that if you understand the sexual implication, you acknowledge that understanding. If you do not understand, you ignore the implied sexual connotation. You never attempt to learn by asking the meaning or definition because this is an age of jokes and secrets. The harder you try to find out what was funny, the more secret the information becomes and *you* become the joke.

There is a wide range of physical growth differential among twelve-year-old boys, but the majority show some evidence of beginning puberty. Growth of the penis and scrotum is common and may precede or succeed pubic hair. Twelve-year-old boys are becoming more interested in sex, especially their own sexuality. They are more fully aware that sex occurs for reasons other than reproduction, and heterosexual boys begin to acquire pictures of nude females.

Boys tend to think of sex as dirty, want accurate information, and would prefer to seek information from a neutral adult. If they do consult with a parent in sexual matters, it will more often be the mother for specific information rather than a full discussion of sex in general. In the absence of a sexual confidant, boys will seek out information from printed sources and have bull sessions with peers to discuss sexual matters to the extent of their pooled knowledge.

Masturbation increases in frequency and may be experienced alone or in groups and may or may not produce ejaculation. Erections occur with or without external cause and may happen spontaneously at inappropriate moments causing embarrassment and anxiety about future situations. Externally triggered erections may also be embarrassing as they are caused by various stimuli often deemed inappropriate by the boy (i.e., sex talk, scuffling or physical contact with male peers, fear, rage, embarrassment, etc.).

Twelve-year-old heterosexual boys are interested in girls, and although most prefer group activities, some fall in love and openly express their affectionate feelings. Kissing is a favorite activity; however, having a girlfriend or boyfriend is more a social phenomenon than an interpersonal one. The assignment of couple status has little or no interpersonal responsibility. It is changed frequently without emotion and is often decided by a group or a "marriage broker" within the group.

A few boys at this age, or seventh grade boys who may be in or closer to their thirteenth year, may actively seek sex with girls. They do not ask permission, thus exempting the girl from verbalizing responsibility, but begin simply to see how far they can go. It is common for junior high girls to stay overnight with a friend and arrange to meet boys who are doing the same. Boys are often aware of girls' slumber parties and make themselves available. When sex occurs between a boy and girl of this age the boy tells his friends who in turn question him for details. He acquires status among peers as they learn about sex acts, sociosexual negotiations, and about their female peers. Girls do not confide in their friends, nor are they questioned by their friends about sexual encounters.

Thirteen-year-old Bob performed cunnilingus on twelve-year-old Fran. He was the first in his circle to have the experience and so he became the "man of the hour" among his curious friends. The information was passed to the girls who were shocked and unbelieving, but none asked Fran for confirmation, denial, or details. This pattern is stable through high school, with boys talking and sharing sexual experiences for knowledge and endorsement and girls gossiping about the sexuality of others but rarely, if ever, sharing firsthand sexual experiences and concerns. One female high school senior remarked, "You don't tell anyone anything about sex that you don't want repeated, not even to your best friend." The result is a large number of sexually naive and uninformed girls, who have misconceptions and misinformation about sexual matters, who depend primarily on experiential learning for sexual knowledge, and who rely on boys to teach them how to be sexual.

Homosexual twelve-year-olds may or may not be involved in sexual activity with peers, even though there is more opportunity for them than there is for many heterosexual youths. Some heterosexual twelves are still engaging in sexual activity and exploration with same-sex peers. Many adult homosexuals retrospectively report gradual awareness of not being turned on to opposite sex peers at this age, but few twelves declare themselves homosexual or bisexual.

ADOLESCENCE

For most adolescent girls, menstrual periods are usually not painful, nor do they usually conform to the adult twenty-eight-day cycle. Girls are ambivalent about others knowing that they are menstruating and most do not want to buy their own sanitary napkins, feeling that it is too embarrassing. Thirteen-year-old Megan started her first period on a Saturday and asked her mother not to tell her father and brother. When Mother replied that she already had, Megan asked with great anticipation, "What did they say?" Her mother replied, "They are both happy for you."

She was delighted and asked if the family could have Sunday dinner in the dining room with the good china and crystal. When her mother agreed that a celebration was appropriate, she asked if she could invite the extended family. Her mother advised that it was pretty short notice, but perhaps one aunt and uncle might be able to come. Megan remarked, "Maybe we shouldn't call them because it would be pretty embarrassing to tell them why they are invited—but we celebrate every other important occasion in our family." As a culture we fail to celebrate fertility and see it rather as a disadvantage, if not an outright danger of adolescence. This contradictory message on the relative merits of maturity is not lost on teens.

Only about half of the boys have ejaculations before their fourteenth year, but most know about them. Masturbation may increase significantly and be accompanied by guilt if they have not learned that it is normal. Nocturnal emission or masturbation are the most common first ejaculatory experiences. Many boys are interested in having sex with girls at thirteen, but are too direct and abrupt to facilitate encounters with any but the most interested and willing girls.

The more sexually popular boys and girls can have important, gratifying relationships with each other. Boys become more interested in selecting girls to "go with" even though couple dating is still a rarity. The group is the most visible social structure and conversation is the major group activity. It is the fortunate thirteen-year-old who has an opposite sex confidant.

By fourteen, most girls are physically mature with all secondary sex characteristics near completion; menstrual cycles are regular (although many are as long as forty-five to fifty days). Many girls have premenstrual symptoms (cramps, headaches, backaches, or general tension or nervousness), and menstrual discomfort the first day causes some girls to lie down for a couple hours, miss a meal, or take medication. Many girls report experiencing a physical response in their involvement with boys. It may be global, rather than genital, and is often confusing to the girl who is poorly informed about sexuality. Girls may begin masturbation in response to this arousal, many for the first time.

Boys, who tend to be maturationally a little behind girls, experience their most rapid growth spurt at fourteen, although it will be another year before they actually look like men. At fourteen the ratio of body fat to muscles decreases, body hair increases and darkens, sideburns elongate, voices may crack suddenly, and what appears to be hoarseness from a cold very often remains. Most boys have ejaculated by the end of their fourteenth year and most develop a regular pattern of sexual activity after their first ejaculation. Many boys are extremely modest, especially about nocturnal emissions and, despite increasing societal tolerance, many experience significant masturbatory guilt. Sex education is needed and eagerly sought by fourteen-year-old boys. They want now to work out their own personal sexual attitudes and need information to do so. They need to know and discuss the broad spectrum of human sexual behavior.

The high school locker room for many fourteen-year-olds is their first experience at public nudity. Most fourteens manage to overcome their shyness and are quickly comfortable in varying stages of undress. A few are so shy that they request to be excused permanently from P.E. or just never show up. This milieu is especially problematic for the homosexual youngster who may be overstimulated by mass nudity of his or her eroticized gender. It is especially traumatic for boys who are more stimulated by visual imagery and whose arousal is visible to all. Physical education instructors need to be reminded that to require a homosexual adolescent to take part in locker room nudity can be every bit as stimulating as expecting a heterosexual boy to dress and shower with the girls.

Most boys by fifteen have established a regular pattern of sexual outlet, have fewer erections to nonsexual stimuli, and may have fewer sex materials around as fantasy alone is sufficient for arousal. Their masturbatory frequency increases and some have regular sex with girls. Gay teens may fall in love, have sex, and understand that they are homosexual.

Management of partner sex is problematic even if the partner is willing. Where and when to find a private place for a sexual encounter is a major concern, as is birth control and venereal disease protection if they are sexually active with a number of partners. Most girls are worried about reputation and fear being found out, but may decide to have intercourse if they are in love, if they trust the boy, and if the relationship seems secure.

Boys, experiencing the sexual urgency of adolescence, attempt to persuade, manipulate, and coerce girls into actual coitus. "If you love me you will let me put it in," "If you don't someone else will," and, "If you let me put it in, I will pull it out in time," are dilemmas the mid-adolescent girl is called upon to deal with as she negotiates the relationship or potential relationship that affords her a social status and a sense of personal worth. Girls have been raised to understand the importance of the primary relationship and to feel responsible for maintaining it. Now they must deal with the needs, expectations, and requirements of the boys who are the necessary other half of the dyad. Culture says, "If you're easy and give them what they want, they will leave you." Boys say, "If you don't give me what I need, I will have to find someone who will." It is a social dilemma.

Actually, coitus with a mid-adolescent boy is rarely the event of a young girl's life. Reminiscent of stories of wedding night disappointments, boys tend not to last long enough or be cognizant enough of their partners to provide the ultimate experience. Boys want sex and often become angry and disgruntled if it is withheld; girls may fall quickly into a pattern of duty sex. Adolescents who delay intercourse and establish patterns of effective petting become more creative sex partners. Boys learn to last longer and girls are more apt to become reliably orgasmic with their partner if foreplay is extensive (Hamilton, 1978).

Girls who only date occasionally may find it easier to delay intercourse. However, some girls use sex in their attempts to secure a steady boyfriend. Boys who don't go steady may have fairly regular partner sex with these girls or girls who have established a casual sex pattern. Some boys just "go for it with every girl," often to the amazement of their peers, and develop sociosexual skills that assure them in increasing number of interested partners. Sexually naive girls may be inordinately attracted to these entrepreneurial boys and may eagerly contribute their virginity in the process (virginity usually does not become a burden until late in adolescence). Nevertheless, more than half the boys and two-thirds of the girls report that they are still virgins at fifteen.

Boys, by sixteen complete their pubertal development; most shave at least once a week and some boys sprout chest hair. Height is about 98 percent complete and bodies have a firmer physique, especially those of boys who are athletically active. Sixteens are interested in work, money, clothes, cars, music, sex, and drugs. Boys' interest in girls increases, and although graphic sex materials are still used, fantasy alone is a reliable and increasing method of initiating the male sexual response cycle. Masturbation continues to be the major sexual outlet for most boys, though kissing and mutual masturbation are favored activities of even informal pairs.

Many girls and some boys at sixteen feel they "are not ready" for sexual intercourse, but few can explain their criteria of readiness. Girls fear pregnancy and their reputation. Birth control is a management problem, especially if they are reluctant to engage their mother's help. Some young couples go to a clinic together to select a birth-control method which reassures the girl's fears of security, reputation, etc.

Older adolescent boys are more interested in relationship sex, see girls as equal partners, and want the security of going steady. Adolescents use the term "cheated on" and feel that it is wrong to have sex outside a committed relationship. There is a characteristic pattern of breaking up and reconciling in relationships which exemplifies the freedom versus security dilemma of mid-adolescence, but both partners believe they should at least try to be honest in their relationship. Cars give sexual privacy, but many sixteens have sex at home, especially if both parents work. Some parents, who value their own sexuality and acknowledge the adolescent need to be sexual, endorse sex at home for their teenagers.

In sexually committed relationships, problems develop; boys want sex usually more than girls and they pressure a girl to have sex when she doesn't want it; they ejaculate too fast and may not effectively stimulate their partner to orgasm; and they deal with the age-old problems of jealousy and possessiveness. Management of an adolescent's sexually active lifestyle is so complicated, (i.e., the decision to have sex, finding a time and place, fear of being caught, fear of pregnancy, no one to confide in, etc.) that there is little or no time spent, or help with learning sexual skills and becoming good sexual partners. Couples who agree not to engage in intercourse, but who continue mutual masturbation, may become highly skilled in foreplay, including oral sex. However, girls, who for one reason or another refuse to have intercourse, often accept oral sex as the forced choice to coitus and resent their involvement in it.

The concept of "sweet sixteen, never been kissed" is nostalgia rather than reality. There is a growing number of stable pairs at sixteen that are characterized by good grades, extracurricular involvement, cooperative attitudes at home and school, responsible behavior, part-time job and/or athletics, and regular partner sex with the use of effective birth control. It may well be that the security needs formerly met at home (family of origin) are being shifted in mid-adolescence toward the intimate bonding of the future (family of choice). Even though autonomy is virtually impossible at this age, it is well to remember that in the first half of this century it was possible at fifteen or sixteen to marry and support the family of choice independently.

Boys are competitive with male peers and seek status by achieving acceptance and recognition from older boys and men. They want money, a car, power at school (student government, athletics, special skills or talent, etc.), and a girlfriend. The girlfriend is a status symbol and signifies success in the sociosexual arena. She is important, but not as important to him as he is to her. Both boys and girls have to succeed with the boys. A male high school senior explained, "Girls are status and security but they can be more trouble than they are worth. If you really want to make it, you have to spend a lot of time with the guys. Girls can hold you back because you have to be on your best behavior and you have to take care of them. You can be crazy and gross with your friends. You can talk about sex, race your car, stay out all night, play practical jokes, learn to drink and dope with the guys, and everyone takes care of himself. You just can't feel free with a girl, it's too much responsibility."

Boys want a girlfriend to take to the dance because going stag is its own form of sociological torture, but they want to go out drinking with the big boys. "As soon as you get your car you try to find someone who can buy" (liquor).

Dating a popular girl is instant status for a boy, but she is expected to "be there," to wait, to come down on the field after the game, to understand when other things take priority. If she becomes possessive and demanding, the relationship is in jeopardy because the boy loses status if he is controlled by a girl. Having a steady boyfriend who has status among his peers is status for a girl. She is considered fortunate if she does not have to worry about a date for important school occasions or Friday and Saturday night. Attractive, popular, achieving girls who are involved in school affairs, have a job and a car, etc., but who do not have a boyfriend devalue themselves in comparison to less talented girls who are able to acquire and maintain a steady relationship. To anxiously wait to be asked to important school events and/or to miss going because no one asked you is a painful adolescent experience. This situation may occur for girls who are so attractive or smart or active that boys assume they are taken or that they would not be interested in them as well as for girls who fall low in the sexual marketplace because of inadequacies.

Girls who are considered "one of the boys" may also have problems with the cultural values of the high school. These girls may be every boy's best friend and confident. Girls who are comfortable with boys, who don't hassle them with unwanted expectations, and who accept them as they are may not develop the sociosexual skills needed for the friendship to become a dating relationship. These girls may even have sex with boys and still be considered a best friend, not a "lover" or a "date."

Conclusion

Although there are many patterns and variation in sexual development, it is evident that sex is much more complicated than function and skill. Sexual needs, gratification patterns, and experiences are the expression of the total self and are intricately woven through the fabric of life as a whole. Psychiatric disorders constitute only a small part of this picture, which in the final analysis has involved us all.

REFERENCES

Barbach, L. *For yourself.* New York: Doubleday, 1975.

Chapman, D. *The sexual equation.* New York: Philosophical Library, 1977.

DeMause, L. (Ed.). *History of childhood.* New York: Psychohistory, 1974.

Dodson, B. *Liberating masturbation.* New York: Dodson, 1974.

Farson, R. *Birthrights.* New York: Macmillan, 1974.

Ford, C. S., and Beach, F. *Patterns of sexual behavior.* New York: Harper & Row, 1951.

Green, R. *Sexual identity conflict in children and adults.* Baltimore: Penguin, 1974.

Haeberly, E. *The sex atlas.* New York: Seabury Press, 1978.

Hamilton, E. *Sex with love.* Boston: Beacon, 1978.

Haroian, L. *Childhood and adolescent sexuality.* (Video Tape Lecture Series.) San Francisco: The Institute for Advanced Study of Human Sexuality, 1980.

Haroian, L. *The development of the erotic response.* (Video tape.) San Francisco: The Institute for Advanced Study of Human Sexuality, 1976.

Haroian, L. *Sexual problems of children.* In C. Walker & M. Roberts (Eds.), *Handbook of clinical child psychology.* New York: Wiley, 1982.

Hass, A. *Teenage sexuality.* New York: Macmillan, 1979.

Hite, S. *The Hite report on female sexuality.* New York: Macmillan, 1976.

Hite, S. *The Hite report on male sexuality.* New York: Knopf, 1981.

Kaplan, H. S. *The new sex therapy, Vol. II: Disorders of sexual desire.* New York: Brunner/Mazel, 1979.

Kempe, R. S., & Kempe, C. H. *Child abuse.* Cambridge: Harvard, 1978.

Kinsey, A. C., Pomeroy, W. B., Martin, C. E., & Gebhard, P. H. *Sexual behavior in the human female.* Philadelphia and London: Saunders, 1953.

Kinsey, A. C., Pomeroy, W. B.,& Martin, C. E. *Sexual behavior in the human male.* Philadelphia: Saunders, 1948.

Langfeldt, T. *Processess in sexual development.* In L. Constantine & F. Martinson (Eds.), *Children and sex.* Boston: Little, Brown, 1981.

Masters, W. S., & Johnson, V. E. *Human sexual response.* Boston: Little, Brown, 1966.

Money, J., & Ehrhardt, A. *Man and woman, boy and girl.* Baltimore: Johns Hopkins, 1973.

National Sex Forum, *S. A. R. guide for a better sex life.* San Francisco: National Sex Forum, 1975

Rekers, G. A. Atypical gender development and psychosocial adjustment. *Journal of Applied Behavior Analysis,* 1974, *7,* 173–190.

Rekers, G. A. *Handbook of treatment of mental disorders in childhood and adolescence.* Englewood Cliffs, NJ: Prentice Hall, 1978.

Silverstein, C. *A family matter: A parent guide to homosexuality.* New York: McGraw Hill, 1978.

Smith, C., Ayres, T., & Rubenstein, M. *Getting in touch.* San Francisco: Multi-media Resource Center, 1972.

Sorenson, R. C. *Adolescent sexuality in contemporary America.* New York: World Publishing, 1973.

Spitz, R. Auto eroticism. *The Psychoanalytic Study of the Child,* 1949, *4,* 55–120.

Stoller, R. J. *Sex and gender.* New York: Science House, 1968.

Stoller, R. J. *Perversions.* New York: Pantheon, 1975.

Tannahill, R. *Sex in history.* New York: Stein and Day, 1980.

Williams, G. J., & Money, J. (Eds.), *Traumatic abuse and neglect of children at home.* Baltimore: Johns Hopkins, 1980.

Yates, A. *Sex without shame.* New York: William Morrow, 1979.

CHAPTER 13

Personality and Conduct Disorders

Charles H. Mahone and Edward C. Budd

Creation of a workable nosology for psychological disturbances of childhood has proven to be a remarkably difficult challenge for mental health professionals. In fact, the numerous classification schemes proposed for these disturbances have been far from uniform, and none has captured the consensual endorsement of psychologists and psychiatrists. DSM-II (American Psychiatric Association, 1968) devoted a scant two pages to diagnoses specifically tailored to children—hardly comprehensive. Other systems, most notably the GAP classification system (Group for the Advancement of Psychiatry, 1966) have been proposed, but none has been universally adopted.

The authors of DSM-III (American Psychiatric Association, 1980) have made some effort to correct this deficiency and devote a fairly large and detailed section to "Disorders Usually First Evident in Infancy, Childhood, or Adolescence." DSM-III uses a symptom checklist or behavioral syndrome approach, emphasizing specific behavioral manifestations of various disorders to the near exclusion of dynamic or theoretically based diagnosis. This strategy represents a thoughtful effort to increase the reliability of diagnosis, a necessary condition for both research and prescriptive clinical assessment.

One general category which is notable for its absence in DSM-III is personality disorders in childhood. This is all the more remarkable because the adult category of personality disorder is regarded as sufficiently important to warrant a separate axis of classification (Axis II) and the detailing of eleven subtypes—avoidant, borderline, compulsive, dependent, histrionic, narcissistic, paranoid, passive-aggressive, schizoid, schizotypal, and a final wastebasket category of atypical/mixed/other.

In the GAP classification system for psychopathological disorders in childhood (1966), a similarly detailed treatment of personality disorders is advocated for children, and thirteen subtypes of personality disorders in childhood are listed: compulsive, hysterical, anxious, overly dependent, oppositional, overly inhibited, overly independent, isolated, mistrustful, tension-discharge disorders, sociosyntonic, sexual deviation, and other. More space is devoted to this group of disorders than to any other major classification.

To understand this striking difference in emphasis between DSM-III and GAP, one must first arrive at a working definition of personality disorder. According to DSM-III, a personality disorder is made up of traits which are inflexible and maladaptive and cause either subjective stress or significant impairment in social or occupational functioning. These traits must be typical of the person's long-term functioning and not limited to discrete episodes. The GAP definition also emphasizes the fixedness and maladaptive quality of the personality traits which constitute the personality disorder, and in addition it points out that the traits are not perceived as a source of intrapsychic distress (though they may be seen as causing adverse external reactions) and hence may be called ego-syntonic.

GAP further suggests that personality disorders may be placed along a continuum. At one end of this continuum are relatively well-organized personalities, in which the pathological characteristics represent mild to moderate exaggeration of healthy personality traits that blend very well with the environment and almost pass unnoticed. At the other end are "markedly impulsive, sometimes poorly organized personalities that dramatically come into conflict with society over their sexual or social patterns of behavior" (GAP, p. 65). This severe end of the continuum may be marked by occasions of severe regression without psychosis and even by episodes of acute psychosis. For psychoanalytically oriented theorists, strong fixations related to conflicts in the narcissistic and oral stages of early childhood are thought to be involved in these disorders.

Most conceptualizations of personality disorder suggest that they originate in constitutional temperamental dispositions and/or early childhood influences or experiences, but do not become manifest in their adult guises until mid to late adolescence. This raises the question of whether it is possible or helpful to delineate childhood versions of these adult personality disorders, and this issue will be considered presently. For those theorists who answer the question affirmatively, most would say that a childhood personality disorder usually does not become evident until the school years. This means that, in addition to constitution and early childhood influences, one might also consider factors such as family dynamics, role models, identification with and modeling after other children, later traumatic learning, and general cultural or subcultural influences. In personality disorders, none of these factors are serious enough to arrest development, but they are important enough to leave a permanent mark on the developing personality of the child. Since we are dealing with a very broad level of personality functioning, it is not expected that any single etiological influence will be predominant, but that there will be complex interactions among the various factors.

The phenotypic description of the personality disorder may vary considerably from one childhood stage to another and from any one of these stages to the adult version. There will be some genotypic continuity across stages, however, though this may only be in evidence if the right issues are brought into focus. This makes it imperative to attend to the central trait(s) which serve as the core of the personality disorder, and to understand that this core "attitude" will organize the perceptions and behaviors of the individual in distinctive ways, even though the behaviors and perceptions themselves may be more similar across individuals within a certain age group than they are similar for a certain type of individual across age groups.

Given the difficulty, it is no wonder that many writers of textbooks in child psychopathology omit any general category of personality (or character) disorder in childhood (e.g., Barker, 1979; Harrison & McDermott, 1972; Knopf, 1979). Metcalf (1977), in his influential review of childhood hysterical disorders, says, "It seems prudent to say from the outset that observation and treatment of children indicates that what is ordinarily meant by character disorder does not occur in children" (p. 225). But he goes on to say that personality "styles" are identifiable in children, and he believes that one of those identifiable styles is the hysterical style. While there may be a good bit of semantic ambiguity in differentiating personality "disorder" from personality "style," he seems to be saying basically that there well may be genotypic continuity in personality dispositions (style), some of which may be sufficiently maladaptive to warrant inclusion in a discussion of childhood psychopathology, but one cannot expect the phenotypic continuity which is characteristic of adult personality disorder. In this chapter the genotypic continuity will be called a childhood *version* of personality disorder.

What are some examples of these stylistic dispositions which may be troublesome from a mental health perspective? Perhaps the most widely recognized of these is the child who is always getting into trouble by flouting rules. The context, the rule-maker, and the kind of rule broken may all vary considerably (phenotypic variability), but the core disposition of rule-breaking represents a (genotypic) continuity.

Another example would be the painfully shy and withdrawn child, who in one context (the classroom) may be described as the model child, because he or she does schoolwork well and faithfully and doesn't bother the other children. In another context (the playground), this child may appear to be quite abnormal because he or she does not participate in activities with other children.

Yet another example is the "show-off" child, who may behave quite appropriately and entertainingly at a party, but may be a chronic disciplinary problem for the teacher. The milder versions of these stylistic "disorders" are often disregarded by parents, teachers, and child clinicians, for most children behave like this at one time or another. It is only when these dispositions become moderately severe that their continuity (and inflexibility) becomes evident, and the clinician can describe them as personality disorders.

The DSM-III classification of childhood disorders does not ignore certain syndromes which GAP includes under the general heading of personality disorder of childhood. However, only one of these syndromes—the oppositional disorder—carries the same label in DSM-III as in the GAP classification. Another DSM-III childhood disorder, the schizoid disorder, is readily recognizable as equivalent to the GAP category of isolated personality disorder. Both the oppositional and the schizoid childhood disorders are listed under the wastebasket heading of "Other Disorders in Childhood" in DSM-III.

A third group of childhood disorders, the conduct disorders, is given more attention in DSM-III. This emphasis was also evident in DSM-II (1968), where three of the seven diagnostic categories specifically reserved for children and adolescents describe behavior patterns which could be diagnosed as conduct disorders in the DSM-III sense. These categories were "Runaway Reaction of Childhood," "Unsocialized Aggressive Reaction of Childhood," and "Group Delinquent Reaction of Childhood."

The GAP personality disorder categories of tension-discharge disorders and sociosyntonic disorders also seem to be basically conduct disorders. The tension-discharge disorders, in particular, seem to represent relatively severe personality disorders on the continuum mentioned above: "Children in this category exhibit chronic behavioral patterns of emotional expression of aggressive and sexual impulses which conflict with society's norms. They act out directly their feelings or impulses toward persons or society in antisocial or destructive fashion, rather than inhibiting or repressing them and developing other modes of psychological defense or symptomatology" (GAP, 1966, p. 73). This description parallels that of the "undersocialized, aggressive" conduct disorder in DSM-III, albeit in psychodynamic terminology.

What, then, is the status of personality disorders as a diagnostic category for childhood psychopathology? Clearly, clinicians have divergent attitudes toward this question, as is evident from the fact that nosological systems range from omission of the category (DSM-III) to emphasis of it as a major class of disorders (GAP). It is equally clear that this divergence does not represent disagreement over the importance of behavioral syndromes which may be described as personality disorders; these syndromes emerge repeatedly in diverse systems of classification. The question is therefore one of conceptual utility. That is, are the behavioral syndromes at issue sufficiently similar (along some dimension) that they constitute a meaningful class of disorders and does the conceptualization of such problems as personality disorders help in planning treatment?

This chapter seeks in part to evaluate the utility of the concept of personality disorders of childhood as a diagnostic category. It does so by discussing personality disorders along several lines, including clinical description, theoretical conceptualization, and empirical research. Conduct disorders are treated as the prototypic personality disorder of childhood, both because such disorders are most universally represented in nosological systems, and because virtually all the empirical research on childhood personality disorders has been on conduct disorders.

Conduct Disorders

The conduct disorders comprise a major diagnostic category of childhood and adolescence in the DSM-III nomenclature. To quote DSM-III: "The essential feature is a repetitive and persistent pattern of conduct in which either the basic rights of others or major age-appropriate societal norms or rules are violated. The conduct is more serious than the ordinary mischief and pranks of children and adolescents" (p. 45). "Antisocial" behavior, in the sense of persistent behavior which ignores or violates societal norms and rules, is thus pathognomic of the conduct disorders.

The conduct disorders are divided into four subtypes: undersocialized, aggressive; undersocialized, nonaggressive; socialized, aggressive; and socialized, nonaggressive. The aggressive-nonaggressive subdivision depends on whether the antisocial pattern of behavior involves direct expressions of hostility (e.g., physical violence against others, vandalism, fire-setting, burglary) or misbehaviors that are nonviolent (e.g., violation of age-appropriate rules at home or school, substance abuse, running away from home). The socialized-undersocialized subdivision is made according to whether the child has established normal interpersonal bonds (socialized), such as friendships, or is characterized by a failure to establish such relationships (undersocialized). This latter dimension often requires a fine distinction which may be based in part on a temperamental pathogenic factor, such as withdrawal tendency. Such temperamental variables may be descriptively useful but, when used in isolation, have been shown to be poor prognostic indicators of antisocial behavior (Thomas & Chess, 1977; Kohlberg, LaCrosse, & Ricks, 1972).

Case Illustration of Undersocialized Nonaggressive Conduct Disorder: Brad is nine years old, bright, but a source of dismay to parents and teachers alike. His biggest problem at home is persistent lying to avoid household responsibilities and rules. He hates any kind of household chore, and he will go to great lengths to alibi his way out of them. He is obese and has agreed verbally to various food restrictions, but he repeatedly violates this agreement and sneaks food whenever he has the opportunity (usually when his parents are out of the home or when he has money to buy junk food). He presses constantly to have his privileges extended (such as curfew), but his handling of current privileges does not warrant an extension. He lies about his homework assignments and works as little as possible at school. He steals small amounts of money belonging to various family members, and engages repeatedly in minor shoplifting. When confronted with his misdeeds, Brad is silent and unrepentant, and he never talks confidingly with anyone. Children at school seem to accept him well enough in their group play, but he is not close to any of his peers. Brad prefers younger children to play with, probably because they are less critical of him and are easier for him to control than are his age-mates. Brad is more of a nonaggressive than an aggressive child, though he does occasionally have temper tantrums when his wishes are thwarted. During those tantrums, he may break things in the home, though he does not become physically aggressive with people.

Case Illustration of Socialized Aggressive Conduct Disorder: Tim, a fourteen-year-old, was picked up several times over a year's period by the police for fighting, vandalism, and breaking and entering. He was charged and found guilty of only one of these offenses, and was placed on probation with the juvenile court. Tim always commits these offenses in the company of one or more companions, to whom he is fiercely loyal and with whom he has long-standing relationships. They are part of an informal gang who roam around town looking for opportunities for mischief. They sometimes fight with other gangs of boys, but they are not organized tightly enough to schedule "rumbles." They are truant from school occasionally, but they mostly get into trouble on weekends and during the summer months. Tim's parents have scolded him for several years about his choice of friends, but they seem unwilling or unable to supervise him closely enough to break up his gang. He does poorly in school, and he has only barely managed to pass. His parents vaguely hope that someday Tim will get a job or a girlfriend to keep him busy and away from his gang friends.

Tim represents a mild to moderate level of conduct disorder, although the aggressiveness of the misconduct could easily escalate as Tim gets older and stronger. Channeling his energy and daring into athletics is sometimes a welcome solution to the problematic pattern that develops in adolescent boys like Tim.

Prevalence

DSM-III offers no figures on the prevalence of conduct disorders, though it does say that the disorder is common. Since this type of personality disorder is so often expressed in delinquent behavior, perhaps it would be useful to note the figures on delinquency. Knopf (1979) estimates that 5 percent of children from ten to seventeen years of age are involved in cases of delinquency in any given year. The male:female ratio here is estimated at 3:1, although DSM-III puts it at 4:1 or higher, except for the undersocialized, nonaggressive type, where it is more equal (1980, p. 47).

Treatment

The literature on conduct disorder is pretty uniformly skeptical about the value of traditional, dynamic psychotherapy for this disorder, especially for adolescents. Incarceration is also of dubious value, for the recidivism rate is quite high (Knopf, 1979). Barker (1979) suggests better alternatives for treatment, which may be subdivided according to the seriousness of the conduct disorder. For the milder disorder, commonsense advice to parents on parental discipline may suffice. If technical treatment is warranted, some kind of behavior modification regime at home and school which emphasizes reward of positive behavior may be instituted (Ross, 1981). For more moderate levels of conduct disorder, family therapy may be the treatment of choice (Alexander & Parsons, 1982). For more serious disorders where the family cannot reach the child, the removal of the child from the home for purposes of resocialization may be warranted. The peer pressure of a day program or residential group home, or the milieu influence of a residential treatment center or a therapeutic foster home, may be preferred agents of resocialization (Quay, 1979).

Theory

According to the ego-analytic understanding of development, persistent violation of societal norms reflects failure in the development of higher-order ego functions. Specifically, conduct disorders are manifestations of the failure to achieve adequate internalized drive control—that is, they reflect inadequate socialization or the ability to conform with appropriate behaviors.

Movement in growth progresses along a continuum from external to internal control of drives and is one of the major developmental tasks of childhood. The behavior of a young infant consists primarily of efforts to fulfill needs or desires immediately; all control over this process is externally mediated. In contrast, older children and mature adults typically display a highly developed capacity for control over impulsive motivations. Indeed, in the words of Anna Freud (1965): "To have the fulfillment of one's drives and wishes, their acceptance and rejection, lodged in external authority equals moral dependency and, as such, is the hallmark of the immature. Almost the whole of personality and character formation, as it is known to us, can be viewed also in terms of remedying this humiliating situation and of acquiring for the mature person the right to judge his own actions" (p. 170).

Socialization, or the internalization of what were external drive controls, is a complex and relatively advanced aspect of ego development. Socialization can occur only if an individual has achieved a certain degree of basic ego development. The basic ego development necessary to support internalization of drive controls essentially involves cognitive maturity, represented by adequate perception, memory, and conceptual competency. In more traditionally psychodynamic terminology, the child must have advanced from pleasure principle to reality principle functioning. Functioning according to the pleasure principle means that one strives primarily for immediate and indiscriminate drive satisfaction regardless of external conditions and environmental norms. Functioning according to the reality principle involves delay and modification of pleasure-seeking in the interest of personal safety and approval. In this way, the adverse consequences that follow maladaptive and unrealistic behaviors may be avoided. "Therefore, the former [the pleasure principle] is linked as firmly with asocial, dissocial, 'irresponsible' behavior as the latter [the reality principle] is essential for social adaptation and the development of law-abiding attitudes" (Freud, 1965, p. 171).

A closely related ability in ego development necessary for socialization is frustration tolerance. The child must be able to tolerate the frustration of drives and wishes, at least to the extent of postponing gratification and being willing to substitute a more socially appropriate satisfaction for another. This tolerance is invariably accompanied by a quantitative reduction of wish fulfillment; the willingness of the child to make this "sacrifice" is regarded by many as a decisive factor in the process of socialization. Submitting to reality-based external drive controls is regarded as a necessary (but not sufficient) condition for the later internalization of such controls.

Once a child has achieved the prerequisite level of basic ego development, internalization of drive controls is dependent on a usually positive, highly energized relationship with parents or other authority figures. The child internalizes injunctions against socially disapproved behaviors and positive valuations of socially desirable behaviors. The three mechanisms by which this process is accomplished are imitation, identification, and introjection. *Imitation* is the earliest and most primitive of these and involves merely the copying of behaviors. *Identification* follows, and it is based on the wish to appropriate desirable characteristics of objects by permanently changing oneself. *Introjection* is a more technical term and refers to the process by which one takes into one's own value system the values and standards of another (usually one or both of the parents, initially). Introjection raises drive control from the status of an externally mediated mechanism to that of a permanent, internal, personal agency—what is called the superego. It does so by rewarding the ego for compliance by feelings of heightened self-esteem and by punishing rebellion with feelings of guilt.

From the psychoanalytic view, the final leap from external to internal drive controls requires that the child have relatively healthy and advanced object relationships with authority figures, generally parents. If the child is insufficiently invested in parental figures, the mechanisms of imitation, identification, and introjection cannot operate. The process will also be blocked if the child's involvement with parents does not include a balance of positive, affectionate feelings (which make identification desirable) and some element of fearful respect (which makes drive control necessary). Finally, internalization of drive controls is impossible if the parent or authority figure with whom the child identifies lacks adequate drive control. Imitation and introjection of sociopathic qualities results in a sociopathic character structure and not in appropriate socialization.

In summary, ego-analytic theory regards childhood conduct disorders as manifestations of impairment of higher-order ego functions—specifically, the internalization of drive controls. This process depends, in very general terms, on (1) adequate basic ego development, emphasizing movement from pleasure principle to reality principle functioning, permitting frustration tolerance and delay of gratification and (2) adequate object relationships with a parental figure or figures who have achieved mature drive control. This theoretical assessment of conduct disorders has several implications regarding both the relationship between childhood conduct disorders and adult pathology and the possible causes of antisocial behavior.

An ego-analytic understanding implies that the presence of a conduct disorder in childhood should be predictive of adult psychopathologies involving inadequate ego development. Obviously, failure to achieve internalization of drive control in childhood should predict patterns of impulsive and antisocial behaviors in adulthood—in a nutshell, many children diagnosed as conduct disorders should become sociopathic adults. Secondly, antisocial behavior on the part of a child should in some cases be predictive of psychosis, since failure of socialization can reflect early and severe impairment of ego development.

Also, the ego-analytic position suggests some possible causes of conduct disorders (and thus, indirectly, of adult sociopathy). First, any characteristic of either the individual or the environment which profoundly impairs basic ego development severely disrupts socialization. Organicity, serious intellectual impairment, and severe maternal deprivation impair ego development, and can thus result in failure to internalize drive control. Such factors can cause other more profound disorders as well, but here our concern is whether their influence may frequently result in patterns of persistent antisocial behavior. Second, failure to form adequate object relations with parents may impair the process of socialization. Loss of a parent or parents, or unresponsiveness on the part of the parents to the child's interpersonal needs, can block internalization of drive controls and result in conduct disorders. Finally, if the parental role model lacks appropriate internal drive controls, antisocial behavior may be expected from the child.

It might be noted here that these three deficiencies at least roughly parallel the three basic elements in the psychopathic personality (lack of impulse control, shallow affect, and unfortunate shaping experiences) (Goldstone, 1983). The lack of impulse control represents a basic ego defect. Shallow affect may stem from poor object relations. Unfortunate shaping experiences may well be represented by identification with a sociopathic parent.

Of course, theoretical viewpoints other

than the psychoanalytic also account for conduct disorders. Most notably, ecological and behavioral perspectives on conduct disorders are quite reasonable. The different behavioral conceptualizations of conduct disorders center on the child's failure to learn negative injunctions due to inappropriate or inconsistent patterns of parental rewards and discipline. A general lack of discipline can of course be a major factor, but a particular style of discipline appears especially suited to the production of antisocial behavior patterns: that is, punishment which is infrequent, severe, and applied without regard to clearly established contingencies. Such disciplinary practices are apt to teach children, not that prohibited actions have aversive consequences, but that interpersonal relationships are potentially highly aversive. This type of discipline therefore tends not to produce socially approved patterns of behavior, but to encourage avoidance of authority figures and development of strategies for avoiding punishment (i.e., it is getting caught, rather than prohibited actions, which become directly associated with aversive consequences).

Other theoretical accounts of conduct disorders abound. Social learning theorists stress the importance of modeling in the etiology of antisocial behaviors. Biological models have provided reasonable accounts of the etiology of adult sociopathy, including the hypothesis that faulty inhibitory mechanisms in the limbic system play a role in sociopathy (Hare, 1970) and the assertion that autonomic hypoactivity on the part of sociopaths interferes with avoidance learning (Skrzypek, 1969).

Clearly, such perspectives are not incompatible with the ego-analytic understanding of conduct disorders. Indeed, models of the etiology of antisocial behavior seem to represent an area of convergence of psychodynamic, behavioral, and biological models of psychopathology. The psychodynamic understanding will be stressed here largely because it directly addresses personality disorders and is the most comprehensive of these theoretical approaches. Though all these models emphasize the failure of the individual to internalize negative injunctions against socially disapproved behaviors, the psychodynamic model represents a broad developmental account of such failure and posits a number of possible mechanisms mediating the failure to internalize drive control. Thus, the behavioral and biological models can be regarded as important additions to the psychodynamic conceptualization and in some sense represent special cases of the general developmental model.

We can now turn to the research in this area and see if these theoretical expectations are supported.

Research

The following survey of research suggests that, at least on a very general level, the ego-analytic position is consistent with empirical data. Specifically, the occurrence of antisocial behaviors in childhood is a significant predictor of adult pathologies involving impairment of higher order ego functions, and analytic inferences regarding the causes of conduct disorders are generally supported.

A good deal of research, including both retrospective and longitudinal studies, suggests that the definitive characteristic of childhood conduct disorders—antisocial behavior—is predictive of adult disorders involving inadequate ego development. In particular, antisocial behavior in childhood is highly predictive of adult antisocial behavior. A broad review of predictability of adult mental health from childhood behavior reported: "The longitudinal research evidence suggests that antisocial behavior—particularly when some estimate of severity is taken into account—is the single most powerful predictor of later adjustment problems of any childhood behavior studied" (Kohlberg, LaCrosse, & Ricks, 1972, p. 1249).

Data bearing on this issue are strikingly consistent in supporting the continuity of antisocial behavior patterns from childhood into adulthood. The landmark study in this area is that of Robins (1966), who examined detailed clinical records of children referred for behavior problems and conducted a thirty-year follow-up of the same individuals as adults. The most striking finding of this study was that childhood antisocial behavior is highly predictive of adult sociopathy. Robins found that 28 percent of children referred for antisocial behavior were later diagnosed as sociopathic personalities, as opposed to only 2 percent of control subjects. Another 8 percent of children referred for antisocial behavior became alcoholics or drug addicts, again as opposed to 2 percent of controls. Moreover, the most severe antisocial behaviors were most predictive of adult sociopathy. Of boys referred for theft or aggression, 37 percent and 39 percent, respectively, were later diagnosed as sociopathic personality. Interestingly, the absence of antisocial behavior patterns in childhood virtually excluded the possibility of adult diagnosis of sociopathic personality. Robins observed that no child without frequent or serious antisocial behavior became a sociopathic adult, and only 4 percent of patients referred for reasons other than antisocial behavior later received a diagnosis of sociopathic personality. It appears on the basis of this study that antisocial behavior in childhood is a necessary but not sufficient (although highly predisposing) condition for adult sociopathy. (This has been recognized in DSM-III by the requirement of a history of antisocial conduct before age fifteen in order to make the adult diagnosis of antisocial personality disorder.)

Moreover, the results of similar studies tend strongly to support these conclusions. For example, Cass and Thomas (1979), in a major longitudinal study of psychopathology, observed that eleven of fifteen children clinically diagnosed as "character disorders" were severely maladjusted in adulthood, and that these individuals were most impaired on social adjustment. Interestingly, they found that the prognosis was far better for children diagnosed as manifesting "neurotic behavior disorders," distinguished from character disorders by the presence of significant guilt and/or anxiety regarding their antisocial behavior.

Early studies by Glueck and Glueck (1940, 1950, 1959) indicated a strong predictive relationship between delinquency in childhood and adolescence and criminal behavior of adults. Fields (1969) reported that antisocial behavior in childhood is highly predictive of later diagnosis of character disorder and of arrests in adulthood. Roff (1974) found that clinicians were able to predict accurately "bad conduct" outcomes in adulthood from records of a child guidance clinic. The cluster of childhood characteristics related to this outcome emphasized such antisocial behaviors as disobedience, defiance of authority, and running away.

Of course, not all studies indicate a strong and simple relationship between childhood conduct disorders and adult sociopathy. Some studies suggest that there may be complex sex differences in the predictability of adult antisocial behavior from childhood misconduct. For example, Mellsop (1972) found that males with personality and conduct disorders were overrepresented in the "unfavorable outcome" group, whereas females with these diagnoses were underrepresented. Nevertheless, the major finding has emerged quite consistently. Both the Kohlberg et al. (1972) and Robins (1979) studies reach this conclusion. In the words of Kohlberg et al.: "In summary, then, childhood severe antisocial behavior is a necessary condition for the prediction of severe adult antisocial behavior, and milder forms of antisocial behavior are relatively good predictors of all forms of adult maladjustment. The predictive power of antisocial behavior does not appear to depend on specific kinds of antisocial behavior or upon particular kinds of aggressive, sexual, or other motives but seems to reflect the fact that distortions of ego development and distortions in the child's relation to his environment are necessary conditions for relatively frequent or severe forms of antisocial behavior" (p. 1253).

The above summary alludes to a second empirical relationship suggested by the ego-analytic perspective on childhood conduct disorders. That is, antisocial behaviors in childhood may, in some individuals, reflect an earlier and more global impairment of ego development. Patterns of antisocial behavior should therefore also be predictive of more serious pathologies, such as psychoses. In fact, data support this conclusion, although the relationship is not nearly so clear-cut as that between conduct disorders and sociopathy. The Robins study provides some support for this relationship. In this study, 11 percent of children referred for antisocial behavior received a diagnosis of psychosis in adulthood in contrast to 6 percent of control subjects. Severe antisocial behavior was, in this study, highly predictive of adult maladjustment in general. Only 5 percent of children with ten or more antisocial symptoms were free of noteworthy psychopathology as adults.

Morris, Escoll, and Wexler (1956) conducted a follow-up study of children referred for antisocial patterns of behavior when they were four to fifteen years of age. Of sixty-six subjects located at follow-up when they were at least eighteen years old, twelve were psychotic, despite the fact that none had received that diagnosis in childhood. Watt et al. (1970) used a retrospective design to investigate the childhood behavior of individuals hospitalized for schizophrenia as adults. Antisocial behavior characterized as "unsocialized aggression" was one of the major factors distinguishing preschizophrenic boys from control subjects. Clearly, the results of such "follow-back" studies are less convincing than those of predictive or longitudinal studies. It bears mentioning that some retrospective studies of adult schizophrenics suggest that preschizophrenic children tend to be actively seclusive, though not disproportionately shy and withdrawn (cf. the review in Kohlberg et al., 1972). This finding is not surprising, since antisocial behavior is only one of several possible manifestations of early and profound disruption of ego development. Also, the combination of anxious withdrawal and delinquent acting-out seems to be a better predictor of psychosis than either one taken alone. In short, the research indicates that antisocial behavior in childhood is predictive of more severe disorders, including psychoses, as well as predicting sociopathic personality. Kohlberg et al. (1979) conclude, "Various forms and dimensions of juvenile antisocial behavior appear to be associated with psychiatric diagnoses of sociopathic personality, alcoholism, hysteria, and schizophrenia and with extent of adult criminal antisocial problems (above and beyond diagnostic categories)" (p. 1249).

A third prediction derived from the ego-analytic account of childhood conduct disorders is that children manifesting relatively severe disruption of higher ego development should only rarely become neurotic adults. Adequate (and usually excessive) internalization of drive control is a necessary condition for development of neurosis; the lack of such internalized control is the major dynamic characteristic of conduct disorders. Little evidence exists to support or refute this prediction, but the limited data available are supportive.

Robins (1966) found that only 14 percent of children referred for antisocial behavior, as compared to 25 percent of controls and 33 percent of patients referred for other reasons, became neurotic adults. The strength of this relationship may be partially obscured by a diagnostic quirk. Women receiving the diagnosis of "hysteria" in the Robins study were strongly characterized by antisocial symptoms, and probably more closely resembled sociopaths than neurotics in a theoretically precise sense. Excluding the hysteria category, 10 percent of children referred for antisocial behaviors were diagnosed neurotic as adults, in contrast to 22 percent of control subjects.

Although most relevant studies do not present their data in forms which make it easy to evaluate this predicted relationship, it appears that their results largely confirm those of the Robins study. In no longitudinal study was antisocial behavior in childhood predictive of neurotic outcomes. In some studies (Roff, 1974), antisocial behavior was the key discriminating element in predicting sociopathic, as opposed to neurotic, outcomes. In short, although existing data are far from conclusive, it appears that severe antisocial behavior in childhood is negatively predictive of adult neurosis.

Another set of expectations deriving from ego-analytic theory has to do with familial factors which impair socialization and therefore engender conduct disorders. One such factor would be prolonged separation from parents. A long series of studies, beginning early in this century, demonstrated that parental deprivation (i.e., absence of normal parent-child relationships due to divorce, loss of a parent or parents, or institutionalization of the child) (see Chapter 9) is associated with antisocial behavior in childhood.

For example, Bowlby (1944) conducted a retrospective study of forty-four children, referred to a child guidance clinic, for whom stealing was a symptom. These children were compared to forty-four controls, matched for age and IQ, who were clinic patients but did not steal. Of the forty-four children for whom stealing was a problem, seventeen had experienced prolonged separation from their mothers or mother-substitutes prior to age five. Only two of the control children had experienced such separation.

Goldfarb (1943) conducted a predictive or follow-up study of the effects of parental deprivation. He studied twenty children who were placed, shortly after birth, in an institution in which infants received minimal affection and handling. Institution children were placed in foster homes around three-and-one-half years of age. They were compared with twenty controls, matched for age and length of time under substitute care, who were transferred to foster mothers directly from the care of their biological mothers—i.e., without the intervening institutional experience. All children were evaluated at between seven-and-one-half and ten years of age. Institution children were more maladjusted than control children on a number of variables, most notably antisocial behavior. These children ranked considerably higher than controls on indices of aggression, disobedience, destructiveness, and dishonesty. In short, the prevalence of antisocial behavior was higher in children who lacked continuous parent-child relationships through early childhood. Bender (1947), Levy (1937), and Beres and Obers (1950) conducted frequently cited studies which support this conclusion. Bowlby's (1951) review of research led him to conclude that parent-child separation is a major cause of delinquency; Morrison (1978) has provided a more recent review.

Despite the apparent conclusiveness of this early finding, more recent research has called into question the connection between separation from parents and conduct disorders. In particular, more precisely controlled studies suggest that this result may be an artifact arising from the association of parental separation with other disruptive factors in a child's development. The study of Rutter (1971) exemplifies this line of research and indicates that the reason for a parent-child separation is more important than the fact of separation per se in producing antisocial behavior patterns. Rutter separately evaluated the effects of transient and prolonged parent-child separations. Transient separations due to marital discord were predictive of antisocial outcomes, whereas transient separations due to illness of a parent were not associated with conduct disorders. Investigation of prolonged separations produced similar findings. That is, the break-up of the family due to divorce or separation of the parents was predictive of antisocial behavior patterns. The death of a parent, on the other hand, was not predictive of antisocial behavior on the part of the child. Reexamination of the data of Glueck and Glueck (1950) and Brown (1966) in the light of these findings reveals that their results do support Rutter's conclusion.

These findings led Rutter (1971) to review in some detail the literature regarding the etiology of delinquency. This review revealed that many studies (Craig & Glick, 1965; McCord & McCord, 1959; Tait & Hodges, 1962) suggest that delinquency is more common in children of intact homes characterized by a high degree of marital discord than in children from "broken" but relatively harmonious homes. Taken collectively, these findings suggest that *it is discord in the home and not separation from the parents which is a critical factor in the development of conduct disorders.* The original findings regarding parental separation may have arisen from the confounding of family break-ups with marital conflict.

From the ego-analytic perspective, it seems likely that this is due to the difficulty of forming healthy object relationships with parents who are unable to maintain a positive marital relationship. Nevertheless, it is important to recognize that antisocial behavior cannot be regarded as a simple product of parent-child separation.

A second factor has to do with the quality of the parent-child relationship. If the parent-child relationship is primarily a negative one, the child is unlikely to identify with a parental authority figure and will therefore tend not to internalize drive control. This supposition has strong empirical support in that children manifesting conduct disorders have frequently been victims of parental rejection and abuse.

For example, Newell (1936) compared eighty-two normal control children with seventy-five children who were rejected by their mothers. "Rejection" was operationally defined by two criteria: (1) the mother explicitly stated that the child's birth was unwanted and (2) the mother's behavior toward the child was predominantly hostile. Newell found that rejected children were significantly more likely than controls to engage in inappropriately aggressive behavior.

Studies by Knight (1933), Bender (1947), Levy (1937), and Baldwin, Kalhorn, and Breese (1945) support this conclusion. Data reported by Schactel and Levi (1945) suggest that brutal treatment of the child engenders antisocial tendencies. McCord and McCord (1956) concluded on the basis of an extensive review of the literature that severe parental rejection is one of the main causes of antisocial behavior. It appears that the father-child relationship is particularly important, and that overt hostility and highly punitive disciplinary practices by the father are especially likely to result in conduct disorders (Shore, 1984).

It is interesting to note that the most assaultive kind of juvenile delinquency comes from individuals who are ordinarily the best behaved and controlled subgroup in the delinquent population (Megargee, 1984). This episodic "explosive" kind of hostility is probably not the result of a failure to internalize parental standards of control of aggressiveness but of the attempt to exercise too much control of hostile impulses (overcontrolled hostility). This subgroup of delinquents seems to come from "good" homes (i.e., homes with adequate nurturance and discipline) and therefore to have good opportunities for internalization (cf. Warren, 1983, on the prevalence of delinquents in subgroups who do show evidence of internalization).

Finally, one would expect that sociopathic parents would produce children who had conduct disorders because, even though internalization might take place, the quality of the internalized drive control could be expected to be low. Robins (1979) found that having antisocial parents or grandparents (i.e., those who as adults had been arrested, drank excessively, failed to work regularly, deserted or neglected the children, beat the children or spouse, or had extramarital sexual relations) considerably increased the chances of a son's dropping out of high school and appearing in police or juvenile court records. This was true in both white-collar and blue-collar families, at about the same rate. Identification with such a role model could well lead to a desire to seem tough and alienated (Hogan & Jones, 1983). This argues, then, for the influence of the familial models, rather than the socioeconomic class.

This review found nothing in the literature which would allow for any etiological distinctions among the four subtypes of conduct disorder discussed in DSM-III. It seems clear, however, that the more "serious" kinds of conduct disorders are most predictive of the antisocial adult personality disorder, and that the seriousness of conduct disturbance is best reflected in the "aggressive" subtypes. As indicated earlier, it is unclear whether the "socialized" versus "undersocialized" distinction is a helpful one empirically, though it would certainly appear to be important conceptually. At any rate, the child who aggressively misbehaves seems most likely to become an antisocial adult, though there are many reasons for, and expressions of, conduct disorders (Harris, 1983).

One additional point has to do with whether these children are capable of experiencing anxiety or guilt about wrongdoing. The evidence is somewhat inconclusive and suggests that it depends upon who defines what is wrong. These children may not feel guilt about violating society's norms, but they may be concerned about going against the code of their group; similarly they may not respond to the usual punishments, though losing what they regard as valuable, such as money, may be an effective deterrent (Achenbach, 1982, pp. 496–500).

Other Personality Disorders

What can be learned from this review of conduct disorders about personality disorders in children generally? The major lesson appears to be that it is reasonable to think that some personality patterning has taken place in an identifiable way by later childhood (let us say, by ten), and that this patterning may be related, conceptually and empirically, to a major personality disorder syndrome in adulthood. How likely is it that other patterns can be found which meet this standard?

PASSIVE-AGGRESSIVE PERSONALITY DISORDER

One candidate for this classification would be the childhood version of the adult diagnosis of passive-aggressive personality disorder. In DSM-III, this diagnosis is viewed as continuous with that of oppositional disorder in childhood, and the latter is described in Chapter 9. Oppositional disorder is chiefly characterized by "a pattern of disobedient, negativistic, and provocative opposition to authority figures" (DSM-III, p. 63). In the passive-aggressive personality disorder, however, the resistance is specifically to demands for adequate performance, and is expressed indirectly rather than directly. The name also implies an emphasis on aggressive inclinations rather than on control issues, though the aggression is expressed indirectly and covertly through resistance to demands (controls from outside).

If this is a meaningful distinction, then it should be possible to identify cases of childhood personality disorder which are more related to the adult passive-aggressive personality disorder than to the childhood oppositional disorder, and indeed DSM-III suggests a consideration of this possibility. It particularly invites us to do so: (a) when resistance is expressed indirectly through procrastination, dawdling, stubbornness, intentional inefficiency, and "forgetfulness"; and (b) when behavior of this sort persists even under circumstances where more self-assertive and effective behavior is possible (p. 329).

In children, one is most apt to see this behavior, as distinct from more overt oppositional behavior, in reaction to expectations about school work, domestic chores, and household routines (such as bedtime routines). The child may not express any direct opposition or defiance, but rather "slow down" or "forget." While this behavior still could be basically the result of a conflict over control or power, this interpretation is weakened by the fact that the child often verbalizes compliance and lack of opposition when questioned. It is as if the child does not want the responsibility of participating in the formulation of rules, but he or she still resents the fact that others are making rules and demands. DSM-III notes that these individuals are often dependent and lack self-confidence, and this lack of autonomy and assertiveness is reflected in the passivity of the passive-aggressive personality.

Finch and Green (1979) may have this personality disorder in mind (though they use the term *oppositional personality*) when they say: "Certain personality organizations are dominated by the issues around compliance with adult requirements. In a certain sense, there are three choices: one can obey all rules and develop a compulsive personality, one can rebel actively and become an antisocial personality disorder, or one can say 'yes' to the rules but never quite follow them and so become an oppositional personality" (p. 243).

Millon (1969), in his discussion of the etiology of the negativistic or passive-aggressive personality style, emphasized the importance of parental ambivalence in the form of inconsistent attitudes and contradictory ("double-bind") family communications. Children imitate the parents' erratic behavior and internalize their conflicting attitudes toward themselves and others, resulting in cognitive ambivalence and occasional affective explosions (usually hostile). This "active-ambivalent" posture is easily recognizable in descriptive accounts of passive-aggressive children, though the ambivalence is more likely to lead to cognitive vagueness and absentmindedness than to temper tantrum explosions.

Early manifestations of negativism are usually represented as normal protective and self-propelling functions that enable the child to overcome infantile dependency. Clinically, however, the later and more extreme expressions of negativism may be enlisted in the service of other dynamics. In the oppositional child, it may be used as a protective device against compliance when there is a strong tendency for the child to be submissive, to yield to the wishes of others. In the passive-aggresive child, it may be used for revenge for rejection or for previous instances of successful manipulation by parents or other authority figures. More serious instances of negativism are reported by Levy (1972) in cases of conversion reaction, anorexia nervosa, and catatonia. He concludes his discussion by suggesting that, in clinical cases, the negativistic mechanism has become "more powerful than motivation" (p. 355), and this statement underlines the strong pull of habit or "style" in cases of personality disorder where the behavior seems to be almost impervious to the claims of enlightened self-interest (or positive reinforcement). If the early negativism persists, children either develop an oppositional or a passive-aggressive personality, depending on the relative strengths of their autonomy and aggressive strivings. In either case, they usually soften their overt negativism as they mature and become more "reasonable." This tends to blur the distinction clinically and perhaps makes the differential diagnosis of oppositional versus passive-aggressive personality even more difficult for adults than for children.

There has been very little empirical work done on either the oppositional or the passive-aggressive child. One study of thirty-six cases seen at the Child Guidance Clinic of the Washington University School of Medicine (Gilpin & Worland, 1976) is perhaps the best such data available. Even here, the *N* was reduced by dividing the thirty-six children into three approximately equal age groups and then focusing on the boys in these groups because of the very small number of girls represented. The first group of boys had a modal age of onset between eight months and two years and probably represents more of the control dynamics associated with the oppositional disorder. The second group of ten boys was first seen at ages ten to twelve, with poor school performance as the most common problem. There were also frequent complaints about lying, stealing, and temper tantrums, showing the aggressive component in the children together with the negativism. The fathers of these boys were often seen as passive or passive-aggressive (seven out of ten), and they tended to identify with their sons but not to express warmth toward them. The mothers tended to be controlling and depressed.

Even though aggression was a big concern for these boys, and they expressed it both overtly and covertly, they were not seen as impulsive. This, plus the fact that they were described as depressed (eight out of ten), might be critical in differentiating these boys from aggressive conduct disorders. Their major distinguishing characteristic, however, was that they were seen as "withholding," and this of course they shared with the younger oppositional group. A somewhat surprising finding was that almost half of this sample, as compared to none of the control group who were chosen at random from the clinic population, were seen as homosexually oriented. However surprising some of these features may be, this group may tentatively be viewed as representing one type of passive-aggressive personality disorder in children, in that the negativistic-withholding factor is blended with the hostile-aggressive one and is expressed by holding back or holding out in school.

Schizoid Disorder of Childhood or Adolescence

Even less is known about the schizoid disorder of childhood or adolescence than about the passive-aggressive disorder. In DSM-III, this childhood syndrome bears the same name and general description as its adult counterpart, the schizoid personality disorder, which is an advantage from a conceptual and classification standpoint. The disorder is considered rare, however, and no etiological clues are provided by the manual.

The DSM-III description emphasizes the preferred social isolation of these children. They are "loners," and they are uncomfortable, inept, and awkward when placed in social situations. They appear aloof, reserved, withdrawn, and seclusive. An associated feature of this disorder is detachment or lack of involvement in external reality generally. "They often appear self-absorbed and engage in excessive daydreaming" (p. 61). This quality seems to anticipate the marginal societal status of many schizoid adults. There is no loss of competence in reality testing, however.

The GAP book makes a helpful distinction between two childhood personality disorders with social withdrawal tendencies. The overly inhibited child is painfully shy about social engagement but yearns for warm and meaningful relationships. This is similar to the DSM-III description of the avoidant disorder of childhood, which is listed under the general category of anxiety disorders. The isolated child, on the other hand, has a restricted capacity for affective experience and seems to prefer detachment.

Both the GAP book and Planansky (1966), in a major article on the early schizoid personality, raise the issue of the extent to which the schizoid personality in childhood is a precursor of schizophrenic disorders in adulthood. Since there are no good data on this question, the GAP book recommends that schizoid personality should retain its traditional connotation of preschizophrenic or latent schizophrenic disposition, while isolated personality disorder should be free of that connotation.

Both GAP and Planansky suggest the strong likelihood of a constitutional tendency in schizoid disorder. If this is true, the tendency would probably bear some resemblance to the Thomas and Chess (1977) "slow-to-warm-up" temperamental constellation, except that one would not expect the child to show gradually "quiet and positive interest and involvement." However, two of the major characteristics—a tendency to negative responses of mild intensity to new stimuli, and slow adaptability after repeated contact—seem to fit pretty well. This constitutional tendency might well interact with parental pressure on the child to make quick social adaptations, especially to nursery or elementary school, to produce a marked avoidant or seclusive reaction pattern in the child.

Perhaps the most penetrating and promising analysis of personality patterning related to the schizoid personality disorder in children is that presented by Millon (1969) in his discussion of the *detached* pattern. "The detached individual typically is introverted, aloof and seclusive; he has difficulty in establishing close friendships, prefers not to become involved with others and seems uninterested in, and tends to avoid, social activities; in general, he gains little gratification in personal relationships" (p. 223).

Millon goes on to divide this detached pattern into two broad subgroups, the "passive" and the "active." The major distinction here seems to be that passive-detached individuals are fairly content with their social isolation because of constitutional factors which naturally inhibit the desire for close interpersonal relationships. Active-detached individuals desire closeness with people, as evidenced by their fantasy life, but avoid it because of generalized interpersonal anxiety. Both of these pathological patterns may well be related to schizoid disorder in childhood, though only the active-detached pattern is related by Millon to the adult schizoid personality.

For Millon, the *passive-detached* (also known as "asocial") personality type is characterized by four general features: affectivity deficit, cognitive slippage, complacent self-image, and interpersonal indifference. The likely constitutional element referred to above would be reflected in a passive, infantile reaction pattern, which includes a low sensory responsivity, motor passivity, and a generally placid mood. Consequently, these infants may be easy to care for, but they are not very responsive or rewarding to parents and therefore may evoke minimal stimulation and affection from parents. The constitutional factors may thus interact with familial factors to produce the asocial pattern in early childhood. The asocial behavioral style serves to maintain social isolation and disengagement very effectively, so the therapeutic prognosis for this personality pattern is not promising, nor is the person expected to "grow out of it."

The *active-detached* (also known as the "avoidant") personality type is characterized by four related but differentiable features: affective disharmony, cognitive interference, alienated self-image, and interpersonal distrust. These individuals are highly alert to social stimuli and are oversensitive to the moods and feelings of others, especially those which are hostile to or rejecting of themselves. The detachment they seek is therefore a protection against the interpersonal stress they anticipate. They may feel their loneliness deeply, but the attendant desire to be accepted is often strongly repressed. To compound the problem, avoidant people also mistrust their own social impulses, aggressive and affectional, fearing that they may prompt others to be rejecting, frustrating, and condemning. They are thus tormented by inner and outer doubts and suspicions.

The likely constitutional elements present in the avoidant child resemble those of the difficult child in the Thomas and Chess (1977) temperament analysis. That is, this type of child has irregular biological functions, negative withdrawal responses to new stimuli, slow adaptability to change, and intense mood expressions which are frequently negative (p. 23). He or she tends to provoke, or interact with, parental frustration, rejection, and deprecation, and this kind of interaction would certainly cultivate the sense of mistrust which is the dominant feature of this personality type. This suspicious attitude may then provoke or interact with peer group alienation in childhood, and the estrangement from others would thus be confirmed both within and outside of the family circle.

Avoidant behavioral strategies are easy to maintain with a minimum of positive reinforcement from the environment, for the avoidance of anticipated hurt and stress is its own reward. In contrast to the passive-detached personality, however, withdrawal from contact with others is self-defeating, for the individual does have a real need to relate to others. This need surely improves the prognosis for the avoidant personality relative to that for the asocial personality (though Millon does not say so). It also introduces a problematic feature into the consideration of this pattern as a personality disorder; namely, the syntonic/dystonic issue. Individuals with a personality disorder should be content with themselves (or at least nonanxious) when their defensive coping strategies are working effectively. Yet here Millon presents a personality type who is frustrated and self-defeating when his or her defenses are working well. Perhaps this part of the description is too close to a classically neurotic picture to be used as a helpful model for the schizoid personality disorder, in children or adults. In this light, perhaps the description should be modified to suggest that a person is content to be avoidant in interpersonal relationships so long as the fantasy life is full of rich and complex involvements with others.

This, then, represents a sketchy theoretical background for understanding the schizoid disorder of childhood or adolescence. Two helpful distinctions are suggested by the literature: (1) We must distinguish between the kind of withdrawal in childhood which is preschizophrenic and which is not. (2) We must distinguish between a "natural" kind of detachment based on constitutionally low affective responsiveness and a defensive detachment based on hypersensitivity and/or parental rejection and deprecation. The latter kind of detachment should be further differentiated from extreme shyness with individuals outside of the immediate family, which is the primary characteristic of the avoidant disorder of childhood in DSM-III.

The empirical literature on this disorder is quite indirect and sketchy, but in the past few years three studies have been published which merit some mention. The article by Wanlass and Prinz (1982) is helpful in differentiating several groupings of behavioral indices which relate to this general category of childhood social isolation. They are: (a) low rates of peer interaction, (b) rejection by peers, (c) social skills deficits, (d) active avoidance of peers, (e) passive-unassertive style, and (f) oversensitivity to criticism or failure, as well as less distinctive combinations of anxiety, unhappiness, and daydreaming.

Among the underlying variables which might be derived from this list are sociability and social problem-solving ability, which have been found to be correlated in kindergarteners and first graders in a study by Rubin et al. (1984). These authors suggest that both social cognition competencies and peer sociability may be undermined by some level of relatively constant social anxiety. For our purposes, this would bring these patterns into closer relationship with the avoidant than with the asocial type of detachment. It would also be necessary to view the hypothesized anxiety as more syntonically experienced than disruptive.

The third study, by Kennedy and Bakeman (1984), is even more distally related to the clinical syndrome in children, but it serves to underline a possibly important early etiological factor. These authors found that amount of mother's attention to her infant was correlated with measures of social competence with adults when the child was three years old. The noteworthy aspect of this study is that the same was not true of the infant's *response* to maternal attention. That is, it would appear that this is not a matter of mother teaching infant how to respond in a socially appropriate way from an early age (a social learning explanation), but just a matter of showing the infant a lot of attention. This leaves unclear what is the effective agent in generating social competency in the young child, but it does not appear to be as simple as reinforcement of early social responses (such as smiling, eye contact, etc.).

Histrionic Personality Disorder

The major feature of the histrionic disorder is an overly dramatic quality, as the name suggests, represented by highly charged emotional reactions. This typically is associated with disturbed interpersonal relationships characterized by undependability, egocentricity, and manipulation. Previously such a syndrome was labeled hysterical personality.

Horowitz (1977) detailed the "core characteristics" of the hysterical personality in a most comprehensive way. He described their typical interpersonal relationships as repetitive, impulsive, and stereotyped, characterized by polarized complementary roles (e.g., victim-aggressor), as well as fantasy roles which are "cardboard" and "caricaturelike." Reality is not real, and the experience of self is that one is not in control and not responsible. Horowitz also described traits of attention-seeking behavior, fluid changes in mood, and episodic flooding with feeling. There often is considerable charm and appeal, but also great inconsistency and provocativeness without conscious recognition of the intent. Their cognitive style is unclear and inhibited, with incomplete statements of ideas and feelings and with a lack of details or clear labels. A shallowness of cognitive processing is exemplified by: (1) nonverbal communications that are not translated into words or conscious meanings; (2) partial or unidirectional associational lines; (3) a short-circuiting approach to apparent completion of problematic thoughts; and (4) the use of language for effect rather than meaning. All of these characteristics, while not peculiar to children, can be found in children.

The Millon (1969) category of active-dependent (or gregarious) personality belongs in this discussion, as indicated by its DSM-II designation of hysterical personality. Etiologically, the roles of excessive early stimulation, parental control by contingent and irregular reward, and parental modeling of histrionic, suggestible, and vacillating traits are emphasized. As children, hysterics may also be endowed with the mixed blessing of a superficially attractive manner (including good looks).

The more extreme hysterical behavior, then, is represented by a wish to court attention and favor (and, perhaps more deeply, to get nurturance/security needs met) by pandering to the more superficial and transient interests of others. Hysterical children try to appear to be whatever the other person would have them be, and in the process they lose their developmental pathway to a more stable and secure self-concept. In the child, as in the adult, this is apt to be most clearly represented in the traits of seductiveness and overweening gregariousness.

Obsessional Personality

A final candidate for a personality disorder of childhood is the obsessional personality type. Obsessional personalities in children have received very little attention in the child psychopathology literature. Relatively few textbooks even address the issue of obsessionality in childhood, and those that do tend to restrict themselves to a discussion of obsessional neuroses. (Judd, 1965, has provided a particularly readable discussion.) However, it seems possible that this omission reflects the overlap of childhood obsessionality with other personality constellations (e.g., the oppositional personality, phobic reactions, and mild manifestations of the detached personality type) and the fact that many obsessional characteristics may be highly valued by parents ("He's such a good child") and therefore may rarely come to the attention of clinicians.

Additionally, obsessional disorders in general seem to be relatively rare. Adams (1973) reviewed epidemiological studies and cited estimates of the prevalence of childhood obsessional disorders—including neuroses—at about 1 percent of clinical contacts. Nevertheless, scattered case reports suggest that obsessional personality constellations may be conceptually important. Unfortunately, the scant attention paid to obsessional personality in children includes an almost total absence of empirical research, so that a discussion of this disorder must be confined to theoretical and clinical information.

DSM-III has an adult category of compulsive personality disorder which provides some guidelines for a discussion of the obsessional personality disorder in children and adolescents. Characteristics of the compulsive personality disorder are: "restricted ability to express warm and tender emotions; perfectionism that interferes with the ability to grasp 'the big picture'; insistence that others submit to his or her way of doing things; excessive devotion to work and productivity to the exclusion of pleasure; and indecisiveness" (p. 326). Further, these individuals are stiff, formal, and stingy in their interpersonal style. They are preoccupied with rules and details, and they are inordinately fearful of making a mistake.

GAP also has a category called compulsive personality, but their description of this childhood category does not always emphasize the same characteristics as the adult DSM-III disorder. The emphasis in GAP is upon orderliness, cleanliness, and conformity. These children are rigid and inflexible, and the achievement of a relaxed state is difficult. In contrast to the general ineffectiveness and emotional stiltedness mentioned for the adult category, the compulsive child is said to perform well and impress others with an emotional maturity.

Millon (1969) discusses the obsessive-compulsive personality under the heading of the passive-ambivalent pattern. This pattern is basically characterized by restrained affectivity, cognitive constriction, conscientious self-image, and interpersonal respectfulness. No particular temperament factors are noted by Millon, but he does focus special attention on two psychogenic factors: parental overcontrol by contingent punishment, and guilt and responsibility training. The child's coping strategy involves overcontrol of self and avoiding vulnerability in relation to others.

The DSM-III and Millon descriptions, though not focused on children per se, are nevertheless relevant to the understanding of a particular kind of child. This child is a "good" child in a formal and conscientious sense, but sensitive observers may well be concerned about this child's lack of spontaneity and warmth. This child is also a hard worker, but one may wonder at the lack of productivity in relation to the effort expended. This child wants to make a good impression on others, but the careful and conformist way in which this is attempted may lead others to overlook this child in favor of others who appear to be more individualized and interesting.

Adams' (1973) book on obsessive children included case material on forty-nine obsessional children, of whom Adams placed ten in the category of obsessional character disorder. Descriptively, such children are most clearly characterized by sadness or relatively flat affect and by a notable lack of spontaneity. They tend to appear intellectually precocious, especially in their style of verbal expression. However, their speech often appears stilted or mechanical and may be used very aggressively—they frequently correct or contradict their peers and even adults. They also tend to be overconcerned with rules and to develop rigid moral codes. They may manifest intrusive obsessional concerns (i.e., repeated emergence of a single theme, such as a concern about disease or death) which have a driven quality. Finally, they may engage in ritualistic behaviors. However, it should be noted that obvious obsessions or compulsions constitute frank symptom formation and usually justify the diagnosis of obsessive-compulsive neurosis. In short, such children tend to appear, at least superficially, mechanical and overcontrolled. Perhaps the most striking quality of these children is that they are decidedly unchildlike.

Dynamically, an obsessional personality structure appears to represent a learned mechanism of overcontrol of relatively regressive drives, centered around conflict between dependency and autonomy. Classic psychoanalytic notions of conflictual toilet training as an etiological mechanism are simplistic and have found little support in either research or clinical experience. However, childhood obsessionality appears to be associated with obsessionality and emotional detachment on the part of parents. A child reared by such parents reaches the toddler stage with unresolved dependency needs. Unconscious attitudes toward parents are therefore ambivalent, charged with both emotional hunger and a component of fear and resentment. Such a child is therefore highly ambivalent about growth toward autonomy.

The development of an obsessional character structure is a learned mechanism of adaptation to this developmental crisis. Parental example, explicit teaching by parents, and some inherent disposition lead the child to control regressive needs and aggressive wishes with intellectual mechanisms. The child develops a characterological style of rigid and mechanistic adherence to rules. This adaptation has the added benefit of winning praise from parents, so that many obsessional children seem motivated to overachieve—their behavior is organized around the attempt to "earn" love. Such children frequently have a rich fantasy life which reveals abundant aggressive themes (Judd, 1965).

Further, careful examination may reveal numerous fears and strong dependency needs which are not superficially apparent. When this characterological adaptation is relatively successful, the child develops an obsessional personality, in contrast to a less successful adaptation which produces more obvious symptoms and is likely to be disguised as a neurosis.

It is important to note that diagnosis of obsessional personality depends on the overall pattern of personality characteristics. Isolated incidents of obsessions or of compulsive behavior can be quite normal developmentally. Much childhood play, both solitary and group play, has a clearly ritualistic quality. Further, some ritualistic behavior (e.g., hyperconcern with cleanliness in a three year old) is phase appropriate.

In short, both psychoanalytic developmental theory and case reports suggest that obsessional personality may be a conceptually important category of psychopathology in childhood. However, such personality constellations—at least in clearly recognizable form—appear to be relatively rare. Further, there is a general lack of empirical information about obsessional personality in childhood.

Conclusions

The preceding discussion presented childhood personality disorders as a diagnostic and conceptual category of potential clinical utility. Conduct disorders, the schizoid disorder, the passive-aggressive personality, the hysterical personality, and the obsessional personality were selected as representing childhood disorders with the best credentials as personality disorders in the traditional sense. As was indicated in the introduction, the very notion of childhood personality disorder is a topic of controversy. Thus, it seems reasonable to seek to evaluate the utility of the concept of childhood personality disorder in light of the material presented.

On the positive side, the notion of childhood personality disorders does appear to organize some important clinical material in a meaningful fashion. The psychodynamic developmental framework, with all its faults, remains a useful general conceptual scheme for the understanding of childhood psychopathology. A particular strength of this viewpoint is that it is general enough to successfully incorporate insights derived from other orientations (e.g., behavioral theories and theories of cognitive development). The behavioral syndromes organized under the heading of personality disorders are of undisputed importance and share the common theme of a relatively stable (i.e., characterological) and ego-syntonic adaptation to the pressures of psychological development.

In a reliability study of the application of the GAP system of psychiatric diagnosis in childhood, Freeman (1971) solicited two case histories from each of twenty-two psychiatrists. These case histories were subsequently resubmitted to the entire group for diagnosis. Fully 22 percent of the cases were diagnosed as personality disorders, suggesting that practicing clinicians find the personality disorder construct to be a conceptually meaningful way of organizing clinical information about children.

Numerous empirical studies exist regarding only one type of childhood personality disorder—the conduct disorders. For the conduct disorders, the concept of personality disorder bears up well under empirical scrutiny. This personality constellation appears to be predictive of adult adjustment. Additionally, its relationship to at least some etiological factors makes sense from a developmental perspective. In short, the notion of personality disorders in childhood appears to have some utility from both clinical and empirical standpoints.

On the negative side, very little empirical information exists regarding childhood personality disorders other than conduct disorders. The absence of good data about the reliability of diagnosis of such disorders is particularly unfortunate. It seems likely that the complex and fluid character of child development makes clear-cut examples of these personality types rare, and that reliable diagnosis may be difficult. The definitions of the various personality disorders are by no means concise; they overlap considerably, and may also be difficult to distinguish from other major categories such as childhood neurosis. Further, with the exception of the conduct disorders, there seems to be no demonstration that diagnosis of a childhood personality disorder is predictive of adult adjustment. There are of course no empirical studies which systematically investigate the treatment of various childhood personality disorders. In short, empirical information regarding childhood personality disorders is sadly lacking.

The task of developing a comprehensive classification for personality disorders in childhood is just beginning. In order to adequately serve the theoretically eclectic world of mental health, such a system must separate itself from the narrow scope of the traditional psychoanalytic viewpoint, as the DSM-III system has done. In order for the system to have coherence and comprehensiveness, however, it must have some underlying conceptual framework, which the DSM-III most assuredly lacks. In the meantime, the task at hand is to look for meaning in the conceptual and empirical work that has been done with existing categories, and to attempt to use that information to refine our conceptualizations of the psychopathology of childhood.

REFERENCES

Achenbach, T. M. *Developmental psychopathology.* 2nd ed. New York: Wiley, 1982.

Adams, P. *Obsessive children: A sociopsychiatric study.* New York: Brunner/Mazel, 1973.

Alexander, J., & Parsons, B. V. *Functional family therapy.* Monterey: Brooks/Cole, 1982.

American Psychiatric Association. *Diagnostic and statistical manual of mental disorders* (2d ed.). Washington DC: American Psychiatric Association, 1968.

American Psychiatric Association. *Diagnostic and statistical manual of mental disorders* (3d ed.). Washington, DC: American Psychiatric Association, 1980.

Baldwin, A., Kalhorn, J., & Breese, F. Patterns of parental behavior. *Psychological Monographs,* 1945, *58,* iii, 75.

Barker, P. *Basic child psychiatry.* Baltimore: University Park, 1979.

Bender, C. Childhood schizophrenia. *American Journal of Orthopsychiatry,* 1947, *17,* 40–56.

Beres, D., & Obers, S. The effects of extreme deprivation in infancy on psychic structure in adolescence: A study in ego development. *Psychoanalytic Study of the Child,* 1950, *26,* 212–235.

Bowlby, J. Forty-four juvenile thieves: Their characters and home-life. *International Journal of Psycho-analysis,* 1944, *25,* 19–53, 107–128.

Bowlby, J. Maternal care and mental health. *World Health Organization Monograph Series,* No. 2. Geneva: WHO, 1951.

Brown, F. Childhood bereavement and subsequent psychiatric disorder. *British Journal of Psychiatry,* 1966, *112,* 1035–1041.

Cass, L., & Thomas C. *Childhood pathology and later adjustment: The question of prediction.* New York: Wiley, 1979.

Craig, M., & Glick, S. *A manual of procedure for applications of the Glueck prediction table.* London: University of London, 1965.

Field, H. Prediction of character disorder and psychotic outcome from childhood behavior. Unpublished Thesis, New York, Teacher's College, Columbia University, 1969.

Finch, S., & Green, J. Personality disorders. In J. Noshpitz (Ed.), *Basic handbook of child psychiatry* (Vol. 2). New York: Basic, 1979.

Freeman, M. A reliability study of psychiatric diagnosis in childhood and adolescence. *Journal of Child Psychology and Psychiatry*, 1971, *12*, 43–54.

Freud, A. *Normality and pathology in childhood.* New York: International Universities, 1965.

Gilpin, D., & Worland, J. Symptomatic oppositionality as seen in the clinic. In E. Anthony & D. Gilpin (Eds.), *Three clinical faces of childhood.* New York: Spectrum 1976.

Glueck, S., & Glueck, E. *Juvenile delinquents grow up.* New York: The Commonwealth Fund, 1940.

Glueck, S., & Glueck, E. *Unravelling juvenile delinquency.* Connecticut: Harvard University, 1950.

Glueck S., & Glueck, E. *Predicting delinquency and crime.* Cambridge: Harvard University 1959.

Goldfarb, W. Infant rearing and problem behavior. *American Journal of Orthopsychiatry*, 1943, *13*, 249–265.

Goldstone, S. The treatment of antisocial behavior. In B. B. Wolman (Ed.), *The therapist's handbook* (2d ed.). New York: Van Nostrand Reinhold, 1983.

Group for the Advancement of Psychiatry. *Psychopathological disorders in childhood.* New York: Aronson, 1966.

Hare, R. *Psychopathy: Theory and research.* New York: Wiley, 1970.

Harris, P. W. The interpersonal maturity of delinquents and nondelinquents. In W. S. Laufer & J. M. Day (Eds.), *Personality theory, moral development, and criminal behavior.* Lexington, MA: Heath, 1983.

Harrison, S., & McDermott, J. (Eds.), *Childhood psychopathology.* New York: International Universities, 1972.

Hogan, R., & Jones, W. H. A role-theoretical model of criminal conduct. In W. S. Laufer & J. M. Day (Eds.), *Personality theory, moral development, and criminal behavior.* Lexington, MA: Heath, 1983.

Horowitz, M. The core characteristics of hysterical personality. In M. Horowitz (Ed.), *Hysterical personality.* New York: Aronson, 1977.

Judd, L. Obsessive compulsive neurosis in children. *Archives of General Psychiatry.* 1965, *12*, 136–143.

Kennedy, J. H., & Bakeman, R. The early mother-infant relationship and social competence with peers and adults at three years. *Journal of Psychology*, 1984, *116*, 23–34.

Knight, E. A descriptive comparison of markedly aggressive and submissive children. Abstracted in *Smith College Studies in Social Work* (Vol. 4). 1933. As reported in McCord & McCord (1956).

Knopf, I. *Childhood psychopathology.* Englewood Cliffs, NJ: Prentice-Hall, 1979.

Kohlberg, L., LaCrosse, J., & Ricks, D. The predictability of adult mental health from childhood behavior. In B. Wolman (Ed.), *Manual of child psychopathology.* New York: McGraw-Hill, 1972.

Levy, D. Primary affect hunger. *American Journal of Psychiatry*, 1937, *94*, 643–652.

Levy, D. Oppositional syndromes and oppositional behavior. In S. Harrison & J. McDermott (Eds.), *Childhood psychopathology.* New York: International Universities, 1972.

McCord, W., & McCord, J. *Psychopathology and delinquency.* New York: Grune & Stratton, 1956.

McCord, W., & McCord, J. *Origins of crime: A new evaluation of the Cambridge-Somerville youth study.* New York: Columbia University, 1959.

Megargee, E. I. Recent research on overcontrolled and undercontrolled personality patterns among violent offenders. In I. Jacks & S. G. Cox (Eds.), *Psychological approaches to crime and its correction: Theory, research, practice.* Chicago: Nelson-Hall, 1984.

Mellsop, G. Psychiatric patients seen as children and adults: Childhood predictors of adult illness. *Journal of Child Psychology and Psychiatry*, 1972, *13*, 91–101.

Metcalf, A. Childhood: From process to structure. In M. Horowitz (Ed.), *Hysterical Personality.* New York: Aronson, 1977.

Millon, T. *Modern psychopathology.* Philadelphia: Saunders, 1969.

Morris, H., Escoll, P., & Wexler, R. Aggressive behavior disorders of childhood: A follow-up study. *American Journal of Psychiatry*, 1956, *112*, 991–997.

Morrison, H. The asocial child: A destiny of sociopath? In W. H. Reid (Ed.) *The psychopath.* New York: Brunner/Mazel, 1978.

Newell, H. A further study of maternal rejection. *American Journal of Orthopsychiatry*, 1936, *6*, 576–589.

Planansky, K. Conceptual boundaries in schizoidness: Suggestions for epidemiological and genetic research. *Journal of Nervous and Mental Disease*, 1966, *142*, 318–331.

Quay, H. C. Residential treatment. In H. C. Quay & J. S. Werry (Eds.), *Psychopathological disorders of childhood.* New York: Wiley, 1979.

Robins, L. *Deviant children grow up.* Baltimore: Williams & Wilkins, 1966.

Robins, L. Follow-up studies. In H. Quay & J. Werry (Eds.), *Psychopathological disorders of childhood.* New York: Wiley, 1979.

Roff, M. Childhood antecedents of adult neurosis, severe bad conduct and psychological health. *Life History Research in Psychopathology,* 1974, *3,* 131–162.

Ross, A. O. *Child behavior therapy.* New York: Wiley, 1981.

Rubin, K. H., et al. Social isolation and social problem-solving: A longitudinal study. *Journal of Consulting and Clinical Psychology,* 1984, *52,* 17–25.

Rutter, M. Parent-child separation: Psychological effects on the children. *Journal of Child Psychology and Psychiatry,* 1971, *12,* 233–260.

Schactel, A., & Levi, M. Character structure of day nursery children in wartime as seen through the Rorschach. *American Journal of Orthopsychiatry,* 1945, *15,* 213–222.

Shore, M. F. Psychological theories of the causes of antisocial behavior. In I. Jacks & S. G. Cox (Eds.), *Psychological approaches to crime and its correction: Theory, research, practice.* Chicago: Nelson-Hall, 1984.

Skrzypek, G. Effect of perceptual isolation and arousal on anxiety, complexity preference, and novelty preference in psychopathic and neurotic delinquents. *Journal of Abnormal Psychology,* 1969, *74,* 321–329.

Tait, C., & Hodges, E. *Delinquents, their families and the community.* Springfield, IL: Charles C. Thomas, 1962.

Thomas A., & Chess, S. *Temperament and development.* New York: Brunner/Mazel, 1977.

Wanlass, R. L., & Prinz, R. J. Methodological issues in conceptualizing and treating childhood social isolation. *Psychological Bulletin,* 1982, *92,* 39–55.

Warren, M. Q. Applications of interpersonal-maturity theory to offender populations. In W. S. Laufer & J. M. Day (Eds.), *Personality theory, moral development, and criminal behavior.* Lexington, MA: Heath, 1983.

Watt, N., Stolorow, R., Lubensky, A., & McClelland, D. School adjustment and behavior of children hospitalized for schizophrenia as adults. *American Journal of Orthopsychiatry,* 1970, *40,* 637–657.

Zetzel, E. The so-called good hysteric. *International Journal of Psycho-Analysis,* 1968, *49,* 256–260.

CHAPTER 14

Disorders Characteristic of Late Adolescence

John Paul McKinney and Mary Ann Reinhart

Before describing disorders characteristic of adolescence it is important to ask whether adolescence in itself is a period of turmoil. Some have argued that by its very nature adolescence is a time of great psychological distress and so the typical adolescent can be expected to be disturbed. This extreme view, taken by many psychoanalysts, sees adolescents laboring under severe pressures and required to make difficult choices with little or no support. Gustin (1961), for example, has argued that "buffeted from within by powerful impulses and pushed from without by a strange and unfriendly world the adolescent must find some new ways to make his life tolerable"(p. 82). According to this view, the storm and stress which is supposed to typify the life of the adolescent carries over to his or her relations with parents and peers, so that rebelliousness is more likely than conformity and impulse expression is more likely than control.

The opposite and equally extreme view of adolescence is suggested by some social learning theorists, who argue that the idea of adolescence as necessarily disruptive is a myth, except to the extent that certain maladaptive behaviors have been learned. These social learning theorists see adolescence as no more stressful than any other period of life. An articulate spokesman for this position is Albert Bandura (1964). He claims that adults have paid too much attention to superficial signs of nonconformity in youth and have, in effect, paid more attention to their fads than to their conformity—to their rebellion and disorganization than to their obedience. According to Bandura the mass media have sensationalized this perception of adolescents and furthermore adolescents themselves may be conforming to this sensationalized view in a self-fulfilling prophecy. The truth about adolescence probably lies somewhere between these two positions.

A brief listing of some of the developmental tasks of the adolescent period will underline the fact that youngsters are indeed under pressure to respond to internal and social demands. The physiological changes of puberty and the psychological correlates of these changes are well known. Increasing independence from the family, turning toward peers and self in making decisions, and emancipation from parents and eventual home-leaving are all characteristic tasks for this age group, as are the identity problems that have been emphasized by Erik Erikson, the psychological response to sexual development and the associated changed peer relations. These are all part of the new developmental scene for the adolescent as are the need for career planning, choice of a college, and finally selection of a mate. It should be clear, however, that not all adolescents turn to their peers instead of their parents in formulating values (Costanzo & Shaw, 1966; Floyd & South, 1972), nor do all adolescents reject their parents. In fact, most research on this topic (Meissner, 1965; Hess & Goldblatt, 1957; Offer, Sabshin, & Marcus, 1965) has suggested that adolescent attitudes toward their parents and other adults tend to be more positive than negative. The same, by the way, is true of parents' attitudes toward their teenagers. The difficulty lies, of course, in communicating these positive attitudes. It appears that neither group is aware of how positively they are regarded by the other group.

Even if we accept the relatively benign nature of the adolescent period and see the difficulties of adolescence as normative crises, we still must acknowledge the rather long list of developmental tasks mentioned above as environmental pressures on the adolescent. Most adolescent pathological response patterns previously discussed in this book have been alleged to be reactions to these pressures and demands of adolescence. We will confine our discussion to identity disorder and substance abuse disorders, two problem areas of great import in our culture.

Identity Disorders

The pressing, lifelong question, "Who am I?" assumes primary importance during the adolescent years. As the late adolescent, who is still attempting to accommodate mature sexual and aggressive urges, severs childhood ties to the family of origin, he or she must face the world and self more or less alone. At this time the need to identify and distinguish self is most pressing (Erikson, 1963a) and, given the likelihood of new, abstract modes of thinking (Inhelder & Piaget, 1958), more possible than ever before. Accordingly, it becomes the task of the late adolescent to integrate these new cognitive capabilities and physiological changes into his or her childhood "self." While doing so the adolescent also must create a more highly individuated self, sufficiently separated from parental identifications so that the new identity comfortably accommodates the familiar child, the current adolescent, the soon-to-be-found adult, and the social world in which the adolescent lives (Erikson, 1968).

Before examining identity theory and the normal and abnormal modes of consolidating identity, we wish to make clear the point that the adolescent's identity formation does not occur in isolation. That is to say, the accomplishment of this developmental task occurs both within a historical context (Erikson, 1959, 1963b, 1968) and a more individual, familial context (Bloom, 1980; Erikson, 1946, 1968; Weiner, 1970). Each adolescent must separate from the family of origin while forming a unique identity within the context of this same family, which has been internalized during previous identification processes and is also an external reality. What the adolescent brings to the process of identity achievement (or diffusion) is intrinsically tied to the family, their mutual and individual histories, and to the current, daily interactions between them (Erikson, 1959; Stierlin, 1974). Just as the adolescent's task is to form a unique identity, consistent with the past, while separating from the current, dependent circumstance, parents must reevaluate their own identities, find satisfaction in the adolescent's newly achieved identity and let go, i.e., separate from the adolescent and recognize the child as independent (Haley, 1980; Stierlin, 1974). Late adolescent separation and identity achievements are both individual and family accomplishments and our discussion of disorders that arise in connection with the adolescent's identity formation task will be centered not only on the adolescent, but also on the adolescent-within-the-family.

The Identity Crisis: Erikson's Theory

Erik Erikson has been the most influential theorist writing on identity since World War II, when he first wrote of "identity confusion" in soldiers who were being treated for emotional disturbances. The identity crisis faced by the adolescent is precipitated, not by an external war according to Erikson (1968), but by an internal war. That is, the precipitation of the identity crisis is a developmental process, normative to the age of adolescence and young adulthood, for it is at this time that the person must face the fact of a rapidly maturing body, complete with adult sexual and aggressive urges, more abstract cognitive functioning, and ever more demanding expectations of assuming adult tasks and responsibilities. The challenge for the adolescent is to form from these changes a new, harmonious sense of psychological well-being, "a feeling of being at home in one's body, a sense of 'knowing where one is going,' and an inner assuredness of anticipated recognition from those who count" (Erikson, 1968, p. 165).

This developing adult identity must be a synthesis of previous childhood identifications and the adolescent's present awareness so that a unique and reasonably unified whole sense of self, consistent with one's past, is created. This major psychological task is accomplished with the help of society and the family, who should allow the adolescent time for role experimentation, firm and consistent guidance during these trials, delay of adult commitments, and recognition of his or her need to find continuity in what is usually a discontinuous stage of development.

This period when the child is granted a time to resolve role confusions and to find his or her own niche in society has been labelled *moratorium* (Erikson, 1968). During moratorium the person is allowed to "practice" various identities and experiment with various roles. If social support is lacking and/or the adolescent's inner war is too fierce, the crisis is not resolved and the youth feels in a state of identity confusion. Until sense is made of the confusion, the adolescent remains in a state of prolonged moratorium, a moratorium that is exemplified not by normative experimentation, but by a state of disorganization and perplexity about what to do and become.

Severe or prolonged identity confusion is considered by Erikson (1968) a serious, if transient, pathological condition of minimal choice and commitment (the adolescent not realizing that refusal to choose is also a commitment). This acutely disordered, developmental state, according to Erikson's theory, is notable for the following four features:

1. Incapacity for intimacy and the associated problem of distantiation, i.e., weakness of ties to others and the quick repudiation of those who are a threat to the adolescent's incomplete identity
2. Diffusion of time perspective, including a disbelief that time brings change and a violent fear that it might
3. Diffusion of industry, which is to say there is an inability to concentrate on required tasks or a self-destructive preoccupation with peripheral tasks and an abhorrence of competitiveness
4. Choice of a negative identity, expressed in snobbish mockery of the roles viewed as desirable and proper in the adolescent's family and wider community

In summary, Erikson's theory posits that identity crisis is a normative developmental phenomenon and the developmental stage of adolescence can be viewed as a psychosocial moratorium during which the adolescent experiments with various identity images. Only in extreme cases, in which the search for an identity has been found to be too demanding, does the identity crisis lead to the nonnormative, or pathological, state of identity confusion. This state of confusion, which shares many symptoms with borderline schizophrenia (Erikson, 1968; Weiner, 1966), recently has been recognized by the American Psychiatric Association (APA) nomenclature as a developmental disorder, most commonly appearing during adolescence, and having a unique set of diagnostic criteria and associated features. It (DSM-III, 1980) is termed identity disorder.

However, before elaborating the criteria and features of identity disorder, we would like to return to Erikson's theory of identity formation and examine appropriate research findings for evidence supporting or refuting Erikson's view that identity crisis is normative during adolescence.

Focusing on Erikson's concept of identity formation as process and the notions of commitment and crisis as integral components of the process, Marcia (1966) defined four stages of identity: (1) identity diffusion, (2) foreclosure, (3) moratorium, and (4) identity achievement. Identity diffusion, moratorium, and identity achievement have essentially the same meanings for Marcia's scheme as they did for Erikson's theory. *Foreclosure* is a term used by Marcia to include those adolescents and adults who have made strong commitments to certain life choices, but did not undergo an identity crisis, i.e., never questioned the choices nor examined others before making final commitment. Identity achievements refer to commitments made after experiencing identity crisis. Moratoria adolescents are in the state of crisis and have made only tentative, somewhat vague commitments. Identity diffusions refer to late adolescents or young adults who have no decided occupational or ideological direction, whether or not they might have experienced a decision-making period.

Marcia (1980) and others (Gilligan, 1977, 1982; Hodgson & Fischer, 1979) found Erikson's theory of identity achievement to be valid mainly for males. Marcia's initial and most successful work was with adolescent and young adult males, but his later work and that of others (Marcia, 1980; Marcia & Friedman, 1970; Schenkel & Marcia, 1972) indicated that males and females establish their identities around different issues and order the tasks of adolescence and young adulthood (identity and intimacy) differently. Therefore, we will divide our discussion of the research evidence according to the gender of the samples, discussing first Marcia's work with males.

Identity and Males. Marcia's Identity Status Interview (1966), a fifteen to thirty minute semistructured interview, is constructed to evaluate each respondent for the presence or absence of crisis and degree of commitment in three areas: occupation, religion and politics, with the last two combined in a general measure of ideology. Marcia (1980) reports average interjudge reliability to be around 80 percent.

Validating Erikson's original theory, the period of late adolescence does seem to be the time when an adolescent male will adopt the identity status that he is likely to keep for the next six to seven years. Marcia (1980) quotes a study by Meilman (1977) in which cross-sectional data indicated that most early adolescents are identity diffusions or foreclosures and the greatest change in status takes place between the ages of eighteen and twenty-one years of age. Meilman's findings are similar to those of Howard (1960) and Munro and Adams (1977), who found more identity achievements among adolescents who went to work following high school than among those who went on to college, validating Erikson's hypothesis (1959) that higher education encourages an extension of the psychosocial moratorium. In a follow-up study investigating changes in identity status over a six- to seven-year period, Marcia (1976) found that those who had been in the statuses of achievement and moratorium had about a 50 percent chance of being in one of those two statuses in the follow-up study. If the student had been in the foreclosure or diffusion status in the original study, he had an 84 percent chance of being in the status of foreclosure or diffusion six to seven years later.

Personality characteristics of the males in the four statuses also tend to confirm Erikson's theory. Those in identity achievement were found to show no conflictual patterns on the MMPI (Oshman & Manosevitz, 1974), had an internal locus of control (Waterman, Buehl, & Waterman, 1970), did the best of the four statuses on a concept attainment task under stressful conditions (Marcia, 1966), were more reflective on a measure of cognitive style than identity diffusions and foreclosures (Waterman & Waterman, 1974), and tended to be in the intimate status of Orlofsky, Marcia, and Lesser's (1973) Intimacy Status Interview.

Moratoria males, like those in identity achievement, had an internal locus of control (Waterman, Buehl, & Waterman, 1970), were reflective in cognitive style (Waterman & Waterman, 1974), and tended to be in the intimate status in the intimacy interview. However, in keeping with Erikson's theory, they tended to be the most anxious of the four statuses (Marcia, 1967; Podd, Marcia, & Rubin, 1970), expressed conflict patterns on the MMPI, changed college majors more frequently than each of the other three statuses (Waterman & Waterman, 1972), and in Podd, Marcia, and Rubin's (1970) prisoner's dilemma game, were less cooperative with authorities than peers, though they tended to follow the opponent's responses with like responses, indicating both rebellion and conformity needs.

Those respondents in the identity diffusion status also seemed to support Erikson's pattern of identity formation. They expressed no conflict patterns on the MMPI, were impulsive (Waterman & Waterman, 1974), tended to leave college, not for self-initiated reasons, but due to negative external pressures (Waterman & Waterman, 1972), and tended to be in the stereotyped relationship status of the Intimacy Status Interview, which is based on criteria of depth, responsibility, and mutuality of interpersonal relationships.

Marcia (1966) describes the young male adult in the foreclosure status as a living extension of his family. He is what others have chosen him to be, and if he chooses to attend college the experience serves only to confirm childhood and family beliefs. The research strongly supports Marcia's description of the foreclosed male. He is the least anxious (Marcia, 1967), but expresses conflict patterns on the MMPI, is the most endorsing of authoritarian values (Marcia, 1966, 1967), and performs the worst on a concept attainment task when placed under stress (Marcia, 1966). He also tends to be impulsive (Waterman & Waterman, 1974), leave college for negative external reasons (Waterman & Waterman, 1972), and to be in the stereotyped relationship status of intimacy (Orlofsky, Marcia, & Lesser, 1973).

Three studies of the relationship of parental patterns to identity status have been reported by Marcia (1980). Jordon (1970, 1971), in the United States, asked parents and their sons to respond to questionnaires eliciting their retrospective perceptions of child-rearing practices, and Matteson (1974), in Denmark, asked parents and their sons to finish a paragraph completion task in a standardized laboratory situation.

The fathers in these studies were found to play a central role in male identity status; both the father's style and quantity of interaction with his son seemed important. Jordon's foreclosure sons saw their parents as accepting and encouraging, and the parents recognized themselves as child-centered and somewhat protective. Matteson found these families to be the most task-oriented and the fathers seemed to be very powerful in the family interactions, making it clear that emotional expression was not encouraged.

Both Matteson and Jordon found identity diffusion parents detached and somewhat inactive in the family interaction pattern. This finding seemed especially true of the fathers; Jordon found these fathers also to be rejecting.

Consistent with Erikson's theory, moratorium sons had rather ambivalent relationships with their parents and were involved in a struggle to free themselves from the family. Also as cited in Marcia (1980), activity and self-expression typified the interaction pattern of the moratorium families in Matteson's study.

Balance, moderation, and some ambivalence characterized the identity achievement of sons and their parents, and while all family members reported positive relationships with each other, the son's greatest ambivalence was directed toward his father.

The foregoing research indicates that identity crisis followed by commitment to occupational and ideological choices leads to psychosocial health for young men and contributes to their resolution of the next task, i.e., intimacy. This research also indicates that the absence of an identity crisis, possible in the identity diffusion status and definitional in the foreclosure status, is associated with a relatively unhealthy psychosocial make-up, again supporting the theory of Erikson. Family patterns associated with the four statuses also are entirely consistent with Erikson's writings, and underscore the role of the family in male adolescent identity formation.

Identity and Females. This clear and consistent picture of identity formation does not exist for females.

The issue for females is commitment to

an identity, i.e., stability of identity, regardless of the presence or absence of crisis. For women, a foreclosure status seems to have the same positive effects that identity achievement has, clearly in contrast to findings for men. Marcia's (1980) review also indicates that identity achievement and foreclosure in women contribute to the same or similar personality characteristics as identity achievement and moratorium in males.

Adding to the problematic nature of the findings of identity achievement in women is a major difficulty in research design in the various studies. The attempt to extend identity status research to females was seriously confounded by different conflict situations used to determine male and female identity status, and different conflict situations used to determine female status in different studies. These inconsistencies make comparisons between the studies difficult.

Nevertheless, the following review of research on continuity/discontinuity in adolescence should help clarify the issue of identity.

Research on Continuity

Erikson (1959, 1968) saw adolescence as a disrupted, i.e., discontinuous, state. Moreover, he also stated that acute confusion indicates a serious clinical syndrome (1956, 1968). The difficulty for professionals lies in how to distinguish between normal identity disruption and acute confusion.

The question of normality of cognitive and emotional disruption in adolescence is certainly not new. Weiner (1970) and Offer and Offer (1971) each have written excellent summaries of the research on the topic. Weiner (1970) summarized his impressive review with the following statement: "Studies of normative and normal samples of adolescents demonstrate that adolescents in general are no more likely than other segments of the population to display features of psychopathology and that there is little basis for anticipating psychological disruption and maladaptive behavior in normal adolescents" (p.68).

Offer and Offer (1971) summarized their eight-year study of adolescents and agreed with Weiner's conclusion: "Our follow-up studies on the adolescents have revealed a continuity of individual personality structures throughout the stages of adolescence. . . . We believe that the development of many adolescents can be better characterized by a concept of gradual shifts than by volcanic eruptions" (pp. 40–41).

To these statements we would like to add the conclusions of two recent studies, both of which were conducted with impressively sized samples and were well executed.

Dusek and Flaherty (1981) used a longitudinal sequential design to study discontinuity/continuity and stability/instability in the development of individual adolescents' self-concepts over the course of either two or three years. Using the factor structures of a semantic differential scale as dependent variables, the authors concluded from the results of year-to-year correlations between individual factor scores and comparisons of group level factor scores that, "The person who enters adolescence is basically the same as that who exits it" (p. 39). That is, the development of self-concept is continuous.

However, the results of year-to-year correlations between individual factor scores indicated that some periods of instability exist in two of the four aspects of self-concept. The authors noted that it may be exactly the adolescents' fluctuations in stability that are misread as evidence of qualitative changes, falsely indicating discontinuity in development of the self-concept. The evidence clearly showed that changes in self-concept do occur, but slowly and continuously, with year-to-year fluctuations.

These fluctuations washed out over a two-year period. Hill (1981) noted in his commentary on the monograph that the most appropriate summary statement might be that the development of self-concept in adolescence "may show periods of instability but is not accurately described as discontinuous" (p. 64).

Offer, Ostrov, and Howard (1981a) continued the adolescent development study begun in 1962 by the senior author and reported the results of over 1,300 respondents to the Offer Self-Image Questionnaire. Respondents included random samples of teenagers replying to the questionnaire either in the 1960s or the 1970s, delinquent, disturbed, and physically ill adolescents, all from the United States, and random samples of adolescents from Australia, Ireland, and Israel.

The results strongly supported those reported by Offer and Offer (1971). The modal young person of the random samples stated that he or she is functioning well, has good relationships with family and friends, and in general accepts cultural values. The one notably negative finding endorsed by the majority of all age groups and both sexes is a high degree of anxiety. The wording of the actual statement eliciting these endorsements is "I am so very anxious." The difficulty in interpretation of the response comes from the fact that approximately 90 percent of each group also endorsed the statement, "I feel relaxed under normal circumstances." The authors concluded that the respondents were referring to situational anxiety when endorsing the anxiety item. We tend to concur and speculate the respondents were telling the researchers they were "so very anxious" when participating in a psychological study. There is no evidence in this monumental study to indicate that adolescence is a period of disruption or discontinuity of self-image.

The findings of this study also allow us to look at contemporary adolescents' self-reports of family relationships. In contrast to the findings of positive relationships reported by the random samples, the delinquent and disturbed samples attest to unhappiness and negative family attitudes. The delinquent sample also indicated rebellion and hostility, and the disturbed sample reported self-doubt and pessimism. Weiner (1970) similarly concluded that "Those adolescents who get along poorly with their families . . . are likely to be deviant youngsters and not normal young people demonstrating developmental vagaries common to their age group" (p. 68).

Contributing to the evidence that normal adolescents and young adults have positive relationships with their families, Moore and Hotch (1981) found college students negatively evaluated "emotional separation" from the family and "dissociation" from parents. Their respondents, who were asked to evaluate reasons that other students had given for saying that they "had left home," thought "economic independence" and "personal control" to be acceptable reasons to separate from the family. However, "emotional separation" and "dissociation" from parents were viewed by the respondents, not as valid reasons for separation, but as negative forms of attachment to the family, again supporting the conclusions of Weiner (1970) and Offer, Ostrov, and Howard (1981a) that normal (modal and healthy) adolescents maintain a sense of relatedness with their families while forming their own identities and separating from them.

Summary. The research reviewed by us and others (Weiner, 1970; Offer and Offer, 1971) indicate no signs of upheaval, disruption, or discontinuity as normative and normal. This finding is consistent for adolescents in various industrialized countries and extends to the relationships between adolescents and their families, where positive relationships, with perhaps some ambivalence, are the normal, actual situation.

Dusek and Flaherty's findings of some instability in self-concept and Offer, Ostrov, and Howard's finding of what seems to be strong situational anxiety might be the phenomena that contribute to the continuing perception by professionals that "adolescent turmoil" is one of the "normal conflicts associated with maturing" (DSM-III, 1980, p. 66). This attitude of contemporary health professionals toward the "*Sturm und Drang*" theory (Hall, 1904) of adolescent development, which is reflected in the notation of DSM-III (1980), was directly examined by Offer, Ostrov, and Howard (1981b). Completing the Offer Self-Image Questionnaire as they believed an average, healthy adolescent would complete it, psychiatrists, psychologists and social workers described the normal adolescent as significantly more disturbed than the normative adolescent described himself or herself on seven out of ten subscales.

Consider again our review of the work on Marcia's identity statuses (1966), the Dusek and Flaherty (1981), and Offer, Ostrov, and Howard (1981a) findings in light of the Offer, Ostrov, and Howard (1981b) finding mentioned above. We concluded that crisis and commitment (identity achievement) lead to the most healthy psychosocial adjustment of young adulthood for men and women, and that the state of crisis and vague commitment in males and commitment with no crisis in females are also healthy, normal statuses during this period. "Crisis" means that the adolescent experiences a decision-making period, perhaps somewhat extensive in length, particularly if the adolescent attends college (Erikson, 1968). "Commitment" implies a pledge to a certain mode of living. The evidence indirectly, although strongly, indicates that this decision-making period and/or period of commitment leads not to discontinuity and disruption, but to some year-to-year instability of self-concept and possibly strong anxiety in unfamiliar situations. Perhaps it has been these signs that have been perceived as indications of discontinuity (Erikson, 1968; Freud, A., 1948, 1958; Freud, S., 1925; Hall, 1904).

Identity Disorder Defined by DSM-III

DSM-III (1980) states that the essential feature of the diagnosis of identity disorder is the adolescent's perception of "severe subjective distress" (p. 65) surrounding the inability to establish a sense of sameness and continuity in his or her sense of self. This subjective distress is reflected in Erikson's (1968) writings about the "central disturbance in severely conflicted young people" (p. 17) and Offer, Ostrov, and Howard's (1981a) delinquent and disturbed samples who described sadness, anxiousness, loneliness, vulnerability, and distorted self-images, which are in strong contrast to their random samples of adolescents who had positive psychological self-concepts and Dusek and Flaherty's (1981) normal sample who showed no disruption in continuity of self-concept.

Elaborating further on the diagnostic

criteria, DSM-III states that this subjective turmoil is associated with uncertainty about "a variety of issues" (1980, p. 65) relating to identity formation, including at least three of the following: long-term goals, career choice, sexual orientation and behavior, religious identification, moral values, friendship patterns, and group loyalties. To meet the criteria for diagnosis, the symptoms should last at least three months, result in impairment of social or occupational functioning, and be perceived by the adolescent as an irreconcilable and permanent aspect of his or her personality. One would suppose many adolescents with substance disorders could also be diagnosed identity disorder.

Indicating further the nonnormality associated with this type of identity difficulty, DSM-III states that identity disorder is often associated with mild anxiety and depression related to inner preoccupation rather than external events, self-doubt and doubt about the future, and negative or oppositional patterns of attempts to form an identity distinct from family or other close individuals, i.e., Erikson's (1968) negative identity. Continuing, DSM-III states these attempts may be manifested as "transient experimental phases of widely divergent behavior as the individual 'tries on' various roles" (1980, p. 66). It is in this last phrase that the key to differentiating the normal status of moratorium from the diagnosis of identity disorder can be found.

As Erikson (1959, 1968) has frequently noted, the adolescent needs permission and approval to experiment with various roles. This includes the moving, perhaps yearly, from one apartment to another, change in college major or the first jobs of a young adult's career, the investigation of differing religions, and altering drastically one's style of dress or hair. This experimental phase of moratorium need not be unhealthy or disruptive and, based on research evidence, apparently is not. When the experimentation is met by a rejecting or denying family or other important individuals, or becomes widely and perhaps consistently divergent, with accompanying disruption of daily functioning, the adolescent is in a state of identity disorder. Turmoil and disruption in adolescence, as in any other developmental phase, is indicative of disorder and the need for professional intervention.

There is, however, one more qualifying remark that must be made concerning the above distinction between the normal process of moratorium and identity disorder. Research has strongly confirmed the normality of the moratorium period for adolescent and young adult males, but not for females. Commitment, with or without crisis, seems normal for adolescent and young adult females, and moratorium is most often, although not always, associated with the same or similar personality, family, and behavior patterns as identity diffusion.

As Erikson (1968) stated in "Womanhood and the Inner Space," women's identity formation seems to be tied to the achievement of intimacy. It seems that intimacy is possible for females along with or even preceding identity, and identity formation in females might not not be possible without intimacy formation (Hodgson & Fischer, 1979). We do not know what direct implications this has for the diagnosis of identity disorder in females, other than the fact that research indicates that the inability to form intimate relationships with important individuals will also be reflected in some inability to make a commitment to an identity. The obvious and broad implication of these two observations is that women who cannot achieve intimacy status might remain in moratorium or identity diffusion status, both of which seem to be unhealthy and costly modes of identity formation.

No reflection of the association of intimacy and identity for women exists in the DSM-III criteria for identity disorder, which is based on what research indicates is a male model of identity formation. Using the DSM-III criteria, it seems possible for a young woman to be diagnosed as an identity disorder, when her problem is actually an "intimacy disorder." It is probable that the DSM-III diagnostic criteria and associated features of identity disorder will, like "both Erikson's theory and the identity status approach, work only more or less, when applied to women" (Marcia, 1980, p. 178).

Incidence. Since identity disorder is a new category, no incidence or prevalence figures are available. However, our discussion would suggest it is not uncommon. Some indication of scope and treatment may also be gained from what follows.

Substance Disorders

According to DSM-III "this diagnostic class deals with behavioral changes associated with more or less regular use of substances that affect the central nervous system" (1980, p. 163). In our society most people use drugs at one time or another that alter mood or behavior. Smoking; drinking alcohol, coffee, and tea; the taking of aspirins, tranquilizers, etc. come under such a broad classification. The taking of substances becomes a disorder when behavioral changes are uncontrollable, socially undesirable, or extreme. Examples of such changes are impaired thinking, inability to function effectively at one's occupation, disturbed social relations, and an inability to control the amount of substance intake or to stop using it.

DSM-III distinguishes between substance abuse and substance dependence. The term *substance abuse* means a pattern of pathological use which impairs social or occupational functioning and lasts for at least one month. *Substance dependence* is defined by either tolerance or withdrawal. Each of these terms also has a technically specific meaning: *Tolerance* refers to the need for a greater and greater dosage of the substance in order to achieve the expected effect. *Withdrawal* refers to a physiological syndrome which follows the cessation of substance use. The type of withdrawal is substance specific; that is, the specific behaviors which characterize the withdrawal syndrome will depend on the particular substance which has been abused.

Another term which should be added to this group is *addiction.* According to Brenner, Coles, and Meagher (1970), "Addiction to a drug takes place when profound changes occur in the chemistry and physiology, or the workings, of the body—profound, but reversible changes." While the mechanism of addiction is not completely understood, and while the term is too often used loosely, it should be clear that we are here referring to physiological changes. Heroin would be perhaps the best example since it is one of the most addictive of all drugs.

It is also helpful to differentiate among the various other levels of drug use. The National Commission on Marijuana and Drug Use (the Shafer Commission) has made the following distinctions among users of psychoactive drugs:

Experimental—short-term, nonpatterned trial of one or more drugs, motivated primarily by curiosity or a desire to experience an altered mood state.

Recreational—occurs in social settings among friends or acquaintances who desire to share an experience which they define as both acceptable and pleasureable. Generally, recreational use is both voluntary and patterned and tends not to escalate to more frequent or intense use patterns.

Circumstantial—generally motivated by the user's perceived need or desire to achieve a new and anticipated effect in order to cope with a specific problem, situation or condition or a personal or vocational nature. This category would include the use of stimulants to relieve tension or boredom.

Intensive—drug use which occurs at least daily and is motivated by an individual's perceived need to achieve relief or maintain a level of performance.

Compulsive—consists of a patterned behavior at a high frequency and high level of intensity, characterized by a high degree of dependency, such as with chronic alcoholics, heroin dependents, and compulsive users of barbiturates (Brill & Winnick, 1980, p. 41).

The classification of drugs which are abused and can create dependence include: (1) alcohol, (2) opiates (or "narcotics"), i.e., drugs which are opium derived, such as heroin, morphine and methadone, (3) barbiturates, tranquilizers, and other sedatives, (4) stimulants (the amphetamines and cocaine), and (5) marijuana. Tobacco is classed by DSM-III as a drug which has the potential for dependence but, surprisingly, not for abuse! Hallucinogens, cocaine, and PCP are drugs of abuse, but do not induce dependence.

Each of the classes of abused substances presents its own characteristic pattern of abuse and toxicity, and of tolerance and withdrawal, in the case of those which induce dependency. For that reason we will present them separately and then deal with the issue of the patterning of drug abuse and the personality of the abuser.

Opioids

The term *narcotic* is generally used to refer to the pain killing drugs: morphine, codeine, and especially heroin. These are derived from opium, which is made from the juice of the poppy fruit. Cocaine, which is made from coca leaves, is legally classed as a narcotic but not chemically. The potential for addiction to the opioids is high. The body develops a tolerance to their use, and withdrawal frequently occurs on cessation of drug taking. It is extremely difficult to treat addiction to narcotics; some estimate that, using heroin as the example, 90 percent of treated users go back to the drug. The problem of acute reactions resulting from the use of the opioids is a serious issue. Overdosing can occur for a variety of reasons. First of all, the novice may not know how much to inject to get the desired effect without overdosing. Secondly, sometimes a user will unwittingly buy almost pure heroin, when he or she has been used to much weaker stuff, which has been cut by the unscrupulous seller with milk sugar. Finally, sometimes after a jail sentence or a hospitalization and withdrawal from the drug, a user injects himself or herself with the former dosage. However, the body's tolerance is now lower and overdose can result. A Blue Shield (1971) publication gives the following example:

In New York, where over half of this country's heroin addicts live, there are thousands of personal tragedies each year. Such as the one involving a young father who could not subordinate the habit to his own family's welfare.

One night the young man left his cheap apartment, where a seven-month-old baby would soon awaken and begin crying for food.

With the money he had been saving for his family, the dark-haired addict purchased a small cellophane package of heroin and quickly ducked into the men's room of a local bar. The door locked behind him, he began to dissolve heroin in a hot spoon, and then shakily injected it into his arm. Shortly afterward he was dead from an overdose.

Prevalence. According to the most recent Comprehensive National Survey on Drug Abuse, conducted by the National Institute on Drug Abuse (NIDA) (Abelson, Fishbourne, & Cisin, 1977) one percent of the nation's youth between the ages of twelve and seventeen have tried heroin. Between the ages of eighteen and twenty-five the prevalence rises to almost 4 percent. While narcotics may be the drugs of least concern to therapists of adolescents by virtue of their relatively infrequent use, they are among the most serious in terms of their potential for addiction, tragic psychosocial effects, and possibility of overdose.

Amphetamines

These drugs were first produced in the 1920s and were used medically as central nervous system stimulants. They ward off sleepiness and fatigue, and have also been used to curb appetite in some medically sponsored weight loss programs. There is a serious question (Ellinwood, 1979) as to whether or not amphetamines should be prescribed as anorectic drugs. However, formulating the cost/benefit equation, one needs to consider the increased mortality and morbidity that might result from obesity if programs involving anorectic drugs are not available. Many investigators feel that amphetamines have questionable medical use. Ellinwood suggests

> One could certainly question whether anorectic drugs, especially those with high stimulant properties, are sufficiently efficacious to warrant their continued use. In fact, the FDA is currently considering removal of the anorectic indication for the labelling of amphetamine products. The FDA action has been conceived as an initial step with amphetamines with the consideration that other substantially abused anorectic drugs will be removed from the anorectic indication. Thus, it is possible that many of the anorectic drugs will be soon removed from the market (1979).

Among the most common stimulants are amphetamine (benzedrine), dextroamphetamine (dexedrine), and methamphetamine (methedrine)—or "bennys," "pep pills," and "speed" to the street user.

Case Illustration: A sixteen-year-old girl had been abused as a child and was now living on her own. Having dropped out of school, Francine was working in a factory on the assembly line. She claimed she was one of the best workers at the plant and could produce more than any of the older employees. Indeed, she did make excellent wages. After a few days in the hospital it was discovered that one of her friends was supplying her with illegal drugs, some of them stolen from the pharmacy of the hospital itself. Needle marks on her feet gave testimony to her habit of injecting speed, the secret of her occupational success, so she thought. In addition, she was taking barbiturates, a combination that could well have proven fatal. Withdrawal from the barbiturates was a difficult and painful process.

Use of amphetamines does not lead to physical dependence or addiction, although the body does develop a tolerance to them, so that larger and larger doses are needed to experience the effect. Some have argued that a "psychological" if not physical dependence develops with these stimulants; that is, the user may develop a habit of relying on drugs for emotional reasons as Francine did.

Prevalence. According to the NIDA (Abelson, Fishbourne, & Cisin, 1977), approximately 5% of U.S. youth between the ages twelve and seventeen have tried central nervous system stimulants. Among eighteen to twenty-five year olds, 21 percent have experimented with this class of drugs. Exact statistics are difficult to obtain. These drugs are relatively easy to get, and are often used by middle- and upper-class adolescents who obtain their first pills through a medical prescription.

There can be a fine line between medical use and drug abuse. It has been estimated that 25 percent of amphetamine abuse derives from legally obtained prescriptions (Ellinwood, 1979), with the other 75 percent coming from street buys, thefts, etc. Indeed, of all medical prescriptions for mood affecting drugs, it is estimated that stimulants account for 20 percent. The housewife who "needs something to keep her going" during the day; the attorney who keeps a few pills on hand for his social parties, as one might serve alcohol; and the athlete who needs something to help him "get up for the game" are examples of misuse, besides the large number of adolescents who are looking for a new kick, or who, like Francine, are trying to prove themselves.

BARBITURATES

The effect of barbiturates (or downers) on the central nervous system is opposite to the effect of amphetamines. The barbiturates or sedatives are used medically to relax the CNS. First produced in the nineteenth century, barbiturates are made from barbituric acid and act as depressants. About 25 percent of all mood changing drugs prescribed by doctors are barbiturates. Like amphetamines, barbiturates are used by the middle- and upper-class who often begin taking the drug via a legal prescription for medical use. According to Smith, Wesson, and Seymour (1979) the barbiturates can be classified into three groups: (1) the ultra short acting (one quarter to three hours), which are used for anesthetic purposes (Thiopental/pentothal); (2) short acting (three to six hours), which are used medically as a preoperative sedative, have a hypnotic affect, and may be injected for rapid seizure control (amobarbital/Amytal, pentobarbital/Nebutal, secobarbital/Seconal); (3) intermediate acting (six to twelve hours), used as a daytime sedative (butabarbital/Butisol); (4) long acting (twelve to twenty-four hours), used for the control of epilepsy, as a daytime sedative, and in the treatment of sedative hypnotic withdrawal (phenobarbital/Luminal).

The barbiturates act directly on the CNS and have an effect called *disinhibition euphoria* in which anxiety, self-criticism, and self-doubt are all reduced, and mood is generally elevated. It is this euphoric or intoxicating effect which make the barbiturates attractive to many drug users. However, some people also experience increased anxiety or fluctuating mood shifts. Barbiturates have the capacity for inducing physical dependence and tolerance. While amphetamines have questionable medical application, it is clear that barbiturates are very important medically. Phenobarbital, for example, is needed to control seizures. Nonetheless, they have become some of the most commonly abused drugs, outside of alcohol, tobacco, and marijuana. According to Smith, Wesson, and Seymour (1979), "Barbiturates are associated with nearly 500 deaths each year and the barbiturate overdose represents a potential major medical emergency with life threatening implications" (1980, p. 236).

Sudden discontinuation or withdrawal from barbiturates can be extremely dangerous, even fatal. Withdrawal needs to be done under careful medical supervision, generally in a hospital (Khantzian & McKenna, 1979).

Prevalence. Four percent of the population of youngsters in this country between the ages of twelve and seventeen have experimented with tranquilizers and three percent have experimented with sedatives (Abelson, Fishbourne, & Cisin, 1977). Eighteen percent of those between the ages of eighteen and twenty-five have experimented with sedatives and over 13 percent with tranquilizers. These percentages are for nonmedically prescribed drug usage. Blum and Richards have suggested that "nonmedical drug use is spreading downward by age so that now in 1978 in many areas it is an elementary school phenomenon" (1979, p. 260). While they mention that amphetamines may more often be the initial illicit drug other than marijuana, it appears from these data that the percentages for the abused barbiturates is nearly as large.

MARIJUANA

Marijuana (weed, grass, mary jane, pot) is made from the resin of the leaves and tops of the hemp plant, *cannabis sativa.* Marijuana can be smoked in a cigarette (joint) or eaten in cakes or cookies for its intoxicating effect. The effect can occur within minutes and lasts for an hour and a half after smoking a joint, and up to six hours if marijuana is ingested. Smoking or ingesting marijuana has a soothing effect; time seems to slow down. Some users report that their sensations are sharpened, their frustrations disappear, and sometimes drowsiness occurs. While some users become garrulous and giggly, others become more introspective and seem to enjoy the solitude of focusing on one object for what seems to be hours. Other users enjoy a group atmosphere and can carry on a seemingly very serious conversation until nobody is quite sure what the point was initially. No matter; a new serious conversation begins.

One can build up a tolerance to marijuana so that greater amounts are needed for the desired effect. While some users become "psychologically dependent," there are no reported cases of overdose or withdrawal. Toxic reactions include panic, frequently with paranoid ideation.

Case Illustration: A sixteen-year-old high school student's parents separated when he was in the eighth grade. After going through an ugly divorce, his father took Jeff to live with him. The father, who was dating heavily and had little time for his son, was a recreational user of marijuana and cocaine. Little by little, Jeff's grades began to slip, and with his father's permission he began to experiment with marijuana. Within the next three years he began to smoke more and more marijuana and to study less and less. His social life became confined to three or four friends who were also regular users of pot. By the time Jeff was in the eleventh grade he was smoking marijuana every day, often beginning before he got out of bed. When asked why he smoked so much, he said, "I couldn't stand school otherwise. All the confusion in the halls, it's impossible." In a sense Jeff had found his own medication. He said that it was easier to laugh when he was on pot and that it was easier to cope with a large high school and the confusing atmosphere within the school.

The relationship between marijuana use and depression has been explored in a study by Kaplan et al. (1980) and will be discussed at length later in this chapter. In Jeff's case, the basis for Jeff's problem was serious depression (see Chapter 9) and the smoking of marijuana was a symptom of this problem and not the major problem itself. Nonetheless, Jeff had become psychologically dependent on the marijuana. It was very difficult, almost impossible, during the time he was seen in psychotherapy to have him refrain, even for a day, from smoking a joint.

Generally, however, marijuana is considered one of the less harmful of the drugs taken by adolescents. According to the *Federal Strategy for Drug Abuse and Traffic Prevention* (1976),

> While marijuana is the most widely used illicit drug, there have been no reported overdose deaths in this country and medical emergency room mentions are two-thirds less frequent than are those for barbiturates, even though the number of youths using marijuana is almost ten times higher, and the number of adults six times higher than those using the barbiturates improperly (Brill & Winnick, 1980, p. 44).

Prevalence. Clearly the most widely used illicit drug, over one-half of U.S. youngsters claim to have experimented with marijuana at some time or other. Regular or occasional use is claimed by 15 million and it has been estimated that as many as 50 million Americans have used marijuana.

Many legislators as well as researchers in the area of drug abuse have urged the decriminalization of marijuana possession, at least for small amounts for personal use. It is believed that controls over the production and sale of marijuana would eliminate the possibility of a user's getting a product whose impurities would be more harmful than the marijuana itself.

ALCOHOL

Although a legal substance, alcohol is a serious problem among teenagers and adults. Fifty-three percent of adolescents between the ages of twelve and seventeen have tried alcohol. Over 31 percent of that group report that they are current drinkers. Among the eighteen to twenty-four year old group, 58 percent say they use alcohol. Alcohol can lead to both dependence and abuse and often does. A tolerance builds up and alcoholic withdrawal symptoms of tremors and anxiety are well-known. It is estimated that in the United States 10 to 15 million adults abuse alcohol and only one-tenth of that number obtain help for their problem (Coleman, Butcher, & Carson, 1984, p. 399).

In an important study dealing with adolescent development and the onset of drinking, Jessor and Jessor (1975) studied 432 junior high school students in grades seven, eight and nine. The subjects were followed over a four-year period. The authors based their findings on several groups: (1) those adolescents who abstained throughout the four years; (2) those who began drinking during the third year; (3) those who began in the second year; (4) those who began in the first year; and (5) those who were already drinkers when the study began. Questionnaire data were collected each year on a large number of variables.

When comparing the abstainers with the transition groups (those who began drinking during the years of the study) a pattern became fairly clear. Abstainers placed a higher value on achievement, a low value on independence, and had higher expectations for achievement. They were less tolerant of deviance, were more religious, and produced more reasons against drinking. The abstainers' perceived environment was also significantly different. They perceived their parents as more supportive and less approving of drinking. Their friends were also seen as less approving of drinking and as less likely to model drinking behavior. Finally, the abstainers engaged less in deviant behavior and were likely to have a higher grade point average than those adolescents in the transition groups. Each of these differences was found both in the responses given at the beginning of the study and again after four years. Furthermore, when comparing the various transition groups it was clear that the earlier the transition to drinking, the more likely deviant behavior, instigation to problem behavior, poor personal goals against transgression, and a perceived environment that approved and modeled drinking.

Abused Substances Not Associated with Dependence

Three classes of substances which do not induce physiological dependence are still classified by DSM-III as substances of abuse because they can lead to impairment in social and/or occupational functioning. These are cocaine, phencyclidine (PCP), and hallucinogens.

Cocaine has been tried by 4 percent of the twelve- to seventeen-year-old group in the U.S. and by 19 percent of the eighteen- to twenty-five-year-old population. Cocaine acts as a central nervous system stimulant that induces "euphoria, confidence, energy, increased heart rate and blood pressure, dilated pupils, constriction of peripheral blood vessels, and rise in body temperature and metabolic rate" (Grinspoon & Bakalar, 1979, p. 241).

While periodic recreational use of cocaine does not induce tolerance, animal studies have demonstrated the effect when the drug is given in high dosages. Also, there is a strong *psychological* craving among those human subjects who have easy access to the drug and use it often. If the drug is taken no more than two or three times per week, it appears to present no serious problems. More frequent usage, in high doses, however, can lead to eating and sleeping difficulties, and some irritability and inability to concentrate, as well as some perceptual disturbances and rarely, paranoid ideation and psychoses. Sometimes mild withdrawal symptoms, like anxiety and depression, have been observed, although physiological dependence has not been reported.

Phencyclidine (PCP) is described as one of the most enigmatic drugs on the streets (Pittel & Oppedahl, 1979). It was first synthesized in 1926 and suggested in the 1950s as a potential anesthetic. Subsequent research, however, uncovered a host of psychological side effects which precluded its use as an effective analgesic for humans. The side effects included disorientation, hallucinations, delirium, and manic excitement. Historians of the drug scene then traced its emergence on the illicit market to Los Angeles (1965), Haight-Ashbury (1967), and New York (1968). Users have often come upon PCP believing they have purchased some more predictable drug such as mescaline or psilocybin. According to some authors (Young et al., 1977; Pittel & Oppedahl, 1979) PCP is one of the least predictable and most problematic drugs on the illegal market. It ranks seventh in U.S. crisis center reports, and cases of PCP poisoning are being reported more frequently than formerly.

There is very little published research on the social context of PCP use. It appears to appeal to a varying group of users for reasons that are not clear. The drug's "high" is neither predictable nor often pleasurable; users often experience confusion, agitation, bizarre, unpredictable behavior, and aggression. Cognitive disorders of speech, perception, and memory can result from chronic use. The call for more research on the psychosocial aspects of PCP use has been issued (Pittel & Oppedahl, 1979) and appears to be essential.

Other hallucinogens also present a problem of illegal drug use among the young. According to the 1977 NIDA report, 5 percent of the twelve- to seventeen-year-old group have experimented with hallucinogens while 20 percent of the eighteen- to twenty-five-year-old group have tried them. Although use of hallucinogens does not lead to dependency, they are classified as drugs of abuse because of their potential for adversely affecting occupational or social functioning.

LSD (lysergic acid diethylamide) is perhaps the most widely known hallucinogen, and goes by several different street names including "acid," "blue heaven," "cubes," "sugar." LSD is a tremendously powerful substance. It is white, odorless, and soluble in water without altering the water's taste. Doses are measured in millionths of a gram. The psychic effect of "tripping" on LSD have been amply documented (Brenner, Coles, & Meagher, 1970; Birdwood, 1969; Goode, 1973; Van Dyke, 1970). Most accounts refer to the illusions, hallucinations, sensory distortions, confusion, and mood alterations as well as to the psychedelic displays, kaleidoscopic illusions, and emotional oneness with the world and God. Some have reported eidetic (pure) imagery, while others have experienced synesthesia (translating sensory input from one modality to another, e.g., "seeing" music). The dangers can be described with equal intensity.

"Bad trips" can result from overdosing, which is easy to do (an ounce of LSD can provide 300,000 doses of 100 micrograms each); from being given LSD accidentally or without the user's awareness; or from wrong "set" (frame of mind) or "setting" (physical and social surroundings). Effects can occur within twenty minutes and last from eight to ten hours. Flight, fight, aggression, and paranoid ideation are some of the reported effects of a "bad trip." Called a *psychomimetic drug*, LSD can induce a psychotic-like state. While physical dependence does not occur, a rapid tolerance does. Some users have experienced post-trip side effects even weeks after an apparently successful trip. These have included severe depression, paranoid delusions, and disturbed schizophrenic thought processes which have led, in some cases, to hospitalization.

According to most reports, the use of LSD and other hallucinogens is declining. Some investigators have optimistically suggested that the profound effects of a bummer have become more widely known. Others provide a more cautious interpretation, namely that a bad trip can be expected periodically and current users may not view it as a condition requiring medical help.

TOBACCO

According to DSM-III, tobacco is a substance associated with dependence, but not abuse, since "heavy use of tobacco itself is not associated with impairment in social or occupational functioning . . . "(p. 166). The manual goes on to indicate that adverse reactions from bystanding nonsmokers may cause social problems, however.

While it may be true that behavioral reactions to smoking tobacco may not cause social or occupational impairment, physical effects surely can. Shortness of breath, a hacking cough, bronchitis, emphysema, coronary artery disease, and lung cancer are among such potential effects.

Dependence more frequently occurs to cigarette smoking than to cigar or pipe smoking or to the snuffing or chewing of tobacco. Three criteria of dependence are suggested by DSM-III: (1) an unsuccessful attempt to stop or reduce smoking, (2) withdrawal symptoms, or (3) smoking despite a serious physical problem which is exacerbated by smoking. The diagnosis is only made if the client has sought help in an attempt to quit, or if the provider believes that the continued use of tobacco is affecting the client's physical health.

Prevalence. Forty-seven percent of adolescents between twelve and seventeen have used tobacco and 22 percent are current tobacco smokers. About 40 percent of eighteen- to twenty-five-year-olds report current smoking.

In studying the personality traits of smoking and nonsmoking high school students, Smith (1969) concluded that smokers score higher on measures of "extraversion" and lower on measures of "agreeableness" and "strength of character" than nonsmokers. In addition, smokers tend to score higher on the traits "crude," "happy-go-lucky," and "frank." Such information about the personality of smokers can be helpful in educational campaigns aimed at helping adolescents reject smoking as a personal habit.

Personality Characteristics of Drug Abusers

A number of investigators of the psychosocial aspects of drug use have attempted to discover a personality profile of the drug user and the addict. Jessor (1979) reported that recent research indicates that the marijuana user tends to score higher on personality attributes related to nonconformity, or nonconventionality. Such attributes include critical beliefs about the norms and values of the culture, a disaffection or alienation from society, and a greater tolerance of deviance in general. Social desirability and achievement motivation, in the conventional sense, are not high values for the marijuana user.

Reporting on research about the etiological aspects of drug addiction, Nurco (1979) discusses both theories and data dealing with the precursors of addiction. Among the theories are: (1) the social learning notion that the costly frustration–agression cycle can be interrupted by heroin, which dampens both feelings; (2) an explanation based on parental deprivation in early childhood, and a consequent inability to delay gratification; (3) inadequate sexual identification and an inability or unwillingness to assume responsibility for expected sex role behavior; (4) inability to obtain personal goals legitimately; (5) a higher "risk-taking" style among addicts; and (6) boredom.

The data, gleaned from several studies, give a picture of the addict as likely having had a dominant overprotective mother and an absent or unavailable father; addicts are also "norm breakers" who defy tradition.

Holroyd and Kahn (1974) compared college nonusers with moderate and heavy users of marijuana, amphetamines, barbiturates, hallucinogens, and opiates. The personality characteristics associated with drug use were distinctly different for males and females. Among males, nonuse was associated with an orientation toward conventional achievement and social approval compared with users, whose orientation could be best described as daring, rash, inquisitive, and nonconforming. Females who were abstainers were more "controlling, nurturant, durable, and cautious" compared with the "nonconforming, ambitious, playful, and inquisitive" users. In each case, both males and females rejected the traditional sex-role attributes assigned to them compared with nonusers.

The importance of boredom as an antecedent to drug use (Nurco, 1979) may provide a clue to a more fundamental problem, namely the problem of depression. Having given the Beck Depression Inventory to eighty high school students, Kaplan et al. (1980) discovered that the students who used drugs other than marijuana were significantly more likely to be depressed than those who did not take drugs. These findings replicated a previous study (Paton, Kessler, & Kandel, 1977) which also demonstrated the relationship between drug taking (except for marijuana) and depression. The question of causality remains, however. Do depressed adolescents medicate themselves with illegal drugs, or do their drug habits lead to depression? The marijuana users are probably too numerous and too variable with respect to motivation for smoking to demonstrate a statistical correlation between their smoking and depression. It is our clinical impression, however, that there is a subset of adolescent marijuana smokers (and they are daily users) who use the drug to ward off depression. Jeff, mentioned above, needed to cope with the confusion at school, so he began his day with marijuana and kept pretty high all through the day. Sam, a fifteen-year-old, said he smoked marijuana because it was easier to laugh, something he could rarely do without his joint.

Nevertheless, the evidence of a relationship between drug taking and psychopathology is unclear (Woody & Blaine, 1979). Some researchers find no serious pathology except character disorder (Beres, 1961), while others suggest that all addicts, ipso facto, have serious personality disorders (see Chapter 13) or identity disorder. The case with depression is clearly established, however (Frederick, Resnick, & Wittlin, 1973).

According to Woody and Blaine (1979), a number of studies have demonstrated the relationship between depression and drug use by using MMPI scores as well as other methods. Possible explanations for the higher prevalence of depression among addicts have included (1) parental loss or abuse among addicts, (2) environmental pressure from the milieu in which the addict lives, (3) intrapsychic conflict generated by drug taking, and (4) biological changes resulting from drug use.

The Treatment of Drug Abusers

Where depression has been associated with drug use, Woody and Blaine (1979) have found three effective treatment procedures. *Antidepressant drugs*, monitored carefully, can be a safe and effective treatment. Where abuse of the medication may result, the authors suggest careful dispensing procedures and/or the use of liquid preparations including methadone.

Psychotherapy, especially of a cognitive-behavioral sort, has proven useful with depressives (Beck, 1977) and with depressed addicts (Rush et al., 1977). Woody and Blaine also recommend *psychoanalytic therapy* for drug abusers, who are inclined to make others feel angry or sorry for them. Analytically trained therapists may be well suited to calmly help the adolescent drug abuser deal with his or her anger, frustration, and demanding, impulsive behavior.

Most treatment for drug abuse is for the older patient or for delinquents who have been diverted by the legal system into counseling. Some of the attempts at treating adult drug users have been summarized recently by Sells & Simpson (1979), who conclude that commitment programs and therapeutic communities appear to be beneficial for narcotics users. Outpatient drug-free programs have been useful for younger substance abusers, particularly polydrug users. Outpatient drug-free treatment can include a variety of effective approaches, such as rap centers, counseling, behavioral approaches, and family therapy. The advantages of each of these have been outlined in an article by Kleber and Slobetz (1979).

Our own view is that, while outcome research is still sparse, some form of family therapy is often indicated for the youthful drug abuser, particularly for the one who is still living "at home." While it is often difficult to get other family members to cooperate with a therapeutic program, it is essential, particularly if the family has some secondary motivation in keeping the adolescent dependent or if some neurotic family function is being served by having a drug-abusing member (Bokos et. al., 1984). In such cases other family members can subtly sabotage treatment efforts. We have found that the individual adolescent's drinking or drug problem is often a symptom of a more pervasive family conflict which requires some sort of family treatment.

REFERENCES

Abelson, H. I., Fishbourne, P. M., & Cisin, I. *National survey in drug abuse: 1977.* Rockville, MD: National Institute on Drug Abuse, 1977.

Bandura, A. The stormy decade: Fact or fiction? *Psychology in the Schools,* 1964, *1,* 224–231.

Beck, A. T. *A treatment manual for cognitive behavioral psychotherapy with narcotics addicts.* Philadelphia: Center for Cognitive Therapy, 1977.

Beres, D. Character formation. In S. Lorand and H. I. Schneer (Eds.), *Adolescents: Psychoanalytic approach to problems and therapy.* New York: Hoeber, 1961.

Birdwood, G. *The willing victim: A parent's guide to drug abuse.* London: Secker and Warburg, 1969.

Bloom, M. V. *Adolescent parental separation.* New York: Gardner, 1980.

Blue Shield publication, *Drug abuse: the chemical cop-out.* U.S.: Blue Shield, 1971.

Blum, R., & Richards, L. Youthful drug use. In R. I. Dupont, A. Goldstein, & J. O'Donnell (Eds.), *Handbook on drug abuse.* Rockville, MD: National Institute on Drug Abuse, 1979.

Bokos, P. J., Lipscomb, S. T., & Schwartzman, J. Macrosystemic approaches to drug treatment. *Personnel & Guidance Journal,* 1984, *62,* 583–584.

Brenner, J. M., Coles, R., & Meagher, D. *Drugs and youth.* New York: Liveright, 1970.

Brill, L., & Winnick, C. *The yearbook of substance use and abuse.* Vol. II. New York: Human Sciences Press, 1980.

Coleman, J. C., Butcher, J. N., & Carson, R. C. *Abnormal psychology and modern life.* Glenview, IL: Scott, Foresman, 1984.

Diagnostic and statistical manual of mental disorders. Washington, DC: American Psychiatric Association, 1980.

Dupont, R. I., Goldstein, A., & O'Donnell J. (Eds.). *Handbook on drug abuse.* Rockville, MD: National Institute on Drug Abuse, 1979.

Dusek, J. B., & Flaherty, J. F. The development of the self-concept during the adolescent years. *Monographs of the Society for Research in Child Development,* 1981, *46* (4, Serial No. 191).

Ellinwood, E. H. Amphetamines/anorectics. In R. I. Dupont, A. Goldstein, & J. O'Donnell (Eds.), *Handbook on drug abuse.* Rockville, MD: National Institute on Drug Abuse, 1979.

Erikson, E. H. Ego development and historical change. *Psychoanalytic Study of the Child,* 1946, *2,* 359–396.

Erikson, E. H. The problem of ego identity. *Journal of the American Psychoanalytic Association,* 1956, *4,* 56–121.

Erikson, E. H. Late adolescence. In D. H. Funkenstein (Ed.), *The student and mental health: An international view.* Cambridge, MA: Riverside Press, 1959.

Erikson, E. H. *Childhood and society.* New York: Norton, 63. (*a*)

Erikson, E. H. Youth: Fidelity and diversity. In E. H.

Erikson (Ed.), *Youth: Change and challenge.* New York: Basic, 1963. (*b*)

Erikson, E. H. *Identity: Youth and crisis.* New York: Norton, 1968.

Floyd, H. H., & South, D. R. Dilemma of youth: The choice of parents or peers as a frame of reference for behavior. *Journal of Marriage and the Family,* 1972, *34,* 627–634.

Frederick, C. J., Resnick, H. L. P., & Wittlin, B. J. Self-destructive aspects of hard core addiction. *Archives of General Psychiatry,* 1973, *28,* 579-585.

Freud, A. Adolescence. *Psychoanalytic Study of the Child,* 1958, *13,* 255–278.

Freud, A. *The ego and the mechanisms of defense.* New York: International Universities, 1948.

Freud, S. Three contributions to the sexual theory. *Nervous and Mental Disorder Monograph Series,* 1925, No. 7.

Gilligan, C. In a different voice: Women's conceptions of self and of morality. *Harvard Educational Review,* 1977, *47,* 481–517.

Gilligan, C. *In a different voice: Psychological theory and women's development.* Cambridge, MA: Harvard Universities Press, 1982.

Goode, E. *The drug phenomenon: Social aspects of drug taking.* Indianapolis, IN: Bobbs-Merrill, 1973.

Grinspoon, L., & Bakalar, J. B. Cocaine. In R. I. Dupont, A. Goldstein, & J. O'Donnell (Eds.), *Handbook on drug abuse.* Rockville, MD: National Institute on Drug Abuse, 1979.

Gustin, J. C. The revolt of youth. *Psychoanalysis and the Psychoanalytic Review,* 1961, *98,* 78–90.

Haley, J. *Leaving home: The therapy of disturbed young people.* New York: McGraw-Hill, 1980.

Hall, G. S. *Adolescence.* New York: Appleton, 1904.

Hess, R. D., & Goldblatt, I. The status of adolescents in American society: A problem in social identity. *Child Development,* 1957, *28,* 459–468.

Hill, J. P. Commentary. *Monographs of the Society for Research in Child Development,* 1981, *46* (4, Serial No. 191).

Hodgson, J. W., & Fischer, J. L. Sex differences in identity and intimacy development in college youth. *Journal of Youth and Adolescence,* 1979, *8,* 37–50.

Holroyd, K., & Kahn, M. Personality factors in student drug use. *Journal of Consulting and Clinical Psychology,* 1974, *42,* 236–243.

Howard, L. P. Identity conflicts in adolescent girls. *Smith College Studies in Social Work,* 1960, *31,* 1–21.

Inhelder, B., & Piaget, J. *The growth of logical thinking from childhood to adolescence.* New York: Basic, 1958.

Jessor, R. Marijuana: A review of recent psychosocial research. In R. I. Dupont, A. Goldstein, & J. O'Donnell (Eds.), *Handbook on drug abuse.* Rockville, MD: National Institute on Drug Abuse, 1979.

Jessor, R., & Jessor, S. L. Adolescent development and the onset of drinking. *Journal of Studies on Alcohol,* 1975, *36,* 27–51.

Jordan, D. Parental antecedents of ego identity formation. Unpublished master's thesis. SUNY, 1970.

Jordan, D. Parental antecedents and personality characteristics of ego identity statuses. Unpublished doctoral dissertation. SUNY, 1971.

Kaplan, S. A., Nussbaum, M., Skomorowsky, P., Shenker, R., & Ramsey, P. Health habits and depression in adolescence. *Journal of Youth and Adolescence,* 1980, *9,* 299–304.

Khantzian, E. J., & McKenna, G. J. Diagnosis and management of acute drug problems. In L. Brill & C. Winnick (Eds.), *The yearbook of substance use and abuse.* Vol. II. New York: Human Sciences, 1980.

Kleber, H. D., & Slobetz, F. Outpatient drug-free treatment. In R. I. Dupont, A. Goldstein, & J. O'Donnell (Eds.), *Handbook on drug abuse.* Rockville, MD: National Institute on Drug Abuse, 1979.

Marcia, J. E. Development and validation of ego identity status. *Journal of Personality and Social Psychology,* 1966, *3,* 551–558.

Marcia, J. E. Ego identity status: Relationship to change in self-esteem, general maladjustment, and authoritarianism. *Journal of Personality,* 1967, *35,* 119–133.

Marcia, J. E. Identity six years after: A follow-up study. *Journal of Youth and Adolescence,* 1976, *5,* 145–160.

Marcia, J. E. Identity in adolescence. In J. Adelson (Ed.), *Handbook of adolescent psychology.* New York: Wiley, 1980.

Marcia, J. E., & Friedman, M. L. Ego identity status in college women. Journal of Personality, 1970, *38,* 249–263.

Matteson, D. R. Alienation vs. exploration and commitment: Personality and family corollaries of adolescent identity statuses. *Report from the project for youth research.* Copenhagen: Royal Danish School of Educational Studies, 1974.

Meilman, P. W. Crisis and commitment in adolescence: A developmental study of ego identity status. Unpublished doctoral dissertation, University of North Carolina, 1977.

Meissner, W. W. Parental interaction of the adolescent boy. *Journal of Genetic Psychology,* 1965, *107,* 225–233.

Moore, D., & Hotch, D. F. Late adolescents' conceptualizations of home-leaving. *Journal of Youth and Adolescence,* 1981, *10,* 1–10.

Munro, G., & Adams, G. R. Ego identity formation in college students and working youth. *Developmental Psychology,* 1977, *13,* 523–524.

Nurco, D. N. *Etiological aspects of drug abuse.* In R. I. Dupont, A. Goldstein, & J. O'Donnell (Eds.), *Handbook on drug abuse.* Rockville, MD: National Institute on Drug Abuse, 1979.

Offer, D., & Offer, J. Four issues in the developmental psychology of adolescents. In J. G. Howells (Ed.), *Modern perspectives in adolescent psychiatry.* Edinburgh: Oliver and Boyd, 1971.

Offer, D., Ostrov, E., & Howard, K. I. *The adolescent: A psychological self-portrait.* New York: Basic, 1981 (*a*).

Offer, D., Ostrov, E., & Howard, K. I. The mental health professional's concept of the normal adolescent. *Archives of General Psychiatry,* 1981, *38,* 149–153. (*b*)

Offer, D., Sabshin, M., & Marcus, I. Clinical evaluation of normal adolescents. *American Journal of Psychiatry,* 1965, *121,* 864–872.

Orlofsky, J. L., Marcia, J. E., & Lesser, I. M. Ego identity status and the intimacy vs. isolation crisis of young adulthood. *Journal of Personality and Social Psychology,* 1973, *27,* 211–219.

Oshman, H. P., & Manosevitz, M. The impact of the identity crisis on the adjustment of late-adolescent males. *Journal of Youth and Adolescence,* 1974, *3,* 207–216.

Paton, S., Kessler, R., & Kandel, D. Depressive mood and adolescent illicit drug use: A longitudinal analysis. *Journal of Genetic Psychology,* 1977, *131,* 267–289.

Pittel, S. M., & Oppedahl, M. C. The enigma of P.C.P. In R. I. Dupont, A. Goldstein, & J. O'Donnell (Eds.), *Handbook on drug abuse.* Rockville, MD: National Institute on Drug Abuse, 1979.

Podd, M. H., Marcia, J. E., & Rubin, B. M. The effects of ego identity and partner perception on a prisoner's dilemma game. *Journal of Social Psychology,* 1970, *82,* 117–126.

Rush, A. J., Beck, A. T., Kovacs, M., & Hallon, S. Comparative efficacy of cognitive therapy and pharmacotherapy in the treatment of depressed out-patients. *Cognitive Therapy Research,* 1977, *1,* 17–38.

Schenkel, S., & Marcia, J. E. Attitudes toward premarital intercourse in determining ego identity status in college women. *Journal of Personality,* 1972, *40,* 472–482.

Sells, S., & Simpson, D. On the effectiveness of treatment of drug abuse; evidence on the DARP research programme in the United States. *Bulletin on Narcotics,* 1971, *31,* 1–12.

Smith, D. E., Wesson, D. R., & Seymour, M. A. The abuse of barbiturates and other sedative-hypnotics. In R. I. Dupont, A. Goldstein, & J. O'Donnell (Eds.), *Handbook on drug abuse.* Rockville, MD: National Institute on Drug Abuse, 1979.

Smith, G. M. Relations between personality and smoking behavior in preadult subjects. *Journal of Consulting and Clinical Psychology,* 1969, *33,* 710–715.

Stierlin, H. *Separating parents and adolescents.* New York: New York Times Book, 1974.

Van Dyke, H. T. *Youth and the drug problem.* Boston: Ginn, 1970.

Waterman, A. S., & Waterman, C. K. The relationship between freshman ego identity status and subsequent academic behavior: A test of the predictive validity of Marcia's categorization system for identity status. *Developmental Psychology,* 1972, *6,* 179.

Waterman, C. K., & Waterman, A. S. Ego identity status and decision styles. *Journal of Youth and Adolescence,* 1974, *3,* 1–6.

Waterman, C. K., Buehl, M. E., & Waterman, A. S. The relationship between resolution of the identity crisis and outcomes of previous psychosocial crises. Proceedings of the 78th annual convention of the American Psychological Association, 1970, *5,* 467–468. (Summary)

Weiner, I. B. *Psychodiagnosis in schizophrenia.* New York: Wiley, 1966.

Weiner, I. B. *Psychological disturbance in adolescence.* New York: Wiley, 1970.

Woody, G. E., & Blaine, J. Depression in narcotic addicts: Quite possibly more than a chance association. In R. I. Dupont, A. Goldstein, and J. O'Donnell (Eds.), *Handbook on drug abuse.* Rockville, MD: National Institute on Drug Abuse, 1979.

Young, L. A., Young, L. G., Klein, M. M., Klein, D. M., & Beyer, D. *Recreational drugs.* New York: Macmillan, 1977.

Index